Psychiatry in Prisons

Forensic Focus Series

This series, edited by Gwen Adshead, takes the field of Forensic Psychotherapy as its focal point, offering a forum for the presentation of theoretical and clinical issues. It embraces such influential neighbouring disciplines as language, law, literature, criminology, ethics and philosophy, as well as psychiatry and psychology, its established progenitors. Gwen Adshead is Consultant Forensic Psychotherapist and Lecturer in Forensic Psychotherapy at Broadmoor Hospital.

other titles in this series

Personality Disorder
The Definitive Reader
Edited by Gwen Adshead and Caroline Jacob
ISBN 978 1 84310 640 1

Therapeutic Relationships with Offenders
An Introduction to the Psychodynamics of Forensic Mental Health Nursing
Edited by Anne Aiyegbusi and Jenifer Clarke-Moore
ISBN 978 1 84310 949 5

Sexual Offending and Mental Health
Multidisciplinary Management in the Community
Edited by Julia Houston and Sarah Galloway
ISBN 978 1 84310 550 3

Forensic Psychotherapy
Crime, Psychodynamics and the Offender Patient
Christopher Cordess and Murray Cox
Foreword by John Gunn
ISBN 978 1 85302 634 8

Forensic Focus 31

Psychiatry in Prisons

A Comprehensive Handbook

Edited by Simon Wilson and Ian Cumming

Jessica Kingsley Publishers
London and Philadelphia

First published in 2010
by Jessica Kingsley Publishers
116 Pentonville Road
London N1 9JB, UK
and
400 Market Street, Suite 400
Philadelphia, PA 19106, USA

www.jkp.com

Library of Congress Cataloging in Publication Data
Psychiatry in prisons : a comprehensive handbook / edited by Simon Wilson and Ian Cumming.
    p. cm.
  Includes bibliographical references and index.
  ISBN 978-1-84310-223-6 (alk. paper)
  1. Prisoners--Mental health services--Great Britain. I. Wilson, Simon, 1970- II. Cumming, Ian, 1962-
  RC451.4.P68P743 2010
  365'.66--dc22
                              2009018366

British Library Cataloguing in Publication Data
A CIP catalogue record for this book is available from the British Library

ISBN 978 1 84310 223 6

Printed and bound in Great Britain by
Athenaeum Press, Gateshead, Tyne and Wear

Contents

Preface and Acknowledgements   8

1.   Introduction – The History of Prison Psychiatry   9
     Simon Wilson and Ian Cumming

2.   The Current Structure of the Prison Service   16
     John Podmore

3.   Delivering Mental Health Services in Prison   24
     Janet Parrott

4.   Health Screening in Prisons   30
     Don Grubin

5.   Mentally Ill Prisoners and Mental Health Issues in Prison   40
     Ian Cumming and Simon Wilson

6.   Suicide, Attempted Suicide and Self-injury in Prison   52
     David Crighton

7.   Managing Substance Misuse in Prison   65
     James Tighe

8.   The Young Offender   77
     Julie Withecomb

9.   Women in Prison   86
     Richard Taylor and Jessica Yakeley

10. Elderly Prisoners   98
     Seena Fazel and Preeti Chhabra

11. People with Intellectual Disabilities in Prison   107
     Kiriakos Xenitidis, Maria Fotiadou and Glynis Murphy

12. Black and Minority Ethnic Prisoners   125
     David Ndegwa and Dominic Johnson

13. Sex Offenders and Vulnerable Prisoners   132
     Rebecca Milner

14. Consent to Treatment, the Mental Health Act, and the Mental
     Capacity Act   144
     Simon Wilson and Raj Dhar

15. Hunger Strike and Food Refusal   155
     Danny Sullivan and Crystal Romilly

16. Psychiatric Reports   172
     Huw Stone

17. The Lifer System in England and Wales   194
     Natalie Pyszora

18. Psychology in Prisons   203
     Graham Towl

19. Prison Therapeutic Regimes   210
     Mark Morris

20. Death in Custody   223
     Andrew Forrester

21. Prisons Inspection   230
     Tish Laing-Morton and Colin Allen

22. International Perspectives (I) – An Overview of US Correctional
     Mental Health   239
     Charles Scott and Barbara McDermott

23. International Perspectives (II) – Delivery of Mental Health
Services in New Zealand Prisons: Context and Approaches   246
Ceri Evans and Phil Brinded

24. Inside–Outside: Ethical Dilemmas in Prison Psychiatry   253
Gwen Adshead

25. Prison Language as an Organisational Defence Against Anxiety 261
Gabrielle Brown and Julian Walker

The Contributors   272

References   276

Legal Cases   305

Subject Index   307

Author Index   313

Preface and Acknowledgements

The development of mental health prison inreach teams across England and Wales has led to a renewed interest in the mental health needs of prisoners, the practicalities of providing mental health services for prisoners, and rather sterile debates about whether such services should be provided by primary care services, general adult mental health teams, or forensic mental health teams. We believe that prison psychiatry presents unique challenges and requires particular skills that are not necessarily provided by training in general adult or forensic psychiatry; it is a sub-specialty of its own. With this in mind, together with the absence of a text bringing together the relevant issues, we decided to embark on this book. That was seven years ago! We both rather underestimated quite what this would involve, and it has had a much longer gestation than either of us wished for. We would like to thank our families, authors and publishers for their extreme patience. We hope you are all as proud of the finished product as we are.

Simon Wilson and Ian Cumming
London 2009

CHAPTER 1

Introduction – The History of Prison Psychiatry

Simon Wilson and Ian Cumming

The history of psychiatry in prisons is the history of the birth of forensic psychiatry, which grew out of the development of psychiatric care for the mentally disordered offender in custody, eventually leading to the establishment of purpose-built hospitals. History seems especially important in forensic psychiatry, in that this has so far largely been a discipline whose development is marked less by scientific advances than by historical landmarks in the form of inquiries, reports and legal statutes (e.g. the Criminal Lunatics Act, the Percy Commission, the Butler Report, and so on).

FILTHY, CORRUPT, AND UNHEALTHY (1750–1800)

There were, of course, prisons in ancient and medieval times, such as the Babylonian *bit asiri* (a prison specifically for foreign captives used as forced labour) and the "Great Prison" of the Egyptian Middle Kingdom (Morris & Rothman 1998). These are not further explored here.

Prisons prior to the late eighteenth century were houses of correction and gaols administered by local justices. They were "filthy, corrupt-ridden and unhealthy" according to John Howard (1784),[1] and largely contained prisoners awaiting sentences of fines, death, corporal punishment, or transportation to the American colonies. They

---

1   John Howard became interested in prisons after being made High Sheriff of Bedfordshire in 1773. He made a tour of prisons in England and continental Europe in 1774–1776, 1781, 1783 and 1785–1786, and published his findings in *The State of the Prisons* (1777).

also contained many mentally ill offenders, as there was nowhere else for such people to go (Walker 1968), Howard (1784, pp.10–11) observing that "many of the bridewells are crowded and offensive, because the rooms which were designed for prisoners are occupied by lunatics". They were corrupt places where the jailers, who were paid by the prisoners for food and drink, would accept bribes to release inmates or to take chains off (Watts 2001). Bridewells, or houses of confinement, introduced in 1556, were an early attempt at reform (Watts 2001). These were intended for vagrants, were self-funded, and staff were paid a wage in an attempt to reduce the levels of corruption. Initially successful, with an Act of 1609 introducing them into every county, their purpose gradually became eroded and they became used as simply another prison, with all the problems that entailed (Watts 2001).

Prison psychiatry might be said to have begun in the eighteenth century with the founding of the Prison Medical Service in England and Wales in 1774 (Sim 1990). The Health of Prisoners Act 1774 (An Act for Preserving the Health of Prisoners in Gaol and Preventing the Gaol Distemper) required the appointment of an experienced surgeon or apothecary to attend each local gaol (Gunn *et al.* 1978). Transportation to the colonies was disrupted by the American War of Independence in 1776 requiring the development of state prisons (Penitentiary Act 1779) and the introduction of the idea of a period of detention in custody as a sentence. Prison "hulks" were introduced on the Thames as a stop-gap measure (ceasing to exist in 1859).

The possibility of transportation to Australia, which began in 1787, removed the need for state prisons, and so the first, Millbank, did not open until 1821 (Walker & McCabe 1973). Transportation ended in 1840 (Smith 1984).

PUNISHMENT, REHABILITATION AND REFORM (1800–1966)

The nineteenth century, with its positivistic preoccupations, saw a rising interest in applying scientific principles to prisons, in terms of the regimen, the punishment, and rehabilitation. Prisons should be places designed to "cure" prisoners of their criminal propensities, and there was a growing awareness of the problems of mentally disordered prisoners. This was associated with a number of legislative changes. The Criminal Lunatics Act 1800 formalised in statute the verdict of not guilty by reason of insanity, and detention until His Majesty's Pleasure be known, following such a verdict. The County Asylums Act 1808 proposed that local asylums be built, which would also house insane offenders. A special wing was given over to this purpose at the Bethlem Royal Hospital in London from 1814. The Insane Prisoners Act 1840 made it possible for mentally ill prisoners to be transferred to an asylum if two doctors and two JPs agreed the prisoner was insane (Walker 1968).[2] Certain prisons and prison hulks

---

2   This principle has continued in English legislation with the Mental Health Acts of 1959 (introduced after the Percy Commission in 1957) and 1983. Many American jurisdictions still require a legal finding of insanity as the gateway to hospital admission, meaning that many mentally ill prisoners remain in prison where they have to be treated by correctional psychiatrists in often very suboptimal surroundings (Green, Naismith & Menzies 1991).

became used exclusively for the "mentally infirm", such as HMP Dartmoor, which in 1852 was designated an "invalid depot".

Elizabeth Fry, Quaker and prison reformer, began to visit Newgate prison in 1813. Appalled at conditions, she began to visit regularly, supplying clothes, and establishing a school and a chapel. She gave evidence to the House of Commons Committee on London Prisons and was instrumental in Peel's introduction of the Gaols Act 1823, which required visiting prison chaplains, payment of gaolers, and the prohibition of irons. These reforms had little effect, however, until the introduction of prison inspectors by the Prisons Act 1835 (Edwards & Hurley 1997), and the centralisation of running prisons by the Prisons Act 1877 (Yellowlees 1987). The latter also created the post of a full-time medical inspector of prisons and a Prison Commission.

The dual pressure of the number of mentally disordered prisoners, along with the growing number of the criminally insane in the county asylums, led to the view that an asylum for the criminally insane was required (Criminal Lunatic Asylums Act 1860), and Broadmoor Hospital was opened in 1863 to take mentally ill prisoners (Walker & McCabe 1973). Broadmoor closed to admissions for male insane convicts from 1874 until the 1880s, as these prisoners were found to be too troublesome. For 11 years these men were sent to a wing at Woking prison (Gunn *et al.* 1978).

LIFE IN PRISON

Prison life in the 1800s was grim. Sir Edmund Du Cane was Chairman of the Directors of Convict Prisons and of the Commissioners for Local Prisons in the 1870s (Edwards & Hurley 1997). He saw prisons as places of punishment and not rehabilitation, and ran them along military lines:

> The diet was intentionally made poor and unpalatable; hammocks were removed from the cells and planks substituted; the crank and treadmill were introduced. In local prisons (where the maximum sentence was two years) solitary confinement was strictly maintained throughout the whole sentence, and in convict prisons it was the rule for the first nine months. Silence at all times was enforced by the use of punishment. (Gunn *et al.* 1978, p.4)

The prison doctor was employed by the state to mediate this use of punishment and to decide which prisoners should be exempt certain aspects of the harsh prison regime. "The prisoner does not consult the doctor, the State pays the doctor and consults him about the prisoner" (Gordon 1922, p.234). Heated debates were conducted in the pages of the medical journals about the management of prisons and prisoners, especially focusing on the role of the prison diet and the doctors' role in determining the minimum food required to sustain life (Sim 1990). This was also the subject of review by the Carnarvon Committee in 1863 which found that there was "an insufficiency of penal discipline" and recommended experiments to "ascertain what might safely be done" in regard to reducing the diet (Sim 1990, pp.34–35). These debates occurred on a background of high death rates in prison, some due to starvation and exhaustion, and some to the high suicide rate (Gover 1880).

In keeping with the scientific spirit of the times, a number of attempts to alter the running of prison regimens were made, with the intention of rehabilitating prisoners. A variety of different systems were tried, usually with the underlying theory that criminal propensities might be contagious, and that solitary, religious reflection might be the cure. The classified system was introduced in 1823, separating male and female prisoners, and subdividing them on the basis of their crimes – for example, separating felony convicts from misdemeanour convicts (Mayhew & Binny 1862). The silent associated system was introduced at Coldbath Fields House of Correction in 1834. No classification of the prisoners was required, as they were allowed no intercourse (hence silent and associated). This required enormous surveillance by the staff. The separate system, introduced at Pentonville in 1842, excluded prisoners from association with other prisoners, it being intended that the prisoner should hold "hold communion with himself" (Mayhew & Binny 1862, p.102). Reverend Kingsmill, the chaplain of Pentonville, held that, "Under this discipline the propagation of crime is impossible – the continuity of vicious habits is broken off – the mind is driven to reflection, and conscience resumes her sway" (Mayhew & Binny 1862, p.102). Mayhew & Binny (1862) noted the tenfold increase in the rate of "lunacy" at Pentonville during the period 1842–1850 under the separate system, and it was discontinued (Watts 2001). The mixed system, used at Millbank, combined aspects of the silent and separate systems. Prisoners would work together in silence during the day, and sleep in separate cells by night (Mayhew & Binny 1862). Finally, the mark system, not used in England, proposed that a prison sentence might be measured by the amount of labour done rather than time served, a series of marks being used to record the former.

PRISON AS REFORMATION

In 1895 the Gladstone Committee reviewed the state of prisons, and started "from the principle that prison treatment should have as its primary and concurrent objects, deterrence and reformation" (Home Office 1895, p.18). This was a shift of perspective, from prison as punishment to prison as rehabilitation. Du Cane resigned after publication of the report and was succeeded by Sir Evelyn Ruggles-Brise (Watts 2001). The Gladstone Committee recommended that prison doctors should have special experience in lunacy, and proposed that prisons should attempt to reform their inmates. They introduced association between prisoners, and less segregation. They also recommended longer sentences for habitual offenders, and the establishment of a juvenile reformatory (Edwards & Hurley 1997). A wing of the convict prison at Borstal was given over to this latter task in 1902, and led to the establishment of Borstal training (Edwards & Hurley 1997).

Sir Alexander Paterson became Prison Commissioner in 1922 and was a force behind many of the reforms recommended by the Gladstone Committee, including phasing out separate confinement, introducing a working day within prison, with prison wages, and encouraging the development of the Borstal system (Edwards & Hurley 1997). The Howard League for Penal Reform was also established in 1922, by Margery Fry (Edwards & Hurley 1997).

In the 1920s a part of Birmingham prison became used for the investigation of the mental condition of remand prisoners (under Dr Hamblin-Smith), and in 1922 Birmingham University began a postgraduate medical course on "The Medical Aspects of Crime and Punishment" (Gunn *et al*. 1978). The first open prison was created in 1930 at Lowdham Grange (Edwards & Hurley 1997). The Dove-Wilson (1932) Committee recommended more psychotherapy in prisons. The year 1933 saw Dr Hubert appointed as psychotherapist to Wormwood Scrubs, and Wakefield prison came to be a centre for psychiatric treatment in 1946. In 1939 criminal psychiatric positivism reached its acme in the East–Hubert Report, finding that "psychotherapy as an adjunct to an ordinary prison sentence appears to be effective in preventing, or in reducing the chance of, future antisocial behaviour" (East & Hubert 1939, p.153) and recommending the creation of a special therapeutic penal institution. Prison psychologists were established in 1950, and Grendon prison finally opened in 1962.

In 1961 the Emery Report (Ministry of Health 1961) recommended the establishment of local secure units, but this had to wait until the Butler Report in 1975 (Home Office, Department of Health and Social Security 1975) before money was identified and ring-fenced for just this purpose, and the medium secure units were born.

The Prison Commission was replaced by the Prison Department of the Home Office in 1963. In 1964 the Gwynn Committee (Home Office 1964) recommended joint psychiatric appointments between prisons and hospitals, and the post of Home Office psychiatrist was created. The death penalty in Britain was suspended in 1965 and finally abolished in 1969.

SECURITY AND DANGEROUSNESS (1966–2009)

The pendulum seems to have swung back from reform and towards a preoccupation with security and dangerousness over the past 40 years. A series of high profile escapes, including that of the spy George Blake, led to a number of reports reviewing prison security (Edwards & Hurley 1997). In 1966 the Mountbatten Report (Home Office 1966) recommended a maximum security prison (Vectis) be built on the Isle of Wight. Although this proposal was subsequently rejected by the Radzinowicz Report (Advisory Council on the Penal System 1968), a large amount of money was redirected into improving security. Closed-circuit television and the prison dog service were introduced, outside working parties were abolished, and security classification of prisoners was started. The Radzinowicz Report recommended, instead of concentrating high-risk prisoners in one maximum security establishment, that they be dispersed in a number of high security prisons. Thus the dispersal prisons were established, renamed the high security estate in 1998.

In a climate of increasing unrest in the prisons in the 1970s with prison riots and poor industrial relations, a Committee of Inquiry into the state of prison services was appointed (Edwards & Hurley 1997). The May Report (Home Office 1979) recommended substantial reorganisation of the prison service, including the appointment of an independent HM Chief Inspector of Prisons reporting directly to the Home Secretary.

The Floud Report (Floud & Young 1981) examined the prediction and prevention of dangerousness in the criminal justice system. It suggested that prediction was poor (33–50% success rate), and that actuarial methods were better than clinical. The Report concluded that sentencing should take account of future risk.

In 1984 the Control Review Committee (Home Office 1984) introduced the "CRC [Control Review Committee] system" for the most disruptive prisoners. There were further reports into prison disturbances and escapes (the Woolf Report (Home Office 1991a) and the Woodcock Report (Home Office 1994)). In 1995 the Learmont Report (Home Office 1995a) again recommended consideration of a "Supermax" facility for the most disturbed prisoners, a control prison for 200 inmates (half thought to need psychiatric attention) and a special security prison for another 200. The Spurr Report (HM Prison Service 1996) introduced the close supervision centre (CSC) system replacing the CRC and continuous assessment scheme (CAS). The CSC system has been well reviewed by Clare & Bottomley (2001).

Prison psychological approaches became much more influenced by crudely behavioural models of human behaviour (rather than the more psychodynamic ideas behind Grendon), and in 1995 the incentives and earned privileges (IEP) scheme was introduced in prisons nationally.

MEDICAL CARE IN PRISONS

The medical care received by prisoners has been heavily criticised in recent decades (e.g. Smith 1984) and a number of documents have been published making clear that the expectation is for an equivalent service for prisoners from the Prison Medical Service to what they would get outside of prison from the National Health Service, with a recommendation that the NHS should take over the health care of prisoners (HM Inspectorate of Prisons 1996). The Prison Medical Service was renamed the "health care service for prisoners" (Wilmott & Foot 2001) following the efficiency scrutiny of 1990 (Home Office 1990a). More recent reports have suggested that the way forward is for a "formal partnership between the NHS and the Prison Service" (HM Prison Service & NHS Executive 1999, p.17), and the NHS took over the responsibility for commissioning prison health services between 2003 and 2006.

The special hospitals and medium secure units were meant, in large part, to move mentally ill prisoners from prison to hospital. Epidemiological surveys have continued to demonstrate a high prevalence of mental illness in prisoners (Fazel & Danesh 2002), and yet the orthodoxy remains that "[p]rison is unsuitable for a person coming within the scope of the Mental Health Act" (Department of Health & Home Office 1992). Seddon (2007) has argued, following Foucault, that the fact that prisons have always contained mentally disordered persons is not an accident of an imperfect system, but tells us something important about the heart of the matter: the "presence of madmen among the prisoners is not the scandalous limit of confinement but its truth; not abuse but essence" (Foucault 1967, p.225).

CONCLUSION

If we are serious about dealing with mentally disordered prisoners, we must understand that the "clearing-out" approach will fail. Psychiatry has failed to address itself properly to the question of what is its role in prisons. Should psychiatry be intimately involved with all prisoners, creating healthy therapeutic prisons (*à la* East–Hubert Report), or should it be more like prison dentistry, simply treating cases of mental illness as and when they arise? Echoes of these polar views can perhaps be seen, on the one hand, in the advancement of the idea of "healthy prisons" (HM Inspectorate of Prisons 1999) contrasted on the other hand with statements like, "[s]pecialist services do not in our view have a place in prison" (Kesteven 2002, p.50).

CHAPTER 2

The Current Structure of the Prison Service

John Podmore

The prison system in the United Kingdom is not one single entity. The Prison Service of England and Wales operates separately from Scotland and Northern Ireland, which each operate their own individual, autonomous systems.

England and Wales has the highest imprisonment rate in Western Europe, at 148 per 100,000 of the population. France has an imprisonment rate of 85 per 100,000 and Germany has a rate of 93 per 100,000. The additional 9,500 places that Lord Falconer announced in June 2007 will take the rate of imprisonment in England and Wales to 166 per 100,000 of population. That is beyond Bulgaria (148), Slovakia (155), Romania (155) and Hungary (156) (International Centre for Prison Studies 2008).

The number of prisoners in England and Wales has increased by 25,000 in the last ten years (Ministry of Justice 2008a). In 1996, the mid-year prison population was 55,256 (Ministry of Justice 2008a). When Labour came to government in May 1997, the prison population was 60,131. Previously it took nearly four decades (1958–1995) for the prison population to rise by 25,000. At the beginning of 2008, the prison population was approximately 82,000 and continuing to rise. There is every indication that this inexorable rise will continue and a population of 100,000 is highly likely in the next five years.

The Prison Service lists its objectives as:

- holding prisoners securely

- reducing the risk of prisoners re-offending

- providing safe and well-ordered establishments in which we treat prisoners humanely, decently and lawfully.

It is this first objective of security that has had the greatest influence on the current structure of the service. More precisely, it is the failures of security during two dramatic periods nearly three decades apart that still leave their hallmark today.

The first period was the mid-Sixties. On 12 August 1964, Great Train Robber Charles Wilson escaped from Winson Green Prison in Birmingham. In the following July one of his fellow train robbers, Ronnie Biggs, escaped from HMP Wandsworth. Wilson remained at large for four years before being recaptured in Canada. Then, on 22 October 1966, one of this country's most notorious spies escaped with equal apparent ease from HMP Wormwood Scrubs. The man in question was George Blake, who five years earlier had been sentenced to what was then the longest determinate sentence ever passed in a British Court: 42 years. He fled to Moscow via East Germany, where he saw out his days.

Nearly three decades later the prison system was rocked by two more high pro-file escapes: on 9 September 1994, six men (five of whom were convicted terrorists) escaped from a special security unit in HMP Whitemoor in Cambridgeshire. All were quickly recaptured, but the organisational and political ramifications were immense. Less than four months later the pressures on the service increased with the escape from HMP Parkhurst on the Isle of Wight (at that time still a High Security Prison) of three more dangerous offenders. They were at large on the Isle of Wight for four days before being recaptured. These two events led to the now infamous exchange between Jeremy Paxman and then Home Secretary Michael Howard, on Howard's alleged involvement with Director General Derek Lewis's sacking of the Governor of Parkhurst.

Both periods saw major inquiries into the security breaches. The year 1966 saw the Inquiry into Prison Escapes and Security headed by Earl Mountbatten (Home Office 1966). Out of this came the security classification system, which remains largely un-changed today and on which much of the Prison Service's operations are predicated. That classification is as follows:

- **Category A** – "Prisoners who must in no circumstances be allowed to get out, either because of security considerations affecting spies, or because their violent behaviour is such that members of the public or the police would be in danger of their lives if they were to get out."

- **Category B** – Prisoners for whom "the very high expenditure on the most modern escape barriers may not be justified, but who ought to be kept in se-cure conditions."

- **Category C** – Prisoners who "lack the resource and will to make escape at-tempts, [but] have not the stability to be kept in conditions where there is no barrier to escape."

- **Category D** – Prisoners "who can reasonably be entrusted to serve their sentences in open conditions."

(Home Office 1966, para. 15, 217)

Years later the Category A classification was modified to delineate high-risk and exceptional-risk Category A prisoners. The numbers fluctuate but remain relatively small.

There was a sharp fall in the number of prison escapes following Blake's, but the 1970s and 1980s saw an inexorable rise, with a peak in 1991. The following decade saw a steep decline in escapes, and whilst the Whitemoor and Parkhurst escapes were high profile, they did not mark any change in the downward trend, which in fact continued following these two events.

The inquiries which followed the Whitemoor and Parkhurst escapes were the Woodcock and Learmont Reports respectively (Home Office 1994, 1995a). In general, they reviewed security in three forms: physical, dynamic and procedural. Physical security is self-explanatory and significant capital investment was made in the full range of security systems, including cameras, alarms and general physical infrastructure. Security procedures were completely overhauled and a stringent security audit system introduced. Dynamic security, essentially the relationship between staff and prisoners, also received an overhaul with training on the conditioning of staff (developed by terrorist prisoners in the Maze in Northern Ireland) becoming a key component of training for those working with high-security prisoners. Procedural security refers to the control of policies and procedures for safe running of the prison. All prisons will attempt to balance these security considerations according to the needs of each establishment and its declared function. Prisons will also attempt to balance security with the need to deliver a constructive regime for prisoners, which will have at its heart the need to reduce re-offending whilst still protecting the public.

This period also saw a review of those prisons housing Category A prisoners. Mountbatten had recommended that all prisoners of high security be housed in one "super prison", Vectis ("white", as he thought it should be located on the Isle of Wight). This approach was rejected, and instead a system of dispersal prisons was set up, with the most difficult and dangerous prisoners spread around the country in designated "dispersals". Post-Woodcock, this was revised into a "high security estate", with some prisons receiving significant expenditure to bring them up to higher security specifications, whilst others, such as HMP Parkhurst, were downgraded, with all Category A prisoners being moved elsewhere.

Of the country's 138 prisons (of which 11 are contracted out), six are within the high security estate. The remainder are divided into local prisons, training prisons and open/resettlement prisons. Local prisons are there to serve the courts, and the vast majority are old and found in the centre of towns and cities. They house a mixture of remand and convicted prisoners, and their role is to ensure that prisoners are taken to court, as and when required, and to categorise and allocate them on to other prisons once they have been convicted and sentenced.

FROM REMAND TO SENTENCE

The remand population is significant and stood at almost 13,000 at the end of 2007 (Prison Reform Trust 2008a). That total comprised 8,000 untried prisoners, with some 5,000 convicted but unsentenced. It is common for there to be a time lag from conviction to sentence as a range of reports are compiled to establish a background picture of the prisoner, covering his or her offending history, health and social background. Nineteen per cent of men and 18% of women held on remand before trial in 2005 were acquitted (Prison Reform Trust 2008a). The vast majority received no compensation for this period of incarceration. Only half of all remanded prisoners actually go on to receive a prison sentence. In 2005, 53% of men and 41% of women on remand received an immediate custodial sentence (Prison Reform Trust 2008a).

At the end of October 2007 there were 957 women on remand, one in five of the female prison population (Prison Reform Trust 2008a). Women on remand have been one of the fastest growing groups among the prison population. There was a 105% increase in the number of women remanded into custody between 1995 and 2005, compared to a 24% increase for men (Prison Reform Trust 2008a).

Once sentenced, a prisoner will be categorised and allocated using a prescriptive algorithm, which incorporates a range of criteria. A prisoner's category will be based on his sentence length, previous convictions and dangerousness (as defined by Mountbatten). Account should also be taken of the need to address a prisoner's offending behaviour, education, training and resettlement needs. However, in a pressured and overcrowded system it would be fair to say that the overall management of the size of the population will inevitably take priority.

If defined as Category A, a prisoner will be located in one of the two local prisons within the high security estate, Belmarsh or Manchester. Category A women are very rare, but it is not unknown for those there are to be placed in improvised units within male prisons. Category B prisoners will move to Category B long-term training prisons, and Category C are similarly moved on. Lower risk prisoners, especially those sentenced to short periods of imprisonment for non-violent offences, may go directly to open prisons. The principle is always to house prisoners in establishments of appropriate security, but most prisons hold a mixture for a variety of reasons. Prisons should never hold prisoners of a security status higher than that of the prison itself. In addition, the security category of prisoners should be regularly reviewed as they progress through their sentence.

Ideally, prisoners are released from open or resettlement prisons. Currently this happens to only a minority, particularly those nearing release on licence from a life sentence. One further drawback to the process is the fact that, for historical reasons, open and resettlement prisons are rarely in the urban locations that most prisoners come from and resettle into.

PRISON ORGANISATION

The prison system operated on a regional system for most of the 1970s and 1980s and then in September 1990 an area structure was brought into being. The arrangements have been modified over the years but there are now 12 Areas with the high security estate standing separately.

The National Offender Management Service (NOMS) was created in 2004, and with it some ten Regional Offender Managers (ROMS), whose original brief was to be commissioners for community and custodial services in the Criminal Justice System. NOMS was designed to be an overarching body covering prisons and probation and was set targets to reduce re-offending by putting into place an "end-to-end" offender strategy. Prison has a poor record for reducing re-offending: 64.7% are reconvicted within two years of being released (Prison Reform Trust 2008a); for young men (18–20) it is 75% (Prison Reform Trust 2008a).

By 2007 ROMS had yet to receive real budgets with which to commission services, and with the creation of the Ministry of Justice in 2007 the whole NOMS strategy was urgently reviewed. In January of 2008, NOMS and the Prison Service were fully amalgamated with the Probation Service, coming under a newly created NOMS Chief Executive who had formerly been the Prison Service Director General. The stated aim was to streamline the headquarters to improve the focus on frontline delivery of prisons and probation, and improve efficiency. The Chief Executive of the restructured NOMS now runs public prisons and manages performance across the sector, through service level agreements and formal contracts with probation boards and trusts, private prisons and other service providers.

Changes to the regional organisation of offender management also began in April 2008 on a phased basis, to merge the roles of Area Manager in the Prison Service and Regional Offender Managers in NOMS. From 1 April 2009 new, regional managers (DOM – Director of Offender Management) were appointed across the nine English Regions and Wales. The high security estate remains a separate functional entity. The role of the DOM is to commission prison and probation services, from public, private and third sector providers, and to manage performance. Each DOM will operate with a common defined structure consisting of regional managers each responsible for custodial services, community services, commissioning, finance and performance, and organisational development.

CHANGES TO HEALTH AND EDUCATION IN PRISONS

The health of prisoners is one of the most significant challenges facing the Prison Service. It is widely accepted that poor physical and mental health are key characteristics of the population (see Chapters 3 and 4). Added to the problems of poor health and educational background are the issues of problematic drug and alcohol use. It is estimated that 70% of the prisoners will have a substance misuse problem on entering prisons, but that 80% of them will not have had contact with drug treatment services

(Social Exclusion Unit 2002). Suicide and self-harm are also major concerns in prison (see Chapters 6 and 20). The suicide rate for men in prison is five times greater than that for men in the community, and boys aged 15–17 are 18 times more likely to kill themselves in prison than in the community (Prison Reform Trust 2008a).

Until 2006, clinicians led by a Senior Medical Officer delivered health in prisons. *Patient or Prisoner?* (HM Inspectorate of Prisons 1996) challenged this approach to the delivery of a key service, but it took until 2003 for the transfer of responsibilities for health from prisons to local primary care trusts to take place. Since then a number of models have developed, with secondary services, such as psychiatric, being contracted out and primary care being delivered through PCTs. Some establishments, such as HMP Wandsworth and HMP Brixton, have contracted out services in their entirety – in the case of Brixton, to a local consortium including local providers and in the case of HMP Wandsworth, to a social enterprise organisation. It is clear that over time commissioning arrangements will continue to develop according to local needs and preferences.

Education programmes have similarly changed. The majority of establishments now let three-year contracts through a commercial tendering process to a range of colleges and education institutions, with oversight and budgetary control coming from the Learning and Skills Council. Most prisoners will have had very poor school experiences, and the majority will have left, often prematurely through truancy and expulsion, and end up therefore with very few qualifications and poor basic skills. Thirty per cent of prisoners will have been regular truants (Social Exclusion Unit 2002). Forty-nine per cent of males and 33% of females will have been excluded (Social Exclusion Unit 2002). Eighty percent will have writing skills, 65% numeracy skills and 50% reading skills at or below the level of an 11-year-old child (Social Exclusion Unit 2002). The whole area of learning disability still needs more urgent attention. Inevitably, the focus of learning and skills in prison is on basic and key skills, and the delivery of qualifications over recent years has been impressive, but the translation of these results into sustained and meaningful employment remains problematic.

THE PRISON JOURNEY

On entry into a prison for the first time a prisoner can expect to undergo what, to some, might be a bewildering array of assessments, including health, drugs and education. Prisoners will also take part in an induction process to ensure that they know how to find their way through prison rules and regulations, benefit as much as possible from the prison regime, and exercise their full rights in relation to access to legal representation, as well as taking forward complaints and grievances. Imparting such information and protecting the rights of individuals in the system, a key task, will be fraught with problems. Prison is a challenging environment at the best of times. Add to this the problems of physical and mental health, literacy, language and culture, compounded with the demands of the judicial system, overcrowding and turnover, and the potential for individuals to have unmet needs is great.

Supporting the processes and procedures for both staff and prisoners is a watchdog body called the Independent Monitoring Board (IMB). Members meet together monthly under an elected Chair. The Board reports directly to the Secretary of State for Justice and members carry out regular rota visits covering all aspects of the prison. Prisoners have the right to meet with them privately and to raise matters of concern. IMB members are also a key part of the review process by which prisoners are kept in, or released from, segregation. All closed prisons have a "segregation unit" where prisoners are kept separately as part of a punishment which can be given as part of the prison disciplinary procedure. They may also be kept there for their own protection, or may opt to go there voluntarily for a variety of different reasons. Whilst some prisoners may see such isolation as a refuge, segregation units remain parts of the prison where prisoners are potentially vulnerable and at risk. Allocation to, retention in, and release from segregation follows strict protocols, which are regularly audited.

Prison governors no longer have the power to effectively add to a prisoner's sentence (referred to as "added days" and seen colloquially as loss of remission). The High Court ruled in the mid-1990s that such power can rest only with a judge, and that for it to be exercised an individual has the right of legal representation (Campbell & Fells v United Kingdom, Ezeh v United Kingdom). Serious allegations of indiscipline are therefore referred to a visiting judge who will carry out a hearing in the establishment. Very serious cases where there is a *prima facie* case for a criminal act are referred to the police.

The Prison Service aims to deliver a constructive and meaningful regime to all prisoners but it is widely acknowledged, not least by Her Majesty's Chief Inspector of Prisons (HMCIP), that there are insufficient resources to provide for the needs of all prisoners. Whilst remand and very short-term prisoners arguably miss out most, there remain serious issues with even longer-term prisoners as the service expands and comes under ever-increasing pressure. The average time out of cell on a weekday for each prisoner was ten hours exactly in 2005–2006, a fall from 11.2 in 1996–7 (Prison Reform Trust 2007).

THE CHANGING POPULATION

The changing nature of sentencing has added to the pressures on the prison estate. Men in prison serving four years or more were the fastest growing section of the population between 1995 and 2005, increasing by 86% (Prison Reform Trust 2008a).

The nature and type of indeterminate sentences is also having a major influence on the system (see Chapter 17). England and Wales has the highest number of life-sentenced prisoners in Europe (Prison Reform Trust 2008b). The new sentence of indeterminate detention for public protection (IPP) is growing rapidly. The number of people serving these sentences now exceeds the number on short sentences of a year or less (Prison Reform Trust 2008b). There were 10,079 people serving indeterminate sentences at the end of October 2007, a rise of 27% on the year before (Prison

Reform Trust 2008b). This compares with fewer than 4,000 in 1998 and 3,000 in 1992 (Prison Reform Trust 2008b). There are now well over 3,000 people serving IPP sentences, more than 300 of whom are being held beyond their tariff (Prison Reform Trust 2008b). It is estimated that there will be 12,500 people serving IPPs by 2012 (Prison Reform Trust 2008b).

As the prison population increases inexorably, the Government is dealing with pressures on the prison estate by building more capacity. Since 1997 the government has increased prison capacity by nearly 20,000 places and a new capacity-building programme has been put in place to deliver 8,000 new prison places by 2012. Just over 4,000 of these places are to be provided by new prisons. The remaining places are to be delivered by expansions at existing prisons. A further 1,500 new prison places were announced on 19 June 2007. In order to ensure rapid delivery of this additional accommodation, a range of build options is to be explored, including quick build units, temporary custodial units and new house blocks. The first new prison in operation under this emergency programme was HMP Kennet. Kennet was financed by NOMS, and HM Prison Service runs the prison. The Government has made a commitment that the operation of new capacity will be shared between the private and public sectors. Many argue that the majority of new establishments will be contracted out, i.e. privately run.

In addition to the emergency building programme, the Government early in 2008 declared its intention to build three supersize prisons, holding about 2,500 inmates each. This followed a report by Lord Carter, who christened them "Titan Prisons" (Ministry of Justice 2008b). The aim was for the first of the three to be operating by 2012, with the other two by 2014. Following widespread opposition to the principle the Government finally abandoned the plans in April 2009 and replaced them with plans for privately run "supersized prisons" holding 1,500 prisoners each. The aim of raising capacity to 96,000 by 2014 remained.

It appears that changes in government are unlikely to change the general trend toward increasing rates of imprisonment and overall capacity. How this increased estate will respond to the demands to reduce re-offending remains to be seen.

CHAPTER 3

Delivering Mental Health Services in Prison

Janet Parrott

INTRODUCTION

Health services in prisons in the UK were subject to much criticism throughout the latter part of the twentieth century. Research on the high prevalence of mental disorder in prisoners (Gunn, Maden & Swinton 1991, Brooke *et al.* 1996) played a crucial role in setting out the need for comprehensive mental health services. Growing concern about deaths in custody, the frustration of prison governors mindful of their responsibilities for the whole organisation, and most important of all, the sustained effort of the then Chief Inspector of Prisons, Sir David Ramsbotham, led to publication of the thematic report on health care in prisons, *Patient or Prisoner?* (HM Inspectorate of Prisons 1996).

Patient or Prisoner? made it clear that prisoners were not being provided with the same standards of health care that would ordinarily be available in the NHS and recommended that the NHS take on responsibility for health care in prisons. Its publication marked a watershed for professionals, parliamentarians and prison management. A joint working group was set up between the Department of Health and the Home Office, culminating in the report *The Future Organisation of Prison Health Care* (HM Prison Service & NHS Executive 1999). Prisoners were to be provided with health care equivalent to that available to other citizens, and a whole system approach was to ensure that this would also extend to those in contact with the courts and criminal justice agencies in the community.

Guidance in *Changing the Outlook* (Department of Health 2001) set out a structure and timetable for commissioning responsibility to transfer to local commissioning groups (primary care trusts), and again emphasised the need for equality of access to health care for prisoners, in line with the principles of the National Service Framework for Mental Health (Department of Health 1999a). These overall changes were hugely significant in bringing prison health care within mainstream commissioning and providing a structure for subsequent health improvement. Funding was allocated for the development of "mental health inreach" teams with the aim of providing equivalence in mental health care for those prisoners with severe mental illness.

COMMISSIONING MENTAL HEALTH SERVICES FOR PRISONS

A health care needs assessment includes epidemiological, comparative and corporate approaches and can be used to establish a baseline of need, current service provision and priorities for action. Prisons and primary care trusts in England and Wales were given joint responsibility for the development of health needs assessments and implementation of local health improvement plans in 2000, with full commissioning responsibility being taken on by the local NHS from April 2006.

NEEDS ASSESSMENT

There is extensive evidence of the substantial burden of treatable mental illness in prison populations. Brooke *et al.* (1996), in a study of 16 prisons and young offenders institutions, found that 5% of the remand population (about 680 men at that time) had a psychotic or affective disorder. Singleton, Meltzer & Gatward (1998) reported that 14% of women and 10% of men in prison had a diagnosis of psychosis and 50% a diagnosis of personality disorder. Co-morbidity between mental illness, substance misuse and personality disorder is the norm. A broadly similar situation prevails in other western countries. In their international systematic review, Fazel & Danesh (2002) found consistent evidence that prisoners were several more times likely to have psychosis or major depression, and about ten times more likely to have antisocial personality disorder, than the general population. Typically, about one in seven prisoners in western countries has psychotic illness or major depression, and about one in two male prisoners and one in five female prisoners has antisocial personality disorder.

UNMET NEED IN MENTAL HEALTH

Using needs assessment instruments, Harty *et al.* (2003) and Thomas (2005) demonstrated that mentally disordered offenders in prison differ significantly from general adult patients living in the community in having both more needs relating to mental health and more unmet needs. The greater unmet needs were in the following domains: psychotic symptoms, psychological distress, welfare benefits, money, daytime activities, company and food. A particular area of unmet need for prisoners in the UK is prompt treatment when inpatient care is considered appropriate. The care pathway from prison to hospital is associated with lengthy delay in the majority of cases (Isherwood & Parrott 2002, McKenzie & Sales 2008).

MODELS OF MENTAL HEALTH CARE

Durcan & Knowles (2006), in a review of mental health services in London prisons, reported a lack of collaborative working and particular difficulties in planning care pathways when other relevant providers of care did not engage. A further review of the care and support of prisoners with mental health needs (HM Inspectorate of Prisons 2007a) considered that there was no clear blueprint for delivering mental health care in prisons based on the assessed needs of the population. Although the requirements for mental health care vary considerably between prisons, the functions discussed below are common to all.

Identification

It is a statutory requirement to assess the health care need of a prisoner on reception (see Chapter 4). However, Brooker, Repper, Beverley *et al.* (2002) found that reception screening fails to pick up about a quarter of those with severe mental illness, and it is usual for it to be followed up by a "well person" review the following day in a less pressured environment. Primary care nursing staff require training in mental health and substance misuse with a level of sophistication in "sign posting" to other services, especially psychological treatment, social support and substance misuse.

Assessment and treatment

Mental health services in prisons should be able to offer comprehensive care plans for those with stable mental illness (see Chapter 5). Active co-operation from non-health-care staff in supporting vulnerable prisoners is also essential, so that the regime does not undermine care. In large prisons with a remand function, a common model of care would include the following options:

(a) Community care
"Community care" is provided to prisoners with moderate mental health needs who can be treated in their usual residential setting. An assessment by a psychiatrist or mental health nurse is followed by either brief intervention, or continuing care under the care programme approach, with support and mental state assessment by a community psychiatric nurse and regular review by a psychiatrist. Successful implementation of the approach has considerable resource implications and requires effective links with the NHS.

For sentenced prisoners with stable mental illness, liaison between the mental health teams (both inside the prison and in the community outside) and prison and probation services is essential for satisfactory pre-release planning. Psychological treatment may form part of the care plan, but in many prisons this is unavailable or ill co-ordinated between the prison and mental health team.

(b) Day care
Some large prisons in the UK enhance "community care" by offering additional support and specific treatment groups through a day programme which may also be available to prisoners in the health care centre. Typical options include cognitive behavioural therapy (CBT)-based groups focusing on anger management, anxiety and depression, and occupational activities to promote social and relational skills, including learning strategies to cope in the prison environment.

(c) Care in the health care centre
Large prisons in the UK generally utilise the option of residential care in the health care centre for those with mental health needs that cannot be met on ordinary location. A significant use of such centres in the UK at present is to accommodate prisoners with severe mental illness who have been referred to outside hospitals for inpatient treatment but experience delay in admission, often of many weeks (Isherwood & Parrott 2002, McKenzie & Sales 2008). Work involved in securing inpatient care for this group remains a prominent part of the work of mental health teams in prison. In some European countries, such as Germany, there is a further option of transfer to a prison with a fully supported psychiatric unit.

(d) Liaison and reporting
Psychiatric teams in prison often play a significant role in liaising with courts and criminal justice agencies. This can include the provision of reports for courts, probation and lifer panels. Prisons with specialist programmes such as sex offender treatment, personality disorder services and units for prisoners with challenging behaviour will have their own particular needs for mental health provision which need to be considered locally.

CHALLENGES TO COMMISSIONING AND DELIVERING MENTAL HEALTH SERVICES

There is considerable variation between prisons with regard to profile of need in mental health, but particular consideration needs to be given to the following factors both in planning, and in funding and delivering services.

Turnover of the population

Busy remand prisons in urban areas in the UK may have in the region of 700 new receptions each year with known morbidity in relation to mental health (Gavin, Parsons & Grubin 2003). This constant flux makes it difficult to develop responsive services that can reliably provide across the range of assessment, acute care, longer term care and psychological treatment. Other parts of the criminal justice system may operate with little reference to health care, and prisoners may be moved with little notice, or fail to return from court, necessitating hasty liaison.

Prisons with a predominantly sentenced and more stable population should provide an environment where the health care needs of individual prisoners can be met in an appropriate manner, provided that small mental health teams in these environments are supported by health facilities outside the prison for acute care.

Integration with local mental health services

Integration with local mental health services is crucial in prisons with a local remand population. In all other prisons mental health team staff require sufficient time to liaise regularly with local services, especially in relation to discharge planning. The extent to which the wider NHS supports the care of prisoners has an important bearing on the demands placed on prison mental health teams. The opportunity to further develop community services within the prison and to enhance work in relation to criminal justice care pathways is often limited by the resource-hungry care required for prisoners with acute needs that could be most appropriately met within hospital services.

Commissioners of services should play an active role in facilitating the support of other mental health services or commissioners for the patient's home area.

Needs for ethnically diverse groups

In a cross-sectional survey of 3,142 prisoners in England and Wales in 1997, Coid *et al.* (2002) found that fewer black men had their psychiatric needs identified in prison than other social/ethnic groups. It is therefore essential for services within prisons to give careful consideration to how access and engagement with services will be monitored and how best they can meet the needs of diverse groups.

Interface with primary care and substance misuse services

In all prisons the nature of the interface with primary care services and their availability and expertise will be a major factor in the demand for specialist mental health provision. Active involvement of primary care services in mental health and substance misuse, at the stages of identification, initial assessment and management and later follow-up of those who do not require secondary services, is essential to allow specialist mental health teams to function efficiently. Careful consideration also needs to be given to the balance and inter-relationships between substance misuse and mental health services, and to how best care is provided for those with dual diagnosis. Closely linked is the ability of the prison as a whole to modify the social stress and isolation inherent in the custodial environment, and the extent to which other staff, voluntary sector groups and prisoners support prisoners in distress.

Clinical governance

The clinical governance framework in the NHS requires clear lines of responsibility and accountability for quality of care, with procedures available to all professionals to improve quality and manage risk. The situation for mental health teams in a prison setting is complex and often frustrating. Usual service outcome measures, such as responsiveness, may be dependent on factors managed directly by the prison or by NHS providers outside the prison.

Commissioners and providers of mental health services need to ensure that at minimum there is clarity about the investigation of untoward incidents and complaints, and that there are structures that support implementation of recommendations of such reviews.

CONCLUSION

There have been considerable improvements in the scope and quality of mental health services in prisons in the UK since implementation of the Mental Health Inreach Initiative and responsibility for provision moving to the Department of Health. However, there are still significant areas of unmet needs, organisational barriers to care, and much variability in quality between prisons. Paradoxically, the move to local commissioning seems to have hindered an overall approach to health improvement and may not have allowed sufficient focus on issues both within and, particularly, across the prison estate, that prove problematic for health care providers.

CHAPTER 4

Health Screening in Prisons

Don Grubin

INTRODUCTION

Morbidity in prison populations is high. The prevalence of psychiatric disorder, substance misuse and infectious disease (including HIV and hepatitis) in particular are greater than in the general population: in western countries, approximately 4% of prisoners are estimated to suffer from psychotic illnesses and 10% from major depression, with the highest rates in remand settings (Birmingham, Mason & Grubin 1996, Singleton, Meltzer & Gatward 1998, Brinded *et al.* 2001, Fazel & Danesh 2002). A large survey of prisons in England and Wales found nearly one half of prisoners to be drug dependent (Singleton *et al.* 1998), and in the United States it is estimated that 20–26% of all people with HIV, 29–43% of all those infected with the hepatitis C virus, and 40% of those with tuberculosis passed through a correctional facility in 1997 (Hammett, Harmon & Rhodes 2002). In addition, in the first few months following release, prisoners are at greater risk of death compared with the general population, mostly owing to drug misuse and self-inflicted causes (Seaman, Brettle & Gore 1998, Coffey *et al.* 2003, Graham 2003, Hobbs *et al.* 2006).

Prison morbidity does not lie only at the more serious end of the spectrum. It has been known for some time that the general health of prisoners is also less good than it is amongst people living in the community (Novick *et al.* 1977, Martin, Colebrook & Gray 1984). An Australian survey with findings unlikely to be unique to that country found that prisoners (particularly younger ones) had a high prevalence of risk factors for cardiovascular disease and diabetes, such as raised blood pressure and elevated blood glucose and cholesterol levels (D'Souza, Butler & Petrovesky 2005). Asthma is also common. In the UK, corrected for age and gender, prisoners consult the prison doctor more frequently than do populations in the community by a factor of three (Marshall, Simpson & Stevens 2001), with similar levels reported elsewhere in Europe (Feron *et al.* 2005). While some of these contacts are for administrative purposes, most are not, with the reason for consultation typically relating to health problems that existed prior to imprisonment.

Although researchers have little difficulty in identifying this significant amount of physical and psychological morbidity when conducting their surveys, they also note that it often goes unrecognised in practice. This is particularly the case in relation to mental health. A study in a large Chicago jail found that about two-thirds of those with severe mental illness did not receive treatment during their first week in prison (Teplin 1990), less than half those with psychotic illnesses or major depression were receiving treatment in a large New Zealand prison cohort (Brinded *et al.* 2001), and in two large English prisons (one male, one female) three-quarters of new remands suffering from severe mental illness went unrecognised (Birmingham *et al.* 1996, Parsons, Walker & Grubin 2001). If missed at reception, the likelihood of mental health problems being picked up at a later stage is not high (Birmingham, Mason & Grubin 1998, Melzer *et al.* 2002).

In respect of suicide risk, internal English Prison Service data from the late 1990s indicated that less than a quarter of those who committed suicide in the weeks immediately following their reception into prison had been recognised as being at immediate risk, suggesting that reception processes failed to identify this group (although the number of at-risk inmates who were successfully identified and for whom effective preventative measures were taken cannot be determined).

Little information is available regarding the extent to which physical health problems are identified at reception into prison, at least in the English system. Because individuals with physical complaints, particularly those for which they are already receiving treatment, are more likely to volunteer the information to prison health staff than is the case for those with mental illnesses or who misuse substances (the latter, of course, depending on the extent to which treatment is on offer), there is probably less of an issue for these types of condition.

The high level of morbidity in the prison population has important implications, both for the individual prisoner whose health is poor, and for the community at large, where the transmission of infectious disease and the future cost of publicly funded health care give rise to clear public health concerns. This, of course, is in addition to the social costs associated with subsequent poor employment prospects, further crime, and the impact on the families of prisoners (Australian Institute of Health and Welfare 2006).

HEALTH SCREENING

If this high level of morbidity in prison populations is to be addressed, it must first be recognised. In busy prisons, carrying out full physical and mental health assessments of all new prisoners is not a practical option. Because of this, it is necessary to employ screening procedures that can identify a smaller group of individuals who are at higher risk of suffering from relevant health problems, with a clear idea of what counts as "relevant", together with systems being in place to assess in more depth those prisoners who screen positive.

The importance of such health screening is well recognised. In a national survey of American prisons it was found that over 80% provided initial screening for mental health problems (cited in Steadman *et al.* 2005), while in England and Wales it is a statutory requirement for all prisoners to be screened for health problems on their reception into prison (and until recently that they all be seen by a doctor within 24 hours) – a tradition dating back to the 1865 Prison Act (Birmingham 2001b). Reception screening is also common elsewhere in Europe, in Australia and in New Zealand.

If the need for screening is recognised and its use widespread, why do prison health screens appear to function so poorly? *First*, perhaps because of its origins in the nineteenth century, the reception health assessment was combined with other tasks that were seen traditionally as being performed by the doctor, such as certifying that a prisoner is fit to be employed in the kitchens. Over the years, a number of other quasi-medical functions were included in the reception health screen, such as confirming that prisoners were fit for work, the gym, and to share a cell. These sorts of assessment, however, distract from health screening generally, and add time to a process that in a busy prison needs to be carried out swiftly. In most instances, health care staff in any case had no clear idea what constitutes "fitness" for these various activities, making for a fruitless exercise.

Second, the distinction between health screening and the more thorough medical assessment necessary for diagnoses was not clearly understood by those responsible for health care on reception, resulting in a confused assessment process. Similarly, the reception health screen confused the necessity of detecting problems of immediate concern (needing attention during the first few days of imprisonment), and those issues that fell into the public health domain and required a less urgent but longer-term approach.

Before recent modifications, the English prison reception health screen was based on a set of health care standards that were introduced in the early 1990s. It comprised two parts: an initial review by a nurse or health care officer (a prison officer with health care training) using a standard questionnaire, followed by a further, less structured evaluation by a doctor, which under prison regulations was required to take place within 24 hours of entry into prison. The questionnaire, which contained 35 questions (with more for women), was a mix of queries relating to current health difficulties, public health issues, and the types of things asked when patients are admitted to hospital. For example, prisoners were questioned about their immunisation status, their family history of medical problems, whether they had ever had an operation, and the number of cigarettes they smoked; there were 13 questions regarding mental health, of which 10 related to suicide and self-harm, the discriminatory value of which was never determined. The doctor, on the other hand, did not have a questionnaire to work from, but was advised to take full medical and psychiatric histories, to examine the cardiovascular, respiratory, abdominal, locomotor, genito-urinary and central nervous systems, and to perform a mental state examination. If carried out properly, it was conservatively estimated that such an evaluation would take about 50 minutes; assuming just ten new receptions a day, the reception health care assessment would require over 8 hours of the doctor's time, his whole working day. Needless to say, doctors did not follow the advice of the health care standards, but neither was it clear what they did that was different from the assessment carried out by the nurse or the health care officer. In the circumstances, it was hard to see what was gained by insisting that all prisoners should be seen by a doctor within 24 hours of entering prison.

Third, there were no protocols advising what to do when positive findings were made during the assessment. Thus, potential problems were recorded but not recognised, or were recognised but not identified as problems, or were identified as problems but no action followed to deal with them. Birmingham *et al.* (1996), for example, noted that in a number of cases symptoms of mental disorder appeared to be elicited during the assessment, but no further evaluation or treatment followed. On occasion, positive findings recorded on the questionnaire as such by nurses went unnoticed by doctors.

Fourth, the physical environment where reception took place in many prisons was not conducive to eliciting information from new prisoners. The surroundings were often cramped and lacking in privacy, with large numbers of inmates arriving at the same time, often just before the prison was due to shut its gates for the night. Staff were rushed, prisoners irritable and tired, and there was competition from other elements of the reception process that needed completion. In addition, few staff were trained specifically in relation to health screening.

It is perhaps not surprising that health screening on reception into English prisons was not effective. It is hard to see how it could have been otherwise.

PRINCIPLES OF EFFECTIVE HEALTH SCREENING

The purpose of health screening is to identify individuals who are at higher risk of having a specific health-related problem, provided that something can be done about it. Screening tests are applied to large populations, aiming to select from them those who require further investigation or more detailed assessment. Screening needs to be quick and simple to administer, and it must be appropriate for use in large groups at reasonable cost.

Effective screening, as opposed to diagnosis, involves the collection of the minimum amount of information needed to indicate higher risk; once an individual is identified as being at increased risk, further information is redundant, particularly if those doing the screening do not have the specialist skills necessary for further evaluation. For example, in screening for cervical cancer, abnormalities in a smear test are sufficient to trigger additional cytological testing, regardless of whether or not other disease markers are present – the answers to questions about bleeding or pain do not influence the need for further testing, do not contribute to the screening process, and hence the questions do not need to be asked. In the case of interview-based screens of the sort employed in prison health screening, questions only need to discriminate between high- and low-risk cases, rather than allow for detailed management decisions to be made.

A large number of screening programmes exist in relation to a range of diseases. Many are criticised for not making proper cost–benefit analyses – for example, regarding whether the programme reduces death or morbidity (as opposed to increasing anxiety amongst those who screen positive); the cost of preventing one death; who should be targeted in respect of age or other risk factors, and the longer term costs to the health care system (Barratt *et al.* 2004). In the UK, a National Screening Committee (2003) has proposed 22 criteria to determine whether a screening programme is likely to be viable, effective and appropriate. Six of these criteria are perhaps most relevant to prison health screening:

- the condition should be an important health problem

- there should be a detectable risk factor or disease marker

- there should be a simple, safe, precise and validated screening test

- there should be an agreed policy on further diagnostic investigation

- there should be an effective treatment or intervention

- there should be evidence that the screening programme is effective.

It should be noted, however, that most screening in the community is targeted at individuals who are either disease-free or who are in the early, non-symptomatic stages of a given condition, and in respect of diseases where the prevalence is usually not particularly high – in breast cancer screening, for example, it is estimated that 5% of women screen positive, of whom 5–6 per 1,000 have cancer diagnosed (Wilson 2000). Prison health screening, on the other hand, is typically intended to identify individuals who are symptomatic and who are well beyond the latent stage, in circumstances where prevalence is high. Furthermore, the screening envisaged is usually little more than an interview, and does not involve any invasive procedures or actions that in themselves carry a risk to health, such as the X-rays or biopsy that are found in screening for cancer. As such, in prison settings it makes more sense to view criteria like those referred to above as guidelines rather than as doctrine.

Balancing false positives and false negatives

The more *sensitive* a screen is, the more likely it is to detect individuals who have the condition of interest, and the less likely it is to miss individuals with the condition – it will have a low *false negative* rate. As sensitivity increases, however, an increasing number of people who do not have the condition will also "screen positive", a rise in the false positive rate. To avoid this, the threshold for screening positive can be raised, making the screen more *specific*, that is, increasing the likelihood that those who do not have the condition are not screened positive, albeit at the cost of a counterbalancing increase in the *false negative* rate.

Because of the implications of missing serious health problems at the time of reception into prison, it can be argued that it is more important for a prison health screen to be sensitive rather than overly specific. There is more to be lost in failing to detect serious illness or health needs than in wrongly identifying individuals who then receive further assessment – false positives are easier to tolerate than false negatives. In the prison context, therefore, sensitivity is more important than specificity. Of course, one must guard against overwhelming the processes that follow on from screening with too many false positives, and prison health screening, like screening in any other setting, needs to determine what are acceptable false negative and false positive rates for its particular circumstances.

What needs to be screened for?

The "community" of individuals coming into prison differs in many respects from the general population. It is younger, it has a lower social class profile, and many are under considerable psychological stress. There is a higher prevalence of serious mental health problems, substance misuse and dependence, blood-borne viruses, and poor health generally. The circumstances associated with being detained in custody carry with them their own special stresses, giving rise to an increased risk of suicide and self-harm. Based on what is known about health care needs on reception into prison, the following conditions would appear to have reasonable claims of being of particular interest for a prison health screen:

- severe mental illness
- alcohol or drug dependence, and risk of withdrawal
- risk of suicide or serious self-harm
- blood-borne infections
- medical conditions requiring treatment
- the need for medication
- pregnancy

- injuries associated with arrest or detention

- unhealthy lifestyles (for example, smoking or poor diet)

- immunisation status.

Clearly, however, while some of these conditions are important to detect in the early days of custody, the detection of others can be delayed, either to a time when advice and counselling is likely to be more effective, or when more lengthy or demanding tasks such as recording blood pressure, height and weight, or taking blood and urine samples, can be more effectively carried out. Screening need not be a one-stage process.

Detectable risk factors or disease markers

In many of the conditions listed above, detecting risk factors or disease markers is a matter of simply asking the individual. The problem in a prison setting, however, is that in some cases the person asked either does not want to disclose the information, or may not be aware that there is a problem to report – the former, for example, can be the case in terms of substance misuse, particularly where sanctions may follow disclosure, while the latter may occur with severe mental illness or the risk of self-harm. Birmingham *et al.* (2000) reported in their study that a considerable number of prisoners admitted they did not volunteer, and often deliberately withheld, information during prison screening assessments because of concern regarding the consequences. In such cases, asking the right questions, rather than asking a lot of questions, is more likely to identify individuals who require more in-depth evaluation.

In terms of mental health, specific screening questionnaires have been advocated. For instance, many prisons in the United States make use of the Referral Decision Scale (RDS), a 14-item instrument with a reported sensitivity of 79% and specificity of 99% (Teplin & Swartz 1989), although researchers different from the developers have described much less impressive figures regarding sensitivity and specificity (Hart *et al.* 1993, Rogers *et al.* 1995, Veysey *et al.* 1998). The advantages of the RDS are that it is said to be quick to administer, easily scored, and contains clear decision criteria, but it has been criticised because it asks about lifetime rather than current symptoms, and some of its questions do not appear appropriate for a prison environment, resulting in the higher false positive rates found in the later studies (Steadman *et al.* 2005).

The Brief Jail Mental Health Screen (BJMHS) is a modification of the RDS comprised of eight items that focus on symptoms experienced over the preceding six months, and is said to take under three minutes to administer (Steadman *et al.* 2005). In a validation study involving over 10,000 prisoners, 11% screened positive for the presence of severe mental illness, with a reported false positive rate of 49% for men and 45% for women, and a false negative rate of 15% for men and 35% for women, giving an overall "accuracy rate" of 73.5% (Steadman *et al.* 2005). The high false negative rate for women is reported to be caused by the screen missing cases of post-traumatic stress disorder (PTSD), and is apparently being addressed in further developmental research (Goldberg & Higgins 2006).

Many of the BJMHS false negatives were associated with prisoners failing to disclose information regarding symptomatology to the screeners. This raises the question of whether a symptom-oriented approach is the best means for detecting individuals with severe mental illness in prison settings, or whether other markers might be more effective. Another largely symptom-focused mental health screen is the Correctional Mental Health Screen, which has separate scales for men and women comprising 12 and 8 items respectively. It is reported to take from three to five minutes to administer, and has a sensitivity of 75% (Ford & Trestman 2005, Goldberg & Higgins 2006). Like the BJMHS, it would benefit from further validation.

There are a number of screening tools available for the detection of substance misuse in prisoners, eight of which are described by Peters *et al.* (2000). The World Health Organisation-derived AUDIT (Alcohol Use Disorder Identification Test) (Babor *et al.* 1992) and the briefer four-item CAGE (mnemonic for the questions asked: Have you ever thought about **C**utting down your drinking? Do you ever get angry if someone **A**sks you about your drinking? Do you ever feel **G**uilty about your drinking? Have you ever had an **E**ye-opener?) (Mayfield, McLeod & Hall 1974) are good examples of such instruments for the detection of problem drinking. Again, however, they are reliant on the co-operation of the person being screened. In a prison sample in which 75 new prison entrants were screened with AUDIT on admission and then two weeks later, it was found that the proportion of men identified as having a probable alcohol problem increased from 19% to 60% between test and retest, and those rated as probably alcohol-dependent increased from 11% to 43%. No prisoner had a lower AUDIT score on second administration (Maggia *et al.* 2004).

THE NEW HEALTH SCREENING PROCESS IN THE ENGLISH PRISON SERVICE

The various issues referred to above regarding screening principles and problems associated with current screening practices were addressed in the development of new health screening procedures for the English prison service. The screening process is divided into two parts. The first is delivered on reception and intends to identify prisoners with health problems who require some form of intervention immediately or in the following few days. The second part deals with broader, but non-urgent, health concerns, and is meant to be carried out during the individual's first week in prison – its aim is to mirror the sort of evaluation that takes place when an individual registers with a new general practitioner in the community, addressing more public health type concerns such as cardiovascular risk factors, immunisation status and unhealthy lifestyles.

The first night evaluation makes use of an instrument comprised of 15 basic questions that screen for severe mental illness, substance dependence, risk of self-harm, significant physical illness, traumatic injury and the need for medication, and takes from five to ten minutes to deliver. The reason that it can be administered so quickly is that the emphasis is on identifying individuals who need further assessment which will take place at a later time, with screeners trained to avoid the temptation of asking additional questions once sufficient information has been collected to categorise the prisoner as "screening positive". This requires the instrument to indicate clearly when an individual has screened positive.

For those who do screen positive, each prison has written protocols that describe what should happen next, the specific protocols themselves differing to some extent between establishments, depending on resources and the views of local prison doctors and health care managers. The protocols remove the requirement for all prisoners to see a doctor within 24 hours; instead, doctors review only those prisoners who require further medical assessment, with a clear reason being given for this – so long as the protocols are followed, heath care staff are protected from the risk of something going wrong, reducing their dependence on the defensive but redundant practice of having all prisoners "reviewed" by the doctor.

In terms of severe mental illness, the first night screen contains just four items, with the presence of any one counting as a positive screen. None involves asking about current symptoms or looking for signs of mental illness. The choice of these items arose from previous research suggesting that a positive response to any one would identify about 80% of those with serious mental illness (Birmingham *et al.* 2000). The items are:

- a charge of murder or manslaughter

- previous treatment by a psychiatrist outside prison

- previous prescription for antipsychotic or antidepressant medication

- a history of self-harm outside prison.

When the four screening items (plus a fifth in respect to homelessness that added little discriminatory power) were tested in one prison over a 15-week period, it was found that the number of prisoners suffering from mental illness identified by the screening questions was in line with expectations of prevalence derived from previous studies of mental illness in remand prisons (Gavin *et al.* 2003).

The functioning of the screen was further reviewed in ten pilot prisons, where it was found that 86% of those with severe mental illness were correctly identified, a rate not dissimilar to the longer mental health screens referred to above. Thirty-three per cent of the sample screened positive for severe mental illness when none was present, but this reduced to 20% when less severe mental health problems were considered as well (Grubin, Carson & Parsons 2002). Overall, over 60% of the sample screened positive for at least one health problem, little in the way of significant physical health problems went undetected, and no cases of drug or alcohol withdrawal were missed. As there were no incidents of serious self-harm during the time of the review, and as it is difficult to determine false positive rates for this indication, given that intervention follows its identification, the screen's efficacy in respect of detecting those at risk of serious self-harm is unclear.

In terms of the general health assessment intended to be carried out later in the week by nurses, it was found that the reorganisation in prison practices that this would have required meant that many establishments simply added it on to the first night reception, to some extent defeating its purpose (although the two types of evaluation were still at least separated out). In prisons where the relevant clinics were offered later in the week, a sizeable minority of prisoners defaulted. It appeared, however, that those who did attend were provided with an opportunity that had not been available previously to address a number of health-related needs.

By the end of 2005 the new health screening procedures were in use in all English remand prisons. An evaluation of their impact and efficacy is awaited.

CONCLUSION

Given the high levels of prison morbidity common throughout the world, and the potential benefits to be gained from good prison health screening programmes, it is perhaps surprising that more research has not been carried out to develop and evaluate effective health screening instruments and procedures. Much of what limited research has taken place has focused on severe mental illness and substance misuse. Perhaps that is in the nature of prison medicine.

It must also be remembered that even an efficient and effective health screen has to negotiate the resistance to change typically found in closed institutions, and in large systems like correctional services. Prisons have many priorities, with security considerations paramount. Even when introduced, new procedures need to be monitored to ensure they are delivered as intended, particularly given high staff turnover rates and the associated drift in implementation. However, if large-scale screening programmes can be successfully introduced and managed in the community, there should be no reason why they cannot also be effectively delivered in the more contained environment of a prison.

CHAPTER 5

Mentally Ill Prisoners and Mental Health Issues in Prison

Ian Cumming and Simon Wilson

INTRODUCTION

Mental health services in prison occur at an intersection between government depart-ments which often have different and competing agenda. Prisons continue to have a low priority and there is often limited public and political support for improvement. *A New Vision for Mental Health* (Future Vision Coalition 2008), the document which heralds the replacement strategy for the National Service Framework (Department of Health 1999a) has only one reference to prisons, commenting that prisoners are an at-risk group. Public discussions dichotomise the issue – the needs of "prisoners" *versus* those of "normal people" – when these are often the same people at different times in their lives. Given that 30% of men have a conviction for a standard list offence by the age of 30 (Home Office 1995d), most prisoners are members of the community who happen to have an address starting with "HMP" for a few weeks from time to time.

The National Health Service tends to have a narrow focus on prisons, tending to apply its own mechanisms and viewpoint to an environment which is singularly differ-ent, and so, whilst health services in prison have improved and changed considerably in recent years, they continue to lag behind and the gap may be widening as the NHS continues to become more complex and separate.

Prison is a good example of a place where the practitioner can work with a very wide range of conditions. Increasingly, outside of prison, practitioners work with delineated patient groups and often lose the skills needed to work with a broader scope of conditions. Prison presents the very widest range of conditions and disorders.

EPIDEMIOLOGY

There have been many epidemiological studies of the prevalence of mental disorder in prisons (see Chapter 4). Mental disorders of every variety (psychosis, neurosis, addictions, learning disabilities and personality disorders) are present at vastly elevated levels relative to the surrounding community. Fazel and Danesh (2002) systematically reviewed 62 surveys of prison studies covering 12 countries and around 22,790 prisoners. They found, amongst men, rates of psychosis – 3.7%, major depression – 10%, and personality disorder – 65%. In comparison to the community, functional psychosis is ten times more prevalent in prisoners (Brugha *et al.* 2005).

The Office for National Statistics (ONS) survey (Singleton, Meltzer & Gatward 1998) aimed to interview 1,200 remand prisoners (one in eight of those in prison), 1,200 sentenced prisoners (one in 34 of those in prison) and 800 female prisoners (one in three of those in prison). Of a total of 3,563 selected, 3,142 (88%) were interviewed (called a lay interview). Every fifth person was selected for a follow-up interview, and of these 76% (505 in number) were interviewed again (called a clinical interview). The later, clinical interview generated most notably data about personality disorder and utilised the SCID (Structured Clinical Interview for DSM Disorders). This showed that the prevalence of any personality disorder was 78% for male remand prisoners, 64% for sentenced prisoners and 50% for female prisoners.

Neurotic disorders in the week prior to interview were assessed in the lay interviews using the CIS–R (Clinical Interview Schedule – Revised). They asked about sleep problems, worry, fatigue, depression, irritability, depressive ideas, concentration, anxiety, obsession, somatic symptoms, compulsions, phobias, worry over physical health, and panic. The findings again showed incidence rates far higher than in the general population, and in most cases double. It was noted that remand prisoners had roughly double the incidence of sentenced prisoners.

The study looked at the relationship between various questions in the lay interview and the results of the SCAN interview and built up a model of what clusters of factors are highly correlated with positive cases of psychotic psychopathology. This model was then applied to the remaining sample to provide an estimate of the likely prevalence of psychoses amongst the sample as a whole, suggesting for men around 10% of the remand and 7% of the sentenced population, and for women 14% for both remand and sentenced.

Treatment implications

Gunn, Maden & Swinton (1990) and Maden *et al.* (1996) in their prevalence studies made recommendations for treatment options for the individuals interviewed, including hospital transfer, and looked at the unmet needs. It was felt that there should be clear policies for the management of mental disorder, and especially for explicit guidance as to when those with psychosis should be transferred out. It also recommended that standards of care for those who remain in prison should be equivalent to the NHS. It was felt that each local prison should expect to transfer about 5% of its remand population to the NHS, amounting to a need for an additional 8–15 beds in high security, 122–244 beds in medium security, 61–122 in local hospitals, and 23–46 beds in prison health care centres. This study took the direct view that the solution to mentally disordered offenders in prison was in the NHS and that equivalence within the prison system was needed.

It is clear that the prison population has high levels of morbidity. What must also be factored in is the turnover of the population, which adds considerably to issues around service design. Most local prisons where the morbidity and risks are high are also subject to a large turnover. If a local prison has around 1,000 prisoners at any one time, several times that amount will pass through its doors each year. Thus average lengths of stay in local prisons can be very short, and although this means that prisoners are not with services for long, it means also that there is a limited window to engage and deliver services.

WHY IS MENTAL DISORDER SO PREVALENT IN PRISON?
Penrose's law

One of the most common assumptions made is that we have mentally ill prisoners because of failures of "care in the community" and "closing the asylums" – Penrose's law that there is an inverse relationship between the mental hospital and prison populations (Penrose 1939). Although these factors might have some relevance, mentally ill prisoners have always been in prison and are a feature in any prison through the world, and through time, and Penrose's law is probably false. (See Gunn (2000) for discussion.) However, many of the severely mentally ill in prisons are not new presentations but are already known to mental health services – about 75% of those transferred to hospital were already known in one recent study (Forrester *et al.,* in press). Given the relationship between mental disorder and offending, it is highly likely that better psychiatric management of a proportion of these cases would have prevented them coming into prison in the first place.

Mental disorder and offending

There is considerable literature on the relationship between mental disorder and crime at all levels. This ranges from those where the offending is incidental, to those whose crime is driven by the underlying disorder, and in a significant group those whose mental disorder is first highlighted by the criminal event. There is a small but significant relationship between mental illness (particularly paranoid schizophrenia) and violent offending. (See Mullen (2006) for a review.)

Prison psychosis

There is a commonly held, but rarely clearly articulated, belief that prisons drive people mad, thus explaining the high prevalence of mental disorder in prisons. Historically this has been implicit in the loose notion of "prison psychosis". There is no clear definition of this term, and it has been used to cover a variety of putative syndromes historically. Whilst it often carries with it an implied taint of deception, it is not a malingered psychosis. Some have referred to Ganser's syndrome, a dissociative disorder characterised by giving "approximate answers", as prison psychosis (e.g. Enoch & Trethowan 1991). However, it is generally taken to be a psychotic response to either the sensory deprivations inherent in a harsh prison regime (Scott 1974) or to the prison environment more generally (Bowers 1913, Karlan 1939). According to Nitsche & Wilmanns (1912), Delbrück considered it to be caused by lengthy sentences, Gutsch by the weakening and inactivity of reproductive life. Typical symptoms were said to include persecutory delusions, particularly about being poisoned by prison food. The psychoses of solitary confinement were said to be characterised by melancholia and an acute onset. Siefert (cited in Nitsche & Wilmanns 1912) provided a proposed subclassification:

1. hysteriform degenerative states

2. simple degenerative forms

3. phantastic degenerative forms

4. paranoid degenerative forms

5. prison psychotic states with simulated symptoms

6. dementia-like states.

Kirn (cited in Nitsche & Wilmanns 1912) suggested that some inmates were psychotic before coming to jail, others were predisposed to mental disorder prior to imprisonment, but that a third group were healthy before coming to prison.

Brugha *et al.* (2005) demonstrated that although there is a higher prevalence of psychosis in prison compared to the community, the nature and clinical presentation of the illnesses are the same. There is no separate prison psychosis. Although the notion of prison psychosis is now largely of only historical interest, the underlying intuition that the prison environment is toxic to mental health continues to influence contemporary prison discourse. The following broad themes are often noticeable, for example: "Prisons cause suicide" – the high rate of self-inflicted deaths and the implication that prisons are causative, although studies with a better comparison group actually suggest that prison may be protective of overall mortality (Sattar 2001); "Prisons cause mental illness" – the indeterminate detention of terrorist suspects (Robbins *et al.* 2005, Wilson 2005), and the harmful effects of solitary confinement (Arrigo & Bullock 2008). Clinically, one also from time to time encounters cases where the psychosis appears to remit quickly on hospital admission and to recur once back in prison.

Foucault

The above explanations for the excess of mental disorder in prisons treat the issue as some kind of administrative or technical problem – the mentally disordered end up in prison because of a failure of health care, because of an increased risk of offending associated with their condition, or because the prison regime is bad for one's mental health. If these explanations are correct, then it follows that if only we had better health care or better prison regimes, there would not be mentally disordered prisoners. However, Seddon (2007) has argued, following Foucault, that the fact that prisons have always contained mentally disordered persons is not an accident of an imperfect system, but tells us something important about the heart of the matter: the "presence of madmen among the prisoners is not the scandalous limit of confinement but its truth; not abuse but essence" (Foucault 1967, p.225). There have always been mentally disordered prisoners because, whilst we may deny it, prisons were always to do with confining the undesirable elements of society, psychiatric patients as well as criminals.

SOLUTIONS
Equivalence of care

In *The Future Organisation of Prison Health Care* (HM Prison Service & NHS Executive 1999), equivalence was promulgated as a guiding principle of prison health care. The World Health Organisation's *Health in Prisons Project* also cites the principle of equivalence (Møller *et al.* 2007), and it is one of the basic principles of the Committee for the Prevention of Torture (2006).

The equivalence of care in a correctional setting is a measure of the extent to which a society practises the principle of equality of citizens (Niveau 2007). The very high morbidity and the reality of the health care spend in prisons make true equivalence unlikely. In 2007, £20.8 million was spent upon prison inreach teams, or 11% of the total health care budget – around a third of what is needed to achieve true equivalence (Sainsbury Centre 2008).

Equivalence was one of the prime drivers behind the dissolution of the prison medical service and prison doctors. Despite being present in prisons for over a decade, and although the NHS now provides medical input, there are no clear training pathways to achieve this. In mental health, there has been a gradual influx of general adult psychiatry into prison establishments, though general psychiatrists receive no formal exposure to prison mental health in their training (unlike forensic psychiatrists). Does this provide the right skill base for the future?

There is no equivalent of a prison health care wing outside of a prison – nowhere else holds extremely psychotic patients, untreated, for many months whilst they wait for hospital admission. Bringing prison hospital wings, suitably staffed and equipped, under the aegis of the Mental Health Act 1983 might provide the best route to equivalence of care for prisoners (Wilson 2004).

Diversion/Transfer

Court diversion services aim to provide appropriate intervention for people with mental disorder charged with a criminal offence, in the least restrictive environment according to risk assessment and the direction of the court, prior to custody. Reviewing these services, James *et al.* (2002) found that although such schemes could improve the detection of mental illness fourfold and could facilitate admission to hospital, they were affected by poor planning, poor case identification and referral procedures, they experienced a lack of commitment from local psychiatric services and were hampered by a lack of access to beds. They also found that the majority of admissions from court were not career criminals who had become mentally ill; most appeared to have offended in the context of mental illness and social exclusion, having fallen through gaps in community care.

Mentally disordered prisoners, in England and Wales, can be diverted to hospital either by the courts or by the Ministry of Justice, medical evidence having been received as to the nature or degree of the mental disorder and the availability of a hospital bed. The relevant sections of the Mental Health Act are shown below (Figure 5.1; see also Table 14.1 on page 146).

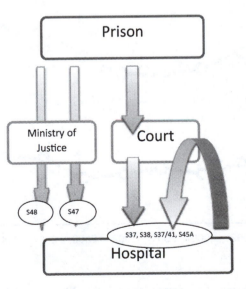

Figure 5.1 Graphical representation of criminal sections of the Mental Health Act 1983

The court sections are used at different points of the criminal justice trajectory, but only Section 37 (hospital order) and Section 45A (hybrid order) are final disposals for the offence concerned. All of the others perform some function, usually in the form of bringing information about the patient into the court. This division is important and also seeks to highlight that a movement to hospital has consequences for the court and that the individual is not considered in isolation. As shown in Figure 5.1, it also applies to non-prisoner defendants (those remanded on bail), unlike the Ministry of Justice sections. Apart from the restriction order, the movement has limited consideration for the level of security required.

In contrast, the pathway to hospital via the Ministry of Justice focuses not just on the mental health needs of the defendant, but also on security and political risks for the Ministry, with less consideration of the issues at court (apart from whether the patient is sentenced or not). From the political point of view, the Ministry of Justice is concerned about the risk of the individual escaping or absconding from hospital, as well as the risks he or she might present to others in that situation. As a result, the Ministry of Justice is often more conservative in its opinion about the level of hospital security required than the clinicians who have assessed the prisoner. Nonetheless, transfer under Section 48 remains the main mechanism to move a mentally disordered remand prisoner to hospital from prison. It reflects the needs of the prisoner rather than the court and is meant to convey urgency and to avoid waiting for a court appearance.

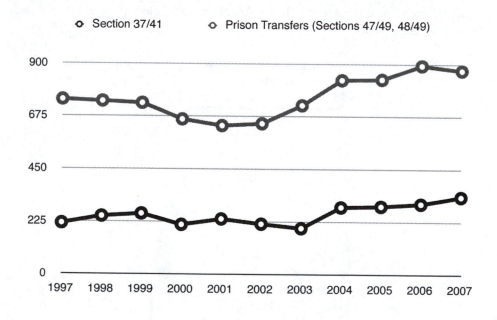

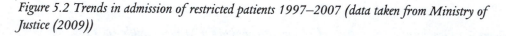

Figure 5.2 Trends in admission of restricted patients 1997–2007 (data taken from Ministry of Justice (2009))

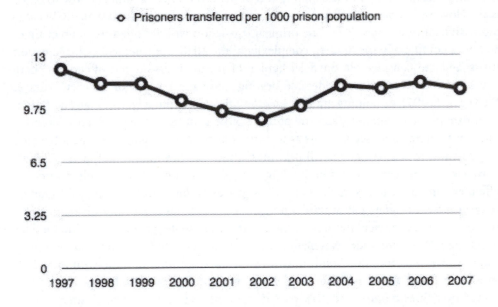

Figure 5.3 Prison transfers as a proportion of the total prison population (numerator data (number of transfers) taken from Ministry of Justice (2009), denominator data (total prison population) taken from the Home Office & Ministry of Justice websites)

At the end of 2007 there were 968 hospital inpatients subject to either Section 47/49 or Section 48/49 of the Mental Health Act 1983, an increase of 21% from 2006 and the largest increase for a decade (Ministry of Justice 2009). In terms of the number of admissions under transfer warrants, there were 873 admissions in 2007, and 333 on Hospital and Restriction Orders (Section 37/41; Ministry of Justice 2009). Although the absolute numbers of these admissions have been increasing since 2003, as shown in Figure 5.2, if one takes into account the increase in the total prison population over this period, there has been little change (Figure 5.3), despite the expansion of hospital beds, and the development of prison inreach services.

The statistical picture presents little information on the process, risks and burden of effecting a transfer under Section 48 or Section 47. The process has changed little since it was originally introduced by the Insane Prisoners Act 1840. Although this is meant to be the mechanism for dealing with "urgent" transfer, in practice most take several months to achieve. Isherwood & Parrott (2002) audited the transfer process at a prison in Southeast London, finding that on average there was a delay of between 103 and 126 days to admit a prisoner to a medium secure unit. The main issue identified as causing delay was the unavailability of beds, although there were also differences in opinion regarding the level of security, legal arguments, and diagnostic disagreements. These factors led to repeated referrals and assessments and long delays to initial assessments.

Since that study the increase in secure beds has continued apace both in the NHS and in the independent sector, so that the physical presence of a bed is unlikely now to be an issue. However, in our experience, transfer from prison to hospital has actually become more difficult (see Figure 5.3). The original legislation was designed for simpler times and does not fit easily the modern complexity of the NHS, the emergence of foundation trusts, and the considerable financial burden of mentally disordered offenders. These issues are likely to have considerable bearing upon the process of transfer. Sales & McKenzie (2007), examining another London prison, identified lack of court diversion, poor care in the community, and the pressure of beds in the acute psychiatric intensive care units and medium secure units as important factors in delaying the urgent hospital admission of seriously mentally ill prisoners. Other issues which are of increasing importance, and perhaps relevant in the light of public concern about mentally disordered offenders, are the lack of step down facilities (places of diminishing secutiry for gradual release) and appropriate pathways of aftercare. The NHS has in recent years implemented changes to try to effect transfer within a more appropriate timsescale (within 14 days of referral). Pilots are under way nationally. A recent study by Forrester *et al.* (in press), auditing transfers from two South London prisons, found little change, with only 20% being transferred within one month, and 38% within three months. Forty-two per cent waited over three months and 10% over six months. It is not known whether London has particular problems, or whether this is a national problem.

MENTAL HEALTH ACT IN PRISON

The Mental Health Act does not apply in prison in the UK, and there are lengthy delays in admitting seriously ill prisoners to hospital for treatment. The result is that prison health care wings contain many seriously ill, untreated prisoners. There is no equivalent to this situation outside of a prison. Would allowing these prisoners to be treated in prison, under the Mental Health Act, be an improvement on the present situation? One of us believes it would. It remains unclear as to why the Mental Health Act is excluded from prisons and whether much consideration was ever given to the matter. It seems likely that this reflects a concern around using psychiatric treatment as a form of social control of prisoners. This topic is discussed in more detail in Chapter 14.

THE MANAGEMENT OF MENTAL ILLNESS IN PRISON

For mental health services in prison the risks of managing mentally ill prisoners whilst waiting for transfer to hospital are considerable. Mental health remains the only area of prison health care which is not the responsibility of local commissioners – while a prisoner with cancer will be managed by the hospital local to the prison, a prisoner with schizophrenia must be managed by the services in the area the patient originates from, and there is therefore no route out to local services if they do not originate from that part of the country.

In general, patients transferred to hospital fall into three groups:

- those acutely ill who require treatment

- those who are complex and require assessment and diagnosis that cannot be delivered in a prison (e.g. for court)

- those who are chronically vulnerable.

Mental illness in prison is detected by a variety of routes and any service should have a good range of strategies to try to identify and prioritise mental illness. We will assume that the prison has a health care centre, though it is to be noted that health care centres with a 24-hour role are in the minority and usually in local urban prisons. It is recognised that mental illness is sometimes not obvious, and indeed it has been noted both anecdotally and in research (Durcan 2008) that prisoners often hide their mental illness, because of issues of insight and/or also because they realise the stigma attached to such a condition within prison. In some cases, patients are already known and court diversion and others will notify prison mental health teams about the arrival of a patient in prison. Not all cases will be flagged up in this way and so a service in prison will need to take into account the various routes into the prison in which they work, and to develop identifying systems accordingly. For example, segregation is often an area where mental health problems are manifested in terms of violent behaviour, and this should be an area of focus for prison mental health services. Forrester *et al.* (in press) found that around 25% of those with mental illness will be detected for the first time in prison.

In addition to the usual mental health assessment, when considering whether a prisoner should be transferred to hospital, the first decision facing the psychiatrist or mental health practitioner in prison is to decide where that individual should be in the prison – should he or she be in the main prison or in the health care centre? In some cases it is obvious, and generally determined by the risk that an individual presents. For others the decision may be complicated by limited or no information on past behaviour (which practitioners outside of prison are often able to draw upon). The development of prison inreach teams means that more support can be given to mentally ill prisoners and there is greater potential for prisoners to remain in the main prison. If remaining in the main prison, are they safe to be in a single cell or should they be in a multi-occupancy cell? The mental health practitioner will also have to consider the issues of safety to other prisoners and there have been a number of high profile deaths in custody in shared accommodation.

In some instances it may not be safe to allow a patient to remain in the main prison and that person will need to be managed in the health care centre. Health care centres are not like hospital wards in psychiatric units – there are a mixture of physical and mental health problems, and there is a focus on containing risk rather than improving health. They are often "a limbo between the community of the prison and the hospital beds of the NHS and independent sector" (Wilson 2004, p.5). It is here that many of the patients who will later be transferred to hospital are located, and where they will wait for several months before receiving the treatment that they need.

What is the solution for mentally ill prisoners?

A combination of treating prisoners the same as the rest of the population, and at the same time being honest about the differences between prisons and other settings, would be a good starting point. Failings in the community treatment of psychiatric patients, and the relationship between mental disorder and offending, may partly explain the high prevalence of mental disorder in prisons. Improving treatment for all mentally disordered people might, therefore, help to reduce the burden in prisons. There will always be mentally disordered prisoners. Improving the quality of services in prisons will also be necessary. Honesty about the total failure of the principle of equivalence as a guide to managing a prison health care centre would be a better place to start considering what to do about this forgotten group of severely ill prisoners.

Health services need to see prison as an opportunity for health improvement rather than a burden. Our society remains troubled by crime, solving it and the economic cost. In the last few years there has been an increased focus upon the links between crime and health and how addressing one can reduce the other, most notably with the links between illegal drugs and crime. It is likely that a greater awareness of and input into offenders' mental health needs and social care will be an increasing priority and also an opportunity to help reduce offending. As an example in the process of resettlement, a good proportion of offenders who leave prison and return to the community do not have a general practitioner. Williamson (2006) found that 50% of prisoners returning to the community had no general practitioner. It is noted that the burden of finding released prisoners a general practitioner falls upon the prison and is outlined within a prison service order on continuity of health care (HM Prison Service 2006b). For many this is the route to accessing mental health. The issues around social exclusion are typified and common to the prison population.

The differentiation between the roles of secondary and primary care is a particular issue. In the community this seems to be far better delineated than within the prison. Recent initiatives are for the development of primary mental health care within prisons. Inreach teams were set up to help people who would, in the community, qualify for help from secondary services because they have severe and enduring problems. In reality most prison mental health services see a far wider spectrum of conditions, often because of a lack of alternatives. Durcan & Knowles (2006) found primary mental health care to be weak in many London prisons, putting extra pressure on inreach teams and diluting the resources intended for those with more complex and severe conditions. HM Inspectorate of Prisons (2007a) found that the boundaries between primary and secondary care were not clear-cut in terms of either diagnosis or service.

The vast majority of prisoners return to their home area or address upon release. The problems facing the offender in the resettlement process are enormous and many are linked – homelessness, employment and financial difficulties, and resuming and repairing relationships. Matters are compounded by short sentences and the unpredictability of release and health needs. Continuity of care is a major difficulty in the transit between the community and prison, and *vice versa*.

Other mental disorders such as learning difficulties are covered in more depth in separate chapters. Only the minority of other mental disorders (such as personality disorder) will be transferred to hospital, although the process is now made easier by the 2007 amendment to the Mental Health Act 1983, providing only one category of mental disorder. In practice, services outside of prison will continue to focus their energies towards the mentally ill population. In the past there has been limited travel of personality disordered patients to medium and high security services, but this is less and less common and typically this group will remain within prison with some flexibility in terms of therapeutic prisons such as HMP Grendon and HMP Dovegate (see Chapter 19). As in health services in the NHS, services for personality disordered patients are being developed, though this is typically for the DSPD group (Dangerous Severe Personality Disorder). Considering the vast sump of prisoners who have a personality disorder of one or more types, these will remain in prison and see out their sentence there. It is to be noted, however, that prison mental health services continue to work with this group, and often this reflects the needs of the prison. Thus, whilst there might be a desire to confine focus to a population of mentally ill prisoners, as in the wider community outside of prison, services are always drawn into working with a non-mentally ill group in addition. In some respects, prison remains the last example of psychiatry being able to work with a wide range of conditions.

As services have been developed and rolled out across the estate, we are witnessing the dawn of a new era in the delivery of mental health services to such a high level of need. Mental health inreach teams have in practice ended up dealing almost exclusively with the severe and enduring conditions that are the focus of secondary services in the community. Four out of five mental health inreach teams felt that they were unable to respond adequately to the range of need (HM Inspectorate of Prisons 2007a). There was no blueprint for delivering mental health care in prisons, based upon the assessed needs of the population.

CHAPTER 6

Suicide, Attempted Suicide and Self-injury in Prison

David Crighton

INTRODUCTION

The study of suicide, attempted suicide and intentional self-injury, both in prisons and outside, is complicated by significant issues of definition. Until 1961 suicide in the UK was a criminal offence. Indeed the legal thinking about suicide remains firmly grounded in criminal law, with suicide verdicts requiring the criminal burden of proof of beyond reasonable doubt. There remains a clear legal presumption against suicide, regularly re-asserted by the superior courts, which have stressed that suicide must be strictly proved and not assumed. This is also reflected in practice, with people still frequently talking somewhat curiously about someone "committing" suicide, as if it remained a criminal act, rather than using more neutral terms such as "completing" suicide (Crighton & Towl 2008).

Official figures therefore represent a significant underestimate of the true rates of suicide, with many self-inflicted deaths being recorded as deaths due to accident, misadventure or unknown causes. Estimates of suicide rates based on official figures are therefore likely to be inaccurate estimates of true rates (Kelly & Bunting 1998, Jenkins & Singh 2000). Epidemiological studies of suicide have thus sought to apply more accurate operational definitions, frequently based on International Classification of Diseases (ICD) categories. Although these have seen detailed changes over time, in the case of self-inflicted deaths they have provided more accurate and internationally comparable baselines than legally defined suicide rates.

Definitions of attempted suicide and self-injury are similarly complex. Legal definitions of such behaviours have generally been restricted to largely tangential areas, as in, for example, the Mental Health Acts or the Female Circumcision Act 1985. A key challenge here is the point at which intentional self-injury or self-poisoning might be defined as attempted suicide and, also, whether there are any clear discontinuities within what is sometimes conceptualised as the continuum from mild to severe injuries (Crighton 2006). In addition, the language used to discuss and define this area has raised concerns. The term "deliberate self-harm" (DSH) (Morgan, Burns, Pococky *et al.* 1975) has gained wide currency, yet the concept of "self-harm" is potentially very broad, logically including a range of seemingly weakly related behaviours such as self-laceration, self-poisoning, drug use, excessive eating, tattooing, piercing and nail-biting (Walsh & Rosen 1988). In seeking to address this, some have suggested more circumscribed notions of DSH which exclude the less severe forms of harm (Pattinson & Kahan 1983), something which has largely occurred in practice. Others have suggested that the term is potentially misleading by describing the behaviours as "deliberate", with the role and extent of deliberation often being unclear or, in some cases, appearing entirely absent. Intentional self-injury (ISI) and intentional self-poisoning (ISP) have been suggested as alternatives to the broad category of DSH, since these recognise the volition of the act without making any assumptions about the degree of associated thought and planning (Towl 2000). Such changes do, however, create a difficulty with comparisons over time, and with epidemiological studies based on the concept of DSH.

Defining attempted suicide and separating this from intentional self-injury and self-poisoning is similarly challenging. Some have suggested the term "parasuicide", largely to describe apparently suicidal acts where there appears to be an absence of suicidal intent (Kreitman, Philip, Greer *et al.* 1969). Such notions gained wide currency during the 1970s and 1980s but have proved problematic. Issues of intent in completed suicides are often unclear, with evidence of frequently confused or conflicting intentions. The term has also become associated with unfortunate notions that those who make unsuccessful attempts at suicide are not at increased risk of ending their own lives, a view which is not supported by the evidence base (Towl & Crighton 1998, Crighton 2006). It has been suggested that, while the term "parasuicide" is tapping into some genuine differences, it may, in terms of identifying treatment needs and prognosis, be simply too broad a diagnostic category. More promising approaches seem likely to involve the separation of self-injury and self-poisoning, along with clearer, probably multi-dimensional, specification of motivation and behaviour.

EPIDEMIOLOGY

The mainstreaming of epidemiological research in this area really only began from the mid-1980s onwards. An early example was a study of self-inflicted deaths in Scottish prisons between 1976 and 1993 (Bogue & Power 1995). In all, 83 deaths had been legally defined as suicide in Scottish prisons during this time and were analysed using information from general prison files. Four-year period cohorts were used to conduct an analysis of trends and this suggested a steady rise in the rate of suicides, which paralleled that being seen in other parts of the UK. The study corrected the then dominant but misplaced view that prisoners on remand were at heightened risk of suicide, with it being noted that this was largely an artefact of death rates being calculated in an overly simplistic way. In general, earlier studies appear to have calculated on the basis of average annual population or average daily population (ADP). For remand prisoners this provides a marked underestimate of the numbers actually placed at risk in the prison environment. In fact annual receptions into prison are a more meaningful basis for estimating population rates of suicide in remand prisoners (Bogue & Power 1995). An analysis of this for prisons in England and Wales yielded similar results to those seen in Scotland. Rates recalculated on the basis of receptions for the period 1988–98 for prisons in England and Wales suggested that when rates were calculated on the basis of receptions, remand prisoners were not at increased risk compared to sentenced prisoners (Crighton & Towl 1997, Crighton 2000a, 2000b). Whilst it is possible that this may be subject to unknown period and cohort effects the central point here is methodological, suggesting that calculation of rates needs to be appropriate to the research question being addressed (Crighton & Towl 2008).

More recently there has been a step change over early research and this has had two major foci. One has involved the introduction of criminological approaches to analysis grounded in sociological theory (Hatty & Walker 1986, Tumim 1990, Liebling 1991), the other has involved the application of mainstream models and methods from medical and public health research (Crighton 1997, 1999, 2000c, 2000d, Crighton & Towl 1997, 2000, Jenkins & Singh 2000, Shaw, Appleby & Baker 2003a). This has resulted in a breaking down of the isolation of prisons from evidence-based research. It has also markedly increased the quantity and quality of research.

Criminological research models

A questionnaire study of 155 self-inflicted deaths in Australian prisons between 1980 and 1985 was conducted, with 77 of the deaths going on to be officially recorded as suicides (Hatty & Walker 1986). The other deaths were recorded as misadventure, accidental death and natural causes. The authors reported higher death rates for women in prison, at 1.7 per 1,000 (170 per 100,000) against 1.2 per 1,000 (120 per 100,000) for men. This, however, was based on very small numbers of women, making the findings very tentative. A pattern in relation to age was also identified, with an over-representation of both younger and older age groups, although for the older age groups this seemed, unsurprisingly, to be largely due to an increased number of deaths from natural causes. Increased rates of suicide were reported for the 20–24 and 25–29 years age cohorts. The 15–19 years age cohort, perhaps more surprisingly, did not appear at increased risk of suicide, although, as with the comparisons made between men and women, the researchers noted a need for caution owing to the small numbers involved. Deaths amongst ethnic minority (aboriginal) Australians were 50% higher in the under-35 age group than for other Australians. This striking finding was not analysed further but was replicated in later research, which has showed continued higher rates of deaths in this socially and economically disadvantaged group (Joudo 2006).

A detailed study of four young offender institutions (YOIs) for men and women in England and Wales built on this work (Liebling 1991). This involved an analogue study of 100 young people who had a recent history of intentional self-injury which had come to the attention of the institution's health care centre. The choice of self-injuring offenders as the basis for an analogue study was predicated on the notion that suicide and self-injury form a continuum of self-destructive behaviours (Liebling 1991). Such views have a long history, traceable as far back as work by Menninger (1938) and Durkheim (1952).

In contrast to previous studies, a matched control group of young offenders from the same institutions was identified. A number of statistically significant between-group differences, using non-parametric tests, were reported. Young people who intentionally self-injured tended to be serving longer sentences, to have fewer positive recommendations in probation reports, and also showed differences in social and family background. Surprisingly the control group self-reported more unstable family backgrounds in some respects, although this finding appeared to conflict with the self-injury group reporting higher rates of placement in local authority care, itself an indirect index of serious family problems. More contacts with mental health services were also evident in those young people who intentionally self-injured, along with higher rates of suicide and "self-harm" within their families. Links between intentional self-injury and drug abuse have long been mooted (Menninger 1938) and this was supported by the finding that young people in the self-injuring group were more likely to have "major" alcohol abuse problems. They also showed higher levels of other drug abuse, with some evidence of consistent misuse in custody and pre-custody.

The actual experience of prison custody also appeared to differ between the two groups of young people, with those who intentionally self-injured being less engaged in activities and being more likely to report a dislike of activities such as physical education. They tended to show a greater preference for cell sharing and to have fewer personal resources, such as literacy, that would let them address feelings of boredom and isolation. The research went on to explain such differences in relation to a construct of "coping" ability, suggesting a profile of individuals who were described using a somewhat circular notion of "poor copers".

This study moved towards more theory-based research, using mixed qualitative and quantitative approaches to research. Largely descriptive to begin with, these criminological studies have marked significant progress, with a level of theory building and hypothesis testing that had been largely absent from preceding research. The work also had a number of methodological limitations. The notion that suicide and intentional self-injury form a continuum remains hypothetical. If correct, this suggests that the study of intentional self-injury and self-poisoning are of direct relevance to the study of suicide. If incorrect, study of these areas becomes less obviously relevant to the study of suicide and may indeed be misleading. A particularly noteworthy finding, echoed by Snow (2006), is that a high proportion of those who engage in self-injurious behaviours do so without apparent intent to complete suicide, but rather report the behaviours as means of managing strong emotions such as anger. Such findings sit uncomfortably with notions of a simple continuum between suicide and intentional self-injury. This has led to suggestions that a simple continuum does not adequately explain the emerging evidence and that a more complex model is required. Alternative approaches using classification tree approaches may, it has been suggested, yield more valid typological models and insights into differences between sub-groups and those at risk of intentional self-injury, attempted and completed suicide (Monahan, Steadman, Silver et al. 2001, Crighton 2006, Crighton & Towl 2008).

The suggested theoretical construct of "coping ability" also raises some issues, particularly in suggesting causal explanations of behaviour. Here other explanations seem equally plausible. The profiles of the intentionally self-injuring young offenders, for example, suggest that for most observers they may have been adapting to more difficult circumstances: longer sentences, lower levels of family support, poor contact with friends and poorer relationships with professional staff. There is a widely recognised bias within human cognition to make internal or dispositional attributions about behaviour and to underestimate the power of situational factors (Connolly, Arkes & Hammond 2000). It might be suggested that notions of "poor coping" and older concepts of "inadequacy" and "manipulation" are, at least partly, examples of this fundamental cognitive bias, and in terms of explanatory power are largely tautological (Towl & Crighton 1998).

Public health research models

The other main focus for the study of suicide, attempted suicide and intentional self-injury in prisons has been built primarily on public health models and methods (Charlton 1995, Crighton & Towl 1997, Towl & Crighton 1998, Crighton 2000a, 2000b, Jenkins, Bhugra, Meltzer et al. 2005). These approaches have generally begun with operational definitions (World Health Organisation 2007), combined with retrospective analyses. This has facilitated meaningful comparisons internationally and allowed for more accurate comparisons of rates in custody with those in the community (Towl, Snow & McHugh 2000).

The largest and most comprehensive analysis of suicides in UK prisons to date used this approach, analysing all the self-inflicted deaths in prisons in England and Wales between 1988 and 1998 (Crighton 2000c, 2006). A retrospective empirical and qualitative analysis of self-inflicted deaths for a decade was undertaken. In all this involved 600 such deaths and, of these, data could be obtained on 525. Analysis was based on written records from formal investigations of the deaths. Over the period a clear upward trend in the rate of suicides was noted, with rates increasing from 80 per 100,000 ADP in 1988 to over 120 per 100,000 ADP in 1998. Calculated on the basis of receptions into prisons, a similar but proportionally greater upward trend was noted, with the rate increasing from just over 20 per 100,000 receptions in 1988 to around 40 per 100,000 receptions in 1998.

Issues of gender in relation to suicides in prison have been contentious, with contradictory results being reported, often on the basis of small sample studies. For the period 1988–98 the overall rate of suicides for men was 94 per 100,000 ADP, compared to a rate for women of 74 per 100,000 ADP. To ensure that this was not largely a facet of the calculation being based on ADP, rates were calculated based on annual receptions, which yielded rates of 30 per 100,000 receptions for men and 16 per 100,000 receptions for women. The data did, however, suggest greater fluctuations in the rates for women, and as a result of this the rates for women were higher for some individual years. A trend analysis was conducted which also showed higher rates for men. A plausible explanation for the variations in the rates for women prisoners' data is one of random statistical fluctuation, given the relatively small numbers involved and the much smaller population of women in prison. This does not rule out the possibility of other explanations but remains a significant methodological challenge in studying gender differences in prisons (Crighton 2006).

Issues of ethnicity have rarely appeared as a focus for research in this area, despite expressed concerns about racism in prisons (Narey 2002). The results of this study replicated findings in the United States (Haycock 1989) with lower rates of suicide amongst black prisoners. In white prisoners the rate was 89 per 100,000 ADP, compared to 84 per 100,000 ADP for South Asian prisoners and 13 per 100,000 ADP for black prisoners. This suggested that black prisoners were at lower risk of suicide, a finding that echoes the lower rates found in community studies (Crighton 2006). The reasons for such findings remain unclear.

Levels of mental disorder and social disadvantage were very high in those completing suicide, with 43% having a documented history of abusing non-prescribed drugs. Over half (55%) had a history of intentional self-injury and 12% had been treated for intentional self-injury during the sentence in which they died. Levels of mental health problems were also evident in terms of the levels of prescribed drugs. Based on a sample of 239 suicides where detailed medical records had been examined, 33% were being prescribed drugs including antipsychotics, antidepressants, painkillers and methadone, often in combination with other drugs. Rates of prescription of antidepressant medication were surprisingly low at 7%, suggesting perhaps low levels of identification and treatment for depressive disorders. This possibility is in line with other evidence which suggested generally poor rates of identification of mental health problems by prison staff (Birmingham *et al.* 1996, Coid, Petruckevitch, Bebbington *et al.* 2003). The qualitative analysis conducted by Crighton (2000c) similarly found high levels of unidentified mental health difficulties, along with failings in detoxification for drug and alcohol misusers.

The study also replicated a number of previous research findings. A link between longer sentences and suicide was noted, with the effect being most marked for those serving indeterminate (life) sentences. Those with index offences of violence or drug misuse were also at increased risk of suicide, whereas sexual offenders were not. Warnings about likely suicide were also common, with 51% of prisoners who killed themselves having a record of having expressed intent generally to staff, relatives or other prisoners prior to doing so. This clearly contradicts the popular myth that those who kill themselves rarely talk about it.

Research in prisons had consistently suggested that the early period of custody is a time of increased risk of suicide (Topp 1979, Crighton & Towl 1997). This was confirmed for the period 1988–98, as illustrated in the graph below (Figure 6.1). The relative level of risk during the first 24 hours after reception is consistently reported to be exceptionally high. Extrapolating the rate of suicides over a year, the rate of self-inflicted deaths was reported to be around 9,500 per annum: from Day 2 to Day 7 the level of risk remained very high compared to a non-prison population, with an annualised rate declining from around 7,000 to 1,500. Days 8 to 30 saw a continued decrease in the level of risk from an annualised rate of around 1,000 to a baseline level. Crucially, the decline in level of risk appears broadly exponential, with baseline levels reached at around two months after reception. This pattern appeared to hold similarly both for new receptions into prison and also for those being transferred between

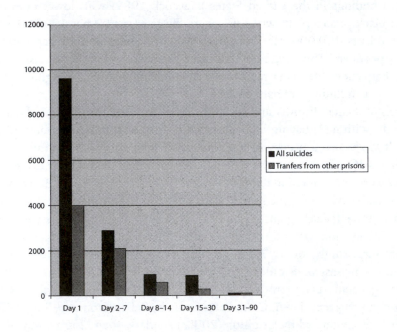

Figure 6.1 Annualised rate of suicide for prisons in England and Wales 1988–98 (Crighton 2000a)

prisons. The effect, therefore, seems unlikely to be an artefact due to those at high risk being transferred between prisons (Crighton 2006). Interestingly this finding in prisons is similar to observed patterns of increased risk noted during the first week of psychiatric hospitalisation and also the first week post-discharge, suggesting that there may be something about novel environments that is associated with markedly increased risk of suicide (Roy 1982, Geddes & Juszczak 1995, Geddes, Juszczak, O'Brien *et al.* 1997, Qin & Nordentoft 2005, Pratt, Piper, Appleby *et al.* 2006). The mechanisms for this are poorly understood but seem a promising avenue for further research both within and outside prison.

Process issues in care management were also analysed via written records in the form of the "F2052SH" system, named after the forms used to record care for prisoners at risk of suicide and self-injury. This provided the administrative framework for management of prisoners assessed as being at increased risk, as well as providing a structured record of support and monitoring. In turn 18% of prisoners had been subject to such procedures at the time of their death, with no level of supervision, including "continuous watches", proving foolproof in preventing suicide. Routine 15-minute checks were the most widely used technique and generally proved ineffective, particularly as they tended to be carried out at rigidly fixed intervals. It seems likely that this predictability of checks undermined the value of such observations in preventing suicides.

It was also suggested that the F2052SH suffered from a number of flaws. Most critically, perhaps, this included the fact that the system had been explicitly based on the assumption that suicide and intentional self-injury were part of a continuum of behaviour. In turn it was assumed that such behaviours could be effectively managed using a common approach. Both these assumptions have been poorly supported by the emerging evidence base and, in terms of practice, the use of a common "one size fits all" approach seems misplaced (Towl *et al.* 2000, Crighton 2006).

Another identified weakness was the reliance placed on prison officers to be instrumental in the detection, monitoring and support of those at high risk of suicide and intentional self-injury. Previous approaches were criticised, often with good reason, for being unduly focused on prison medical services, which were themselves, at that time, becoming increasingly professionally isolated from, and out of step with practice in mainstream NHS primary care services. With the benefit of hindsight there was perhaps an excessive focus on reducing the role of health care practitioners, as this often resulted in low and decreasing levels of specialist support and guidance for prison officers. This occurred despite prison officers often being inadequately equipped to detect, support and manage such behaviour.

During the 1990s the role of psychologists significantly decreased in the management of suicide and intentional self-injury. Psychologists progressively withdrew from this area of work, instead focusing on work intended to reduce the risk of re-offending. This shift was largely at the expense of work in relation to health and welfare. The work of primary and secondary health care teams additionally tended to become more and more focused on those with mental disorders falling within the Mental Health Act 1983. Such changes were noted in a report by the Royal College of Psychiatrists (2002) and to an extent in the earlier thematic review of suicide by the Chief Inspector of Prisons (HM Inspectorate of Prisons 1999). It was argued that increases in input from specialist staff, in parallel with the mainstreaming of services in prisons, were essential in effectively managing suicide. The Royal College response was also critical of misunderstandings over the role and nature of professional confidentiality and the failings of professional staff to give appropriate support to prison officers, in such complex and difficult areas of work. It is gratifying that significant progress has been made in delivering these objectives (Crighton & Towl 2000, Cinamon & Bradshaw 2005). Since April 2007 the F2052SH system has been replaced with Assessment, Care in Custody, and Teamwork (ACCT). This marked a number of clear shifts in policy, with a reversal of trends to withdraw health care practitioners from managing suicide and intentional self-injury. ACCT sets out clear requirements for mainstream mental health assessment and support. It has also, to a large extent, moved away from assumptions about suicidal and self-injurious behaviours being a simple continuum, with associated moves away from a single approach to assessment and intervention (HM Prison Service 2007a, National Offender Management Service 2008a).

In this respect research specifically into intentional self-injury has yielded interesting results which have shaped policy (Snow 2006). In this study of prisons in England and Wales a mixed range of negative emotional states including boredom, stress, anxiety, depression and loneliness were reported at elevated rates in those who intentionally self-injured. Interestingly, those who reported frequent depressed mood appeared at higher risk of suicide and attempted suicide than those who reported infrequent depression (Snow 2006). In addition it appeared that individuals differed in terms of being "active" or "passive", suggesting different presentation and responses to distinct negative emotional states. The findings from this study suggest much greater complexity in intentional self-injury and attempted suicide than has previously been recognised. In turn, such differences seem likely to require differing assessment and intervention approaches (Crighton 2006).

Overall much of the research on suicide and intentional self-injury can be criticised for an unduly empirical emphasis, at the expense of theoretical models and understanding (Crighton 1999, 2000a, Sattar 2001, Fruehwald *et al.* 2003). This has been placed in stark relief with the further development of the empirical evidence base and the development of large-scale case control studies (Shaw *et al.* 2003a). There have, however, been initial attempts at theoretical model building (Plutchik 1980, 1997, Crighton 2006, Snow 2006). In seeking to explain suicide and intentional self-injury, fundamental research into the development and regulation of emotions has been drawn on extensively (Plutchik 1980, 1997, Crighton 2006) and these studies have clear advantages. They facilitate scientific research that goes beyond empirically descriptive work, replacing this with testable explanatory models. They also have practical advantages in suggesting more accurate specification of observed behaviours and more targeted interventions to reduce risk.

One clear and testable hypothesis emerging from these models is that those who show high levels of violence towards others will, when prevented, be more likely to be violent towards themselves. This is consistent with the finding that those convicted of violent offences tended to be at greater risk of suicide than those who were not (Crighton 2006). The model also suggests that there are a number of points at which intervention might be effective within what may be termed a "biopsychosocial" approach. These could include efforts to intervene in ways that are not immediately obvious – for example, with interventions to improve self-regulation of emotions such as anger. Equally, interventions might be made earlier in the process to reduce levels of perceived threat and unnecessary loss of control experienced in the environment.

REDUCING SUICIDE AND INTENTIONAL SELF-INJURY: EVIDENCE-BASED PRACTICE

Evaluating the evidence for interventions intended to reduce the risk of suicide, attempted suicide, intentional self-injury and self-poisoning in prisons presents considerable ethical and practical problems. These include difficulties with conducting methodologically rigorous and randomised studies. Despite this, there is an emerging and improving evidence base to draw from.

In relation to suicide and attempted suicide, significant efforts have been focused on attempts to produce structured risk assessment tools to identify those at risk. Such efforts have understandably been the focus of extensive criticism (Fitzgibbon & Green 2006). Indeed, efforts to develop structured risk assessments to identify those at risk of suicide, or efforts to use existing structured assessments for this purpose, are likely to present severe challenges. Even in prisons suicide and attempted suicide have statistically low base rates. Accordingly even assessments with very high levels of specificity and sensitivity are likely to result in large numbers of false positives. As with other very low frequency events, the most accurate prediction, based on an undifferentiated population, is that someone is not at risk (Gigerenzer 2002). Indeed, suicide and attempted suicide provide good illustrations of areas where such shortcut replacements for competent and systematic assessment and management are at their most ineffective (Crighton 2006, Crighton & Towl 2008).

Efforts to reduce the risk of suicide have also become increasingly evidence-based. This has resulted in efforts to address and improve the broader social environment within prisons as a means of reducing such behaviours. It has also led to an increased focus on identified correlates and risk factors seen in suicide, in particular mental health problems, poor education and difficulties in effectively regulating emotions. Other efforts have been directed to reducing opportunities to complete suicide, including removal of easily accessible ligature points, sharp blades and toxic materials. Efforts have also been made in some prisons to improve reception and the initial period in custody with, for example, "first night" units. Whilst these efforts are intuitively appealing, they have yet to be adequately evaluated, with the exception of the evidence base for interventions to address depression (Crighton 2006). Here there is evidence to support modest statistically significant positive effects from cognitive behavioural therapy (CBT), interpersonal therapy (IPT) and antidepressants in reducing symptoms and achieving remission (National Institute for Clinical Excellence (NICE) 2007a).

Research into interventions to reduce intentional self-injury is similarly challenging, but there are some promising developments. One difficulty in the prison context is that studies have often pooled incidents of intentional self-injury and intentional self-poisoning. This is problematic in itself, as it is unclear to what extent there are significant differences between these behaviours. In turn, this complicates analysis and interpretation of the evidence base in this area. This is especially marked in prisons where intentional self-poisoning is comparatively uncommon.

It has been suggested that there is little evidence *per se* that hospital admission reduces the risk of repetition of intentional self-injury or self-poisoning (Waterhouse & Platt 1990). This tentative conclusion needs to be tempered by high exclusion rates in this study, with only 15% of referred patients eligible for inclusion. All participants needed to be assessed as "low risk" and without immediate medical or mental health needs, and all were subject to a relatively short follow-up period. This suggests a more conservative conclusion that hospitalisation has little effect for these low risk groups (Crighton & Towl 2008).

Five community-based studies comparing problem-solving interventions with standard care were identified and evaluated in a review by Hawton, Townsend, Arensman *et al.* (2007). All five reported a reduction in levels of "self-harm" but the summary odds ratio suggested no statistically significant effect (OR 0.70 95% CI 0.45 to 1.11). Excluding one study with relatively weak allocation concealment again yielded a result that was not statistically significant. Examination of studies that included those who repeatedly "harmed" themselves and only those studies with mixed allocation were also negative. A number of studies have been reported looking at intensive intervention and outreach compared to standard care, but again suggest no positive effect (OR 0.84 95% CI 0.62 to 1.15). Inclusion of only those studies with the highest quality allocation and concealment made little difference to these results (Hawton *et al.* 2007).

A study into the effects of therapist continuity on follow-up reported that repetition was significantly higher for those seeing the same therapist on follow-up (OR 3.70 95% CI 1.13 to 12.09). However, despite being a random allocation study, the researchers found differences between the groups prior to intervention, with the same therapist group showing higher levels of pre-existing risk factors. Those who saw the same therapist were also more effectively retained in treatment, with 71% attending at least one outpatient appointment compared to 47% for the control group (OR 2.75 95% CI 1.37 to 5.52) (Torhorst, Moller, Schmid-Bode *et al.* 1988).

There is some evidence to support the use of dialectical behaviour therapy (DBT) in reducing the frequency of incidents, with small but significant differences in self-injury and suicide attempts at 6- and 12-month follow-up (n=63, RR 0.81, 95% CI 0.66 to 0.98, NNT 12, 95% CI 7 to 108). DBT has also been compared with a combination of comprehensive validation therapy and a 12-step substance abuse intervention, with no significant difference reported (n=23, RR 1.09, 95% CI 0.64 to 1.87) (Hawton *et al.* 2007). In a comparison of DBT and client-centred therapy, no statistical difference in admissions to hospital was found (n=24, RR 0.33, 95% CI 0.08 to 1.33), although fewer of the DBT group intentionally self-injured or attempted suicide (n=24, RR 0.13, 95% CI 0.02 to 0.85, NNT 2, CI 2 to 11) (Hawton *et al.* 2007). In a comparison of dialectical behaviour therapy (DBT) with standard aftercare, a significantly lower rate of repetition of "self-harm" was found (OR 0.24, 95% CI 0.06 to 0.93) (Linehan, Armstrong, Suarez *et al.* 1991). In assessing this positive outcome it is worth noting that the comparison was based on a sub-group that was smaller than the number entering the trial, creating the risk of selection bias. DBT was also delivered by a highly motivated and skilled group of practitioners and, as such, the extent to which these results might generalise to mainstream prison and indeed community settings requires some caution.

Overall the striking characteristic of the current evidence base is its moderate quality. The evidence that exists generally involves small sample studies with associated risks of sampling biases. Studies have also tended to be statistically low-powered, reducing the scope to identify modest positive and negative treatment effects – and indeed, there has been little reported evidence on adverse effects associated with interventions. Substantial amounts of data have also often been lost through unclear reporting. Even so the evidence is moderately encouraging, suggesting that existing psychosocial interventions warrant further study.

The evidence on drug-based interventions is similarly limited, but again there are a number of interesting findings. A comparison of flupenthixol and placebo found a statistically significant reduction in the levels of repetition of "self-harm" (OR 0.09, 95% CI 0.02 to 0.50). However, this result was based on a small number of individuals and included only a sub-group who repeatedly "self-harmed". As such the clinical utility of flupenthixol and the extent to which this finding might be generalised is unclear (Hawton *et al.* 2007).

Antidepressant drugs have been a major focus of research, largely on the basis of associations between depression, self-injury, self-poisoning and suicide (attempted and completed). A number of comparisons of antidepressant drugs with placebo have been reported, with generally disappointing results. One study of paroxetine compared to placebo, using a sub-group analysis of "minor repeaters" (fewer than five acts) and "major repeaters" (five or more acts), reported a statistically significant reduction. This was found for "minor repeaters" but not for "major repeaters". The clinical significance and implications of this finding remain unclear (Verkes, Van der Mast, Hengevald *et al.* 1998). Overall the evidence base for the use of such interventions is surprisingly limited when compared to other areas of mental health research. There is clear evidence of the efficacy of drugs in treating some of the risk factors associated with intentional self-injury, self-poisoning and suicide – most notably in the treatment of severe depression. Direct evidence is far more limited, with current studies suggesting no reduction in repetition of intentional self-injury and self-poisoning. Indeed, it has been suggested that some forms of antidepressant drugs may serve to disinhibit aggression and result in an increased risk of intentional self-injury (Bregin 2004).

Arguably what is needed is more focused and theory-based research looking at tightly defined, specific sub-groups of those who engage in intentionally self-injurious and self-destructive behaviours (Crighton 2006). Given the current state of knowledge, it is probably most accurate to say that both biological and psychosocial interventions in this area are best seen as promising but still largely experimental in nature.

CHAPTER 7

Managing Substance Misuse in Prison

James Tighe

HISTORY

There is very little mention of the role of substance misuse in authoritative histories of the prison service. In the US, Roberts' (1994) work, and in the UK, Sim's (1990) on the Prison Medical Service make no mention of substance misuse. However, a number of historical works on substance misuse mention the role of incarceration, and a rough narrative can be constructed.

In sixteenth-century England "bridewells", or "houses of correction", were established as part of the welfare system. Those too poor or too infirm to support themselves were the responsibility of their local parish, which could raise taxes from which to provide relief. However, some "honest" tax payers clearly felt that not all cases of parish relief were deserving. The bridewell was established, originally in London, as "the stick to balance the carrot of parish relief" (Dillon 2002, p.158). The idea soon spread across England as a way of dealing with the indolent, drunk or lunatic. Any person whose poverty was seen as self-perpetuated or whose behaviour offended public morals or order could find him- or herself confined to the bridewell under a system of laws which, in retrospect, appear draconian.

The running of bridewells was a business. Prisoners were provided with bread, water and, of course, board for free. The provenance of both the bread and water was often suspect. However, a prisoner's conditions could be substantially improved for the right fee. This included the provision not only of better living conditions, but also of food and drink. This was a lucrative business. The post of warden was often passed from father to son or could be sold on for thousands of pounds. While public drunkenness was as good a reason as any to incarcerate a person in a bridewell, a more common reason, by the early eighteenth century, was debt.

This changed after the second Gin Act was passed in 1736. It severely restricted the sale and production of gin. Unlawful production could be fined up to £100, selling could lead to a fine of £10. Many producers, once caught, could afford the fine; however, small time sellers often could not, as £10 was more than a year's wages for many. These people went to the bridewell. News sheets of the day recount street traders lining up at the magistrates, ready to go to prison, with bottles of gin hidden in their clothing (Dillon 2002). Such was the level of civil disobedience produced by the Act that many people were opting to go to the bridewell as a protest, knowing full well that their supporters outside would keep them provided for. This led to overcrowding of the bridewells and a very open internal market in alcohol, often supplied by the attendants. One visitor recounted being shocked by the boldness of some women prisoners, who persuaded him to part with a few shillings for brandy. By 1741 the number of deaths in the bridewells was high enough for the Middlesex magistrates to launch an investigation. They found gin shops existing within the bridewell walls, and one estimate was that around 120 gallons were sold weekly (Dillon 2002). In 1743 a new Gin Act ended prohibition, and taxation and licensing were reintroduced. It was slowly but surely realised by the governments of the eighteenth and nineteenth centuries that legislating against gin and other liquors was self-defeating. Instead, a system of regulation and taxation was used to control the use of alcohol. By 1784 the provision of beer by gaolers to prisoners was prohibited (Creese, Bynum & Beam 1995), though given the standard of drinking water in the eighteenth century, beer was often the healthier alternative (Porter 2001).

The Temperance Movement that developed in the nineteenth century was most rapt by the concept of "social degeneration" and its connection with alcoholism. This included ideas from eugenics and could take on a distinctly racial slant (Sournia 1990). Criminal behaviour was central to this argument, with the full range of offending behaviour being attributed to alcohol at various times. Occasionally statistics were produced to support the argument: for example, two-thirds of the 600 young offenders in Massachusetts being found to have a family member who was alcoholic. This kind of figure was produced, not to suggest a direct connection between alcohol and crime, though they would not deny that such existed, but to demonstrate the impact of alcoholics on those connected with and dependent upon them.

In the UK, by 1878 the Habitual Drunkards Act confirmed the dominance of a medically led treatment approach to the social problems caused by alcohol. The impact of this on the prison population has not been assessed, but the expense of treatment was outside the reach of most poor people. During the debates about the Mental Deficiency Act 1913, there was a clear drive by those who favoured guardianship-type arrangements under medical supervision. They won the day, and for the first time other intoxicating substances, i.e. morphine and its derivatives, were included. However, it was not until the Defence of the Realm Act 1917 (DORA 1917) that narcotic substances actually became illegal.

We do not know the incidence of drug use in prison prior to DORA 1917. One isolated fact is that in 1896 the Scottish Prison Service reported treating two prisoners for morphia addiction in Glasgow (Berridge & Edwards 1987). From this it is reasonable to suppose that drug use in prisons in the UK was not a big problem during the nineteenth century. DORA 1917 did not have the impact on the prison population that the Gin Acts had in the eighteenth century (Dillon 2002). Addicts and dealers did find their way into prison, but not in sufficient numbers to cause the kinds of social concern that gin did. Nonetheless, Charlie Chaplin's film *Modern Times*, about the evils of an industrialised society, hilariously commented upon the problem of cocaine smuggled into prisons. High profile cases like those of Edgar Manning (an Afro-Caribbean man) and Brilliant Chang (a Chinese man), both convicted of trafficking, fuelled salacious concerns about foreign nationals using drugs to seduce British women (Kohn 1992).

It was not until 1971 that a Home Office working party produced the report *Habitual Drunken Offenders* (Home Office 1971), recommending what would now be referred to as seamless and integrated post-discharge support services. When it came to illicit drugs the 1960s saw a boom in use that led inevitably to arrests and convictions. Setting up drug services in the community proved to be an uphill struggle (Whynes & Bean 1991). Policy makers did not get around to prisons until 1979 with the Advisory Council on the Misuse of Drugs (ACMD 1979) report on *Drug Dependants within the Prison System in England and Wales*; thus began the long established call for specialist units in prisons with options for both abstinence and maintenance-based treatments and the involvement of voluntary and other external agencies. In the 1990s the ACMD produced three reports on substance misuse in the criminal justice system. The third (ACMD 1996) addressed prisons. It recommended a harm minimisation approach. Before this, however, the government's White Paper *Tackling Drugs Together* (Home Office 1995c) had raised the issue of mandatory drug testing, in the hope that a true picture of use in prisons might be obtained. This proved controversial, with some workers arguing that it drove prisoners to change their use to more difficult-to-detect drugs with possibly greater potential for addiction, i.e. from cannabis (which can remain detectable in urine for more than a week) to heroin (which remains detectable for only two to three days). Despite this, during the 1990s treatment programmes such as Compass and Rehabilitation of Addicted Prisoners Trust (RAPt) did begin to make inroads into the prison system, and in 1999 the Counselling, Assessment, Referral, Advice and Throughcare (or CARAT) Teams were introduced across the prison estate as part of a co-ordinated drug strategy.

EPIDEMIOLOGY

Illicit drugs

Estimates of the annual percentage of 16–24-year-olds using five of the most common illicit drugs between 1996 and 2006 show declining amounts of cannabis and amphetamine use, fairly constant levels of Ecstasy and cocaine use, and a continuing, comparatively small but important minority of opiate users (Chivite-Matthews *et al.* 2005). There is a similar pattern when these figures are plotted for 16–59-year-olds; however the percentages amongst 16–24-year-olds are substantially higher. Illicit drug use remains a greater problem amongst those who would mostly be termed "young offenders" within the UK prison system. It is also important to bear in mind the actual numbers that each percentage point represents in a population of over 60 million people. Estimated numbers for heroin use in 2002–2003 were approximately 45,000 people, 12,000 of those in the 16–24-year age range. Annual reported drug use amongst younger age groups (10–24-year-olds) appears to be associated with being in one or more vulnerable groups, including ever having been in care, homeless, truant, excluded from school and having committed an offence (Chivite-Matthews *et al.* 2005).

More men than women appear to use each type of drug (Chivite-Matthews *et al.* 2005). However, while the general trend is downwards, the gap between the genders appears to have narrowed. When data are analysed by ethnicity and gender, real differences appear to emerge. First, it seems that more females than males use drugs in certain ethnic groups, i.e. black and mixed. Second, almost as many white females as males use drugs. This data was taken from 11–15-year-olds (NHS Health & Social Care Information Centre 2006). Given the vulnerability associated with drug use in this age group, a possible pattern of drug use being associated with social marginalisation of groups defined by ethnicity and gender seems a genuine reality. However, it does appear that there are higher numbers of male substance misusers dying annually (Office for National Statistics 2007), peaking in the early 2000s; this, though, is taken from raw data. It is not clear whether there is a difference between the proportion of drug users dying within each gender.

What can be drawn from the existing data is that, while overall levels of use may be in decline, there are still demographic groups who remain at greater risk of drug use and the social and psychological problems that accompany this. Being young (under 24), socially vulnerable, female, and from a black or mixed race heritage appears to be a profile that particularly raises risk. Tailoring interventions to meet the needs of specific groups is a particular issue for prison services.

Alcohol use

Alcohol is known as "our favourite drug" (Royal College of Psychiatrists 2008a) and its popularity appears to be increasing from an estimated average of 5 litres of alcohol per person (over 14 years old) per year in 1956 to an estimated 11 litres in 2007 (Institute of Alcohol Studies 2007). This is to some extent associated with a creeping increase in potency. For example, table wine in 1994–95 had an average of 11.4% alcohol by volume (ABV). This rose to 11.85% ABV in 2003–2004. Similarly, normal strength beer rose from an average of 4.06% ABV in 1994–95 to 4.19% ABV in 2003–2004 (NHS Scotland 2005). As a nation we are consuming more alcohol. Paradoxically, however, it does not appear that there is more harmful drinking. The Office for National Statistics (2005) estimates overall declines in the number of people drinking in excess of the recommended amounts per week.

However, just as with illicit drugs, these figures can obscure the presence of a vulnerable minority, especially in the case of what are known as "binge drinkers". Taking the Home Office Youth Lifestyle Survey (Richardson *et al.* 2003) definition of binge drinkers as "those who get drunk at least once a month", 39% of 18–24-year-olds fulfilled the criteria (48% of men, 31% of women). This group were more likely to have committed an offence in the previous 12 months (39% of binge drinkers v 14% of regular drinkers), particularly a violent crime (17% of binge drinkers v 4% of regular drinkers). Getting drunk on at least a weekly basis made the probability of getting into a fight five times higher than for regular drinkers. Violence was associated not with the amount of alcohol consumed overall, but with episodes of drunkenness; the regular drinkers group could have been consuming more alcohol than their binge-drinking peers. Similarly, when offences, rather than drinkers, are studied, there does appear to be a clear association between alcohol use and crime. The British Crime Survey (Home Office 2008) found that 45% of violent incidents involved a victim or assailant under the influence of alcohol, and 39% of domestic violence cases involved alcohol.

Drug and alcohol use in the criminal justice system

Although heroin users constitute the smallest number of drug users in the general population, they are the largest and fastest growing group within the prison population (Ahmad & Mwenda 2004). While there may be fewer female drug users overall in the population, they constitute a greater proportion of *prisoners* within their gender than men.

Counting drug convictions can miss those prisoners whose substance misuse leads to their offending, but whose conviction falls into another category. The disproportionately high incidence of substance misuse in the prison population in comparison to the general population was the focus of a recent review by McSweeney, Turnbull & Hough (2008). Alcohol abuse is in danger of being overlooked because it is not illegal. Fazel, Bains & Doll (2006) conducted a useful systematic review of prevalence studies of drug and alcohol use problems presenting at reception, and found that alcohol abuse and dependence in male prisoners ranged from 18% to 30%, and in women prisoners from 10% to 24%. Estimates of prevalence of drug abuse and dependence were for male prisoners 10% to 48%, and for women prisoners 30% to 60%.

One needs assessment has attempted to address the needs of women, ethnic minorities and young people in prison (Borrill *et al.* 2003). It is clear that for all three groups cannabis is a commonplace, particularly amongst young prisoners (94%). This is concerning, given cannabis' role in raising vulnerability to psychosis, and may go some way to explaining the differing levels of psychotic symptoms between the groups. There is a clear racial split, with crack cocaine being a main substance after cannabis for both men (85%) and women (36%) from black and ethnic minorities. Amongst white women, while crack is also a concern (48%), heroin is a main drug (59%), with the attendant raised incidence of injecting (41%). It is possible that some of the heroin use is in response to the need to "come down" after using crack. Alcohol can also be used for this, and the report raised real concerns about co-morbid alcohol problems for black crack cocaine users (29% women, 48% men). It is notable that co-morbid psychiatric problems split more along gender than racial lines, depression being the most prevalent problem amongst women (53% white, 40% black and ethnic minority), while for black and ethnic minority men anxiety (38%), mania (35%) and sub-clinical psychotic symptoms (30%) predominate. Young prisoners present a highly heterogeneous group regarding drug use and co-morbid symptoms. There were high levels of addiction for white women (60%), black and ethnic minority men (80%) and young people (76%), though black and ethnic minority women appear to have been more resilient (29%).

Borrill *et al.* (2003) noted inconsistencies in detoxification regimens between prisons, the difficulty all three groups had in accessing therapeutic community treatment, and the need for programmes that are sensitive to issues raised by substance, race and gender. In practical terms, it might therefore be useful to develop programmes that address issues as much related to crack and alcohol as heroin, and that address themselves equally to the emotional problems that can both cause and be caused by substance misuse (i.e. depression, anxiety and psychotic symptoms).

Mortality statistics regarding drug use and prison are truly grave. Substance misuse is a major predictor of suicide in custody, especially in the first 28 days (Palmer 2006). On release, Singleton *et al.* (2003b), from a sample of 12,438 prisoners released over six months in 1999, found that 95 had died within a month of release. Likelihood of death in the first week after discharge was 40 times greater than that in the general population. Ninety per cent of these deaths were due to drug use. However, it was not younger but older prisoners (25–39 years old) using opiates who were most at risk.

MANAGING SUBSTANCE MISUSE IN PRISON

Drugs in prison

While there have been prevalence and intervention studies of drug use within prison, to date there has only been one study examining the dynamic relationship between security, therapy and supply of drugs in a prison setting (Penfold, Turnbull & Webster 2005). A qualitative study using 121 subjects (current prisoners, recently released prisoners, and staff) in six prisons, it examined how drugs get into prisons, how drug markets work in prisons, the impact of drug treatment regimens, and of security procedures. Social visits were by far the most commonly identified route for drugs to get in, though mail, newly received prisoners, prison staff, throwing over the wall and during court visits were also identified. Three levels of dealing were described: altruistic or reciprocal sharing between cell mates and friends; currency dealing where drugs were used to purchase canteen items; and organised dealing by prisoners with external contacts.

This latter group held no drugs or money themselves; they employed runners within the prison to deliver drugs once it was confirmed that the appropriate monies had been deposited to associates outside the prison. The amounts that could be bought were much smaller than outside: £10 in prison bought the equivalent of £2.50 worth of heroin on the street.

Drug treatment was inconsistent across the prisons. A particular problem was diversion of medication and bullying that could be associated with this and, while the psychosocial interventions that were available were positively viewed, there was general agreement that provision was inadequate. There were also inconsistencies in security procedures and the rigour with which these were carried out. In one prison a drug supply reduction team had proved remarkably efficient; however, this prison's poor treatment regimen led to high levels of bullying to obtain the few prescribed drugs available.

Treatment literature

A number of treatment approaches are commonly used in prisons:

- **therapeutic communities (TC)** – a group therapy-based approach in which participants live together in a community, take decisions democratically and can be subject to honest feedback from peers and recovering addicts

- **12-step programmes** – another group-based approach based on the philosophy of Alcoholics and Narcotics Anonymous. It can be delivered in a TC format as in the Rehabilitation of Addicted Prisoners Trust (RAPt) programmes or as a regular group within the prison

- **cognitive-behavioural therapy** – an approach that focuses on the person's evaluations of situations and the accompanying feelings. It places a strong emphasis on identifying and dealing with cues to relapse. These would include the Prison-Addressing Substance-Related Offending (P-ASRO) course

- **pharmacotherapy** – this can include a number of different detoxification regimens (methadone, buprenorphine, lofexidine), or stabilisation, or maintenance prescribing (usually on methadone or buprenorphine)

- **boot camp** – "short, sharp shock" approaches, usually involving some form of military style programme designed to instil self-discipline, reliance and esteem in participants, beloved of the right-wing press and politicians.

Perry *et al.*'s (2006) Cochrane review mostly focuses on court-sanctioned and probation interventions. However, one meta-analysis was carried out of two studies (Wexler *et al.* 1999, Sacks *et al.* 2004) that examined the impact of therapeutic community (TC) treatment on re-incarceration. The results favoured TCs: odds-ratio (OR) for re-incarceration for TC graduates was 0.37 (95% CI: 0.16 to 0.87). Thus non-graduates of TCs could have a probability of re-incarceration about 2.7 times greater than their TC graduate peers. However, another Cochrane review of TCs generally (Smith, Gates & Foxcroft 2006) is less optimistic about this form of treatment.

One study of pharmacological interventions for prisoners made it through the Cochrane process into the Perry *et al.* (2006) review: that by Dolan *et al.* (2003). This was a comparison of methadone maintenance with a waiting-list control for drug use in a prison population in Australia. Results were assessed using hair testing. Odds-ratios for use were 0.67 (95% CI 0.36 to 1.25) at two months, 0.46 (95% CI 0.25 to 0.82) at three months, and 0.66 (95% CI 0.37 to 1.21) at four months follow-up. Only the three-months figure was found to be statistically significant. Thus those on the waiting list for methadone maintenance could be about 1.5 times more likely to be using illicit drugs.

The UK Drug Policy Commission Report (UKDPC 2008), which was based on the literature review carried out by McSweeney *et al.* (2008), found "reasonable evidence to support" TCs, RAPt style programmes and opiate detoxification and maintenance programmes, but "no evaluations of the effectiveness of" CARAT interventions, drug-free wings and short-term CBT (i.e. P-ASRO). The general paucity of data on the effectiveness of prison-based treatment, especially given the money spent (£77 million per year (Prison Reform Trust 2007)), was one theme of this report. However, while this is a cause for concern, a greater concern may be the even more parlous state of alcohol treatment programmes in UK prisons. The first accredited programme, run by RAPt, did not commence operation until 2006 and was described as the first of its kind. Until then alcohol services were acknowledged to have developed on an *ad hoc* basis. Another theme of the UKDPC literature review and report was the increasing need to integrate prison-based treatment with community treatment.

Both of these reviews identify effective community-based criminal justice interventions with substance misusers that are effective, such as Criminal Justice Integrated Teams (CJITs), Drug Treatment and Testing Orders (DTTOs) and drug courts. In addition, there are systematic reviews specifically addressing the efficacy and effectiveness of community-based intervention on reduction of offending and substance use (Lipton *et al.* 2002, Holloway, Bennett & Farrington 2005, McMurran 2007). While the place of meta-analytic and systematic reviews in developing treatment cannot be disputed, slavishly restricting the options for a service to such recommendations may lead to prisoners missing out on treatment options that could prove helpful. For example, cognitive-behavioural therapy (CBT) has an increasingly rich evidence base supporting both its efficacy and effectiveness in a number of settings with a number of conditions. However CBT-based programmes such as P-ASRO are yet to receive the close scrutiny that RAPt has undergone, and so the effectiveness of CBT approaches in prison venues remains to be established.

Current services

Current standards for the provision of treatment to incarcerated drug users are set out in *Clinical Management of Drug Dependence in the Adult Prison Setting* (Department of Health 2006). For drug users generally, reference should also be made to the National Institute for Clinical Excellence (NICE) Guidelines numbers 51, *Drug Misuse: Psychosocial Interventions* (NICE 2007b) and 52, *Drug Misuse: Opioid Detoxification* (National Collaborating Centre for Mental Health 2008). In 2003 HM Prison Service's Drug Strategy Unit stated that there were 60 treatment programmes within the prison system (43 CBT, 13 12-step and 4 TCs), all meeting quality criteria set either by the Correctional Services Accreditation Panel (CSAP) or by Prison Service Order 4350, *Effective Regime Interventions* (Drug Strategy Unit 2003).

CARAT

The Counselling, Assessment, Referral, Advice and Throughcare (CARAT) service was established in 1999 across the prison establishment. It provides assessment of treatment need, advice to prisoners and staff and onward referral for treatment. It also provides a limited amount of formal treatment. Statistics for CARAT's performance remain focused on throughput, not outcome (May 2005). Their statistics more than any others outline the level of need that they face on a daily basis. In 2003–2004 they saw 34,037 cases, in 2004–2005 this had risen to 46,263 cases. The most common main drug was crack cocaine (55% of cases 2003–2004, 49% of cases 2004–2005). In addition it is usually CARAT's staff who actually deliver some of the most accessible CBT-based treatment programmes for prisoners, such as P-ASRO and the Short Duration Programme (SDP), a 20-sessions over four weeks harm minimisation group for short term prisoners.

RAPt

The Rehabilitation of Addicted Prisoners Trust (RAPt) currently runs treatment programmes in nine UK prisons, in addition to a number of CARAT and community services. Its philosophy is based on the 12-step approach that also underlies Alcoholics Anonymous and Narcotics Anonymous. From its beginnings in 1992 it has engaged in a number of evaluations. These were reviewed by Martin, Player & Liriano (2003). They found that about 48% of referrals managed to complete the programme (with 18% dropping out, and 35% not starting the programme). Of those that completed the programme, 95% remained drug-free in prison, as did 51% of the drop-outs, and 76% of the non-starters. Thus it is possible that failing to complete the programme raises the likelihood of relapse in comparison to not engaging at all. On release from prison, RAPt graduates were compared to a group of similar age and offence profile and the rates of reconviction after one year were ascertained for the two groups. Of the RAPt graduates, 25% had been reconvicted within one year. Of the comparison group, the figure was 38%. At two years, the figures were 40% and 50% respectively. Both differences are statistically significant. Analysis of reconviction by main drug use shows the programme to be most effective with users of opiates, and crack and polydrug users.

FUTURE DEVELOPMENTS

When the UKDPC Report (2008) was published with the need for better links with health and community services as one of its themes, the Integrated Drug Treatment System (IDTS) for prisoners had already been piloted in 53 prisons. IDTS is designed to improve the clinical and psychosocial services offered within prisons. The objective of IDTS is to expand the quantity and quality of drug treatment within HM Prisons by:

- increasing the range of treatment options available to those in prison, notably substitute prescribing

- integrating clinical and psychological treatment in prison into one system that works to the standards of Models of Care and the Treatment Effectiveness Strategy and works to one care plan

- integrating prison and community treatment to prevent damaging interruptions either on reception into custody or on release back home.

(National Treatment Agency for Substance Misuse 2009)

The IDTS has to work closely with the government's Drug Intervention Programme (DIP) in particular to ensure that offenders receive seamless support and are retained in treatment after release. There is a central project team comprising Prison Service, Prison Health, Care Services Improvement Partnership and National Treatment Agency (NTA), that has the task of managing the roll-out of the programme over a series of staged implementation waves as increasing funding becomes available. The NTA now has lead responsibility for this task. The first wave was a roll-out in 49 prisons (approximately a third of prisons in England). There is an IDTS regional development manager based in, or working closely with each regional NTA team.

The third wave of this policy was being rolled out to a further 38 prisons in 2008–2009. The aims of IDTS are: first, to integrate criminal justice system agencies both in prisons (i.e. CARAT) and outside of prisons (i.e. Criminal Justice Intervention Teams (CJITs)) with health service interventions via links with primary care trusts (PCTs) and other health service providers, to link prison-based treatment services (i.e. RAPt, etc.) with community-based treatment services (i.e. community drug teams) provided by PCTs and other health service providers (see Figure 7.1). It also aims to deliver evidence-based best practice interventions to prisoners and allow services to develop to come into line with the practices described in *Clinical Management of Drug Dependence in the Adult Prison Setting* (Department of Health 2006) and the National Institute for Clinical Excellence Guidelines. If this is achieved, the inconsistencies in approach across the prison estate would have been resolved. Also, if the problems of communication between criminal justice and health care agencies in both prisons and communities are addressed, at the very least the high mortality rate of newly released prisoners may be reduced.

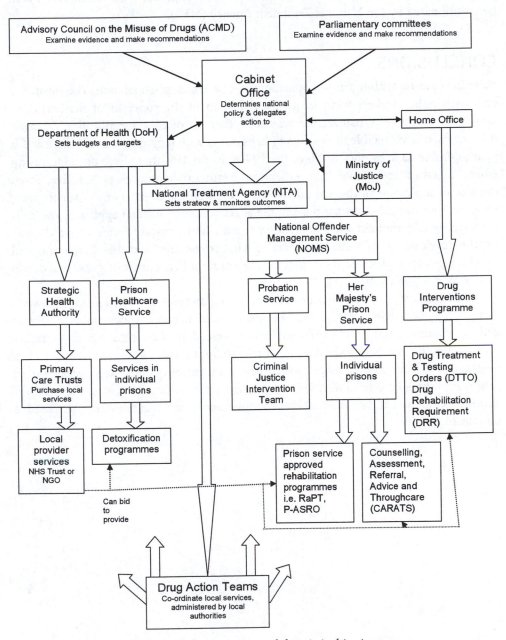

Figure 7.1 Overview of substance misuse services and the criminal justice system

This is to be achieved by the provision of extra funds, via both the NHS and the National Offender Management Service (NOMS) to PCTs and prisons. However, all monies provided under this scheme are to be kept on a separate budget line and spending is to be approved under joint agreements between PCT chief executives, prison governors and local Drug Action Team (DAT) Chairs. Nationally the whole IDTS is to be co-ordinated by the National Treatment Agency (NTA).

CONCLUSIONS

Substance misuse within prison populations is a perennial phenomenon. The substance on which policy makers focus is often a reflection of the concerns of the particular society at that time. Whatever the substance, there is often a socially disadvantaged minority that is vulnerable to developing behaviours with regard to the substance and is seen as problematic by society. Since the 1970s, in the UK, there have been increasing efforts to address these issues from a therapeutic rather than punitive perspective. Given the size of the problem, this led initially to a focus on the numbers of prisoners seen, which in turn has led to criticism about the effectiveness of such an approach, and calls for focus on effectiveness. Meta-analytic, systematic and literature reviews have allowed for the development of a clearer picture of what is effective, and this literature is still developing. Meanwhile the RAPt programme has set a benchmark of good practice in its rigorous self-evaluation.

In addition to this, there has been an increasing awareness of the tensions between being simultaneously custodial and therapeutic, and between treatment in custodial and community settings. These issues have coalesced into concerns about mortality through suicide in prison and overdose on release from prison. As a result the IDTS has been established to provide more consistently therapeutically based approaches within prison settings, establish more community-based interventions to reduce the need for custodial sentences, and ensure that care continues in the most seamless manner possible on release.

CHAPTER 8

The Young Offender

Julie Withecomb

INTRODUCTION

England and Wales continue to detain large numbers of young people in secure settings, with 3,209 places purchased in the secure estate by the Youth Justice Board in 2005 (Youth Justice Board 2005) and 2,663 under-18s in custody in April 2009 (Youth Justice Board 2009).

This chapter aims to explore the kinds of psychological difficulties presented by the population of young people detained by the criminal justice system. The management of mental health within the secure estate will be described in the context of what is known generally about child and adolescent mental health, the structure of the secure estate, and the current legislative frameworks that govern custodial settings for young people.

THE PSYCHIATRY OF CHILDHOOD AND ADOLESCENCE

Child psychiatry differs from adult psychiatry in that a) the prevalence of the various psychiatric disorders is different and b) the presentation of some conditions is altered by the developmental stage that the young person has reached.

The overall prevalence of mental disorder severe enough to cause distress or impairment is 10% in 5–15-year-olds in the general population, with higher rates as age increases, and (for most conditions) higher rates in boys (Meltzer *et al.* 2000).

The most commonly occurring condition is conduct disorder, found in 5% of young people (Meltzer *et al.* 2000), defined by the presence of a "persistent pattern of behaviour in which the rights of others are violated" (American Psychiatric Association 2000). Adolescent conduct problems have repeatedly been shown to predict later offending and mental disorder in adulthood, the common diagnoses in adulthood being substance misuse or personality disorder (Kratzer & Hodgins 1997). The earlier the onset and the wider the range of antisocial behaviours, the greater the later risk.

Conduct disorder has a significant co-morbidity, frequently occurring alongside hyperkinetic disorders and substance misuse, both of which also carry independent additional risks for offending (Cohen & Brook 1987, Rutter, Giller & Hagell 1998). This group of disorders is often characterised by a particular pattern of distorted cognitions and affect that includes hostile attributions, a focus on aggressive cues, poor verbal problem-solving and labelling one's own arousal as anger (Bailey & Marshall 2004).

Schizophrenia occurs in only 0.03% to 0.05% of 15–19-year-olds, but does increase the risk of aggression (Milton *et al.* 2001) and substance misuse (Cantwell *et al.* 1999). Current evidence shows that early intervention improves outcome, but this can prove difficult to deliver, partly because the onset of schizophrenia can be insidious, with behavioural and cognitive problems occurring for some time before psychotic symptoms become obvious. The evidence that cannabis use in young people increases the risk of schizophrenia is now strong (Arsenault *et al.* 2002).

Bipolar disorder, occurring in up to 1% of 14–18-year-olds (Lewinsohn, Klein & Seeley 1995), can also prove difficult to diagnose, especially when there is an early onset during or even prior to puberty. Some of these younger children present with a rapid-cycling condition, where irritability occurs alongside symptoms suggestive of hyperkinetic or conduct disorders. This means that bipolar disorder can be "misdiagnosed" as delinquency.

Pervasive developmental disorders (PDD), including autism and Asperger's syndrome, occur in around four children in every 10,000, although the apparent incidence is increasing with improved awareness and diagnostic skills. Most young people with PDD are law-abiding, some to the point of obsession, but offending can occur, including extreme acts of violence. Inhibition of violence is decreased by lack of empathy for the intended victim and specific acts may be triggered if the young person with autism has his or her rituals or routines disturbed.

THE MENTAL HEALTH OF YOUNG PEOPLE IN CUSTODY

Hagell, in her 2002 review, *Bright Futures*, states that the prevalence of mental health problems in young people in custody is likely to be at least three times that of the general population. This figure is supported by a number of sources, including the Chief Inspector of Prisons' thematic review (Home Office & HM Inspectorate of Prisons 1997), which cites rates of diagnosable mental disorder of 50% in remanded young people and 30% in those who have been sentenced.

Lader, Singleton & Meltzer (2000) interviewed 590 young offenders (aged 16–20). A substantial proportion had been treated for a mental health problem in the 12 months prior to custody–11% of sentenced males, 13% of remand males, and 27% of females. The prevalence of personality disorder was 84% of the male remand population. The prevalence of functional psychosis was around 10%. Sixty-two per cent of the male remand, 70% of the male sentenced, and 51% of the female populations had a history of hazardous drinking. More than 70% had used street drugs prior to custody. These figures are much higher than previous epidemiological studies (e.g. Gunn, Maden & Swinton 1991).

Harrington and Bailey (2005) provided information on a group of 300 young people in contact with six youth offending teams and six custodial units (a mixed group of young people from both community and secure residential settings, therefore). Thirty-one per cent were identified as having mental health needs, with the most frequent diagnoses being depression (18%), anxiety (10%), post-traumatic stress disorder (9%) and hyperactivity (7%). The same study also found that 25% of the group had learning difficulties.

Of over 500 young people held in the secure estate, 97% had used an illegal drug at some point in their lives, 72% had used cannabis on a daily basis for 12 months before their arrest, and 40% had been dependent on a substance (Youth Justice Board 2004). For this latter group, it was concluded that a significant number had been self-medicating on the basis that 30% reported that they had taken drugs just to "feel normal" and 38% gave the reason for their drug use as the wish to "forget everything".

Several authors, including Zeitlin (1999), have commented on how those showing evidence of mental illness are at a greater risk of substance misuse, and vice versa. It has also been established that offenders are disadvantaged across a range of physical health, social and occupational factors.

Taken together, these different studies suggest not only that independent rates of occurrence of mental illness, learning problems and substance misuse are high in this population, but also that co-morbidity with cumulative negative effects of these various problems is likely.

Although prevalence studies of young people in the community find higher rates of most mental health problems in boys, Harrington and Bailey (2005) reported significantly higher rates of some conditions in young female offenders. In a mixed sample of those on community and custodial sentences, it was found that nearly three times as many girls as boys reported depression, more than twice as many deliberate self-harm, and more than three times as many had post-traumatic stress disorder.

Young men from black and ethnic minority groups are more likely to be incarcerated, and may also show higher levels of mental health problems, with Harrington and Bailey (2005) finding a higher prevalence of post-traumatic stress disorder in this group.

There have also been a number of studies exploring why it should be that certain young people are vulnerable to both mental illness and offending. First, the predisposing factors for mental disorder and offending in young people are the same (Hagell 2002).

Second, young offenders are likely to have witnessed violence (Vermeiren, Clippele & Deboutte 2000), indulged in high-risk behaviours (Dolan *et al.* 1999) and experienced the loss of loved ones (Hagell & Newburn 1994), all of which may contribute to higher levels of stress, and so predispose to psychological difficulties. It has also been shown that imprisonment itself has a negative impact on the mental health of young offenders (Mental Health Foundation 1999).

The process of placing young offenders in custody is one which involves taking some of the most vulnerable young people in society, already disadvantaged by a complex interplay of mental health needs, substance misuse and poor educational achievements, and placing them in an environment which is potentially stressful and may in itself trigger psychological problems. Given that the Youth Justice Board's stated aims for secure establishments for young people include to "safeguard and promote their health, both physical and mental" (Youth Justice Board 2005, p.6) it might be thought wise to add the proviso that this target be achieved "to the greatest extent possible".

DETAINING YOUNG PEOPLE

There are three statutory routes to restricting young people's liberty:

- remand and sentencing through the criminal justice system

- detention under the Mental Health Act

- Secure Accommodation Orders.

In England and Wales children of ten years and over are regarded as criminally responsible, and so can be charged and sentenced. The majority of offences will be dealt with by the Youth Court, a specialist branch of the Magistrates' Court, which allows for some consideration to be given to the welfare of the child, handing down a variety of community and custodial sentences (Detention and Training Orders, described below). More serious sexual and violent crimes are dealt with by the Crown Court, which has additional powers described under Section 90/91 of the Criminal Justice Act 2003 to detain young people up to the maximum adult sentence for that offence, which includes life sentencing.

Detention and Training Orders, introduced by the Crime and Disorder Act 1998, provide for custodial sentences of 4–24 months for:

- 10–11-year-old persistent offenders, where public protection is an issue, and only handed down with the approval of the Home Secretary

- 12–14-year-old persistent offenders who have committed an offence serious enough to justify custody

- 15–17-year-olds for any offence serious enough to justify custody.

The Mental Health Act 1983 (amended 2007) has no lower age limit, and so civil and criminal sections are applicable to young people in the same way as to adults.

Secure Accommodation Orders are described in Section 25 of the Children Act 1989. They allow for the detention of children up to the age of 18 years, who are already looked after or accommodated by the local authority, to be held in a secure setting if:

a) they are likely to abscond from any other kind of setting

b) they are likely to injure themselves or others if accommodated elsewhere.

The types of institution where young people can be held in the UK include:

- NHS and private health facilities for those detained under a Section of the Mental Health Act

- Young Offender Institutions (YOIs) for those remanded or sentenced under criminal law

- secure training centres (STCs) also for those remanded or sentenced, usually being those who are younger or considered vulnerable

- local authority secure children's homes (secure units) for both remanded and sentenced young people, especially where there is vulnerability and for those on Secure Accommodation Orders.

In April 2000 the Youth Justice Board was made responsible for the commissioning of custodial placements for 10–17-year-olds, and as of April 2005 made use of 3,209 beds in YOIs, STCs and secure units (Youth Justice Board 2005). These placements are collectively referred to as the secure estate.

In practice, the route that a particular young person takes into a locked facility and the type of institution in which he or she is housed depends on a range of factors including age, psychological and intellectual functioning, cost, bed availability and luck, although there have been improvements in provision arising from specific strategic aims set by the Youth Justice Board.

Since April 2000, the Youth Justice Board has worked to establish separate facilities for younger detainees, albeit sometimes on the same sites as the accommodation for older offenders. Boys aged 12–14 and girls aged 15–16 are now predominantly housed in STCs and secure units rather than YOIs. Young men aged 15–17 are deemed "juveniles" and are increasingly housed in separate accommodation, and there are also 94 beds now available for 16–17-year-old young women in five specially developed units. This strategy is driven by the identified need for specialisation within the secure estate, with further work now under way to provide input to young pregnant detainees and identified units for older young men recognised as having special needs.

Those who require assessment or treatment for mental disorders can be transferred from the secure estate to psychiatric units, using the Mental Health Act. However, there remains a significant shortage of adolescent medium secure beds, although there has been a recent increase in private provision and there is ongoing expansion of NHS beds (see below).

THE CHILDREN ACT AND CHILD PROTECTION FOR YOUNG PEOPLE IN CUSTODY

The establishment of the Youth Justice Board in 1998 at first appeared to herald a new era in the management of children in custody. Based on *Regimes for Juveniles* (HM Prison Service 2004c), a child-centred approach was described, that included directives such as access to a "full, purposeful and active day" (p.24) with at least ten hours out of cell time. However, this Order was voluntary, and in practice appeared to be making little difference to the lives of the children looked after in prison.

In 2002 the legal department of the Howard League for Penal Reform (2002) challenged the Home Office in court on the basis that the Children Act 1989 should apply to young people in custody in the same way as it did to other young people looked after elsewhere. The outcome was a finding that the Act did apply to such children, with young detainees being entitled to the same services under the Children Act as their counterparts in the community, though with the proviso that this was subject to the requirements of imprisonment.

The welfare principle described in the UN Convention and European Charter, requiring the best interests of the child to be put first, was deemed an enforceable obligation on the Prison Service, as were Articles 3 and 8 of the European Convention on Human Rights, requiring that children be protected from ill treatment either by staff or by other inmates. The translation of this legislation into day-to-day practice remains controversial.

It has been accepted that Child Protection Investigations are now obligatory for those aged 15 years and under in YOIs and STCs, just as they would be for children not in custody. There is also the principle of these young people being regarded as "children in need" for the purposes of the Act, with a consequent requirement for a formal needs assessment.

The establishment of social work posts within YOIs is viewed by some as problematic, with concerns that such workers may become institutionalised and not able to meet the young people's welfare needs in the same way that a social worker from an external team might. The definition and development of the social work role within prison inreach teams is continuing, however, and the impact of such work on provision for vulnerable young people in custody is already experienced as highly valuable within the multi-disciplinary team.

Now that the range of psychological difficulties experienced by young offenders and the routes to their detention have been explored, the mental health provision to YOIs can be considered in context. This provision can be divided into that provided to young people within the prison setting (inreach), and that within hospitals into which remanded and sentenced young people can be transferred under the Mental Health Act.

MENTAL HEALTH SERVICES FOR YOUNG PEOPLE IN CUSTODIAL SETTINGS

As recently as 1999 there was virtually no provision from properly trained and net-worked practitioners for adolescents held in custody, with input being provided either by prison doctors with no adolescent psychiatry training, or by isolated mental health workers with a special interest in the field but little in the way of support or pathways for the long-term management of young people across organisational boundaries. The situation now is somewhat improved, but still far from the gold standard of young peo-ple held in custody having the same access to mental health services as young people in the community.

As with the adult population, some difficulties arise in the context of trying to pro-vide a service to a potentially shifting group, and adequate continuity of care is almost impossible when the clinician cannot tell from one day to another whether remand prisoners will remain in the same institution. Most services are under-resourced, espe-cially when the high morbidity is taken into account, and mental health professionals may have to work to lower standards in order to ensure that all those with needs get at least some input. Essentially, there is a tension between the security requirements of the prison setting, and the child-centred approach that would be the natural focus for mental health workers; this requires a robust but sensitive approach to merging the dif-ferent cultures of prison and health staff.

Each establishment has its own strategy for provision of mental health services, leading to huge disparity in accessibility. The wide variation in competencies of those working with the young people is currently under scrutiny by policy makers, and it is likely that statutory training and targets will be set.

An example of a working service model is that provided at Brinsford YOI and Remand Centre in Staffordshire from 2005 to 2008. In line with recognised best prac-tice (Banerjee et al. 1995) the team comprised workers who had a base in a national health setting, accessing supervision and clinical governance procedures through that base and regularly working sessions within a hospital unit as well as in the prison. For a population of approximately 460 young men between the ages of 15 and 20, the Brinsford inreach team had provision of one day a week of psychiatry, two days of psychology, the equivalent of one full-time psychiatric nurse and a full-time psychiatric social worker, with roles for occupational therapy, art therapy and speech and language therapy. The YOI itself employed six mental health nurses and two nurses with a special responsibility for those with alcohol and substance misuse problems. These staff as-sessed and managed those with mental health problems, either within the 11-bedded prison hospital or in the "community" settings of the general wings, the unit for vulner-able inmates and the segregation block. The nature of the work was diverse, with the aim of providing input over a spectrum of problems, from the treatment and transfer of those with illnesses such as schizophrenia, through cognitive skills for management of anger and poor impulse control, to counselling for post-trauma symptoms. The social work role aimed to provide a link with the outside world, helping in information gathering from families and the professional network, and smoothing the path of the young person into community services at the time of release.

The YOIs Feltham (in West London) and Huntercombe (in Oxfordshire) also have adolescent forensic inreach teams linked to forensic child and adolescent mental health services, as does the Orchard Lodge secure unit in Southeast London. Other institutions, such as the Medway STC in Kent, have arrangements outside the forensic child and adolescent mental health services network to access mental health services, and some units have no regular input.

Services for those with substance misuse problems is improving (Harrington & Bailey 2005), with CARAT (Counselling, Assessment, Referral, Advice and Throughcare) having the aim of providing support for those in custody, as well as ensuring appropriate onward referral to those leaving the institution. However, there is still lack of integration between mental health and substance misuse services, described as essential for this group in *The Substance of Young Needs* (Gilvarry 2001); these services are separately commissioned and provided.

The number of young sex offenders held in custody is small but recently increasing, with sexual offences as a percentage of total offences leading to a police or court disposal rising from 0.6% in 2006–2007 to 0.8% in 2007–2008, according to statistics published in the Youth Justice Annual Workload Data (available at www.yjb.gov.uk/publications). The same legislation and statutory frameworks, such as MAPPA (multi-agency public protection arrangements), apply to the under-18s, albeit with additional age and sentence criteria in some cases; for example, an offence of sexual assault by someone under the age of 18 needs to attract an additional custodial sentence of at least 12 months before sex offender registration is required. Treatment programmes for young sex offenders remain sparse both in the community and in custody. The Lucy Faithfull Foundation provides programmes in a small number of young offender institutions, but assessment alone takes three months and there are obvious limitations in providing input such as joint family sessions.

ADOLESCENT FORENSIC MENTAL HEALTH – MEDIUM SECURITY AND BEYOND

The National Adolescent Forensic Network is a group of medium secure units within the National Health Service (NHS) that provides inpatient care under the Mental Health Act on criminal and civil sections for 10–18-year-olds. Those admitted usually show evidence of both offending behaviour and mental illness.

Together, the units in Manchester, Newcastle, Birmingham, Southampton and West and Southeast London provide around 80 beds accessed through a single referral system. The cost of maintaining the inpatient service is currently met by the National

Commissioning Group (NCG), which has allowed the ongoing expansion of bed numbers. There is also some provision within the private sector, including St Andrew's Hospital in Northampton, the Huntercombe group and the Oakview Unit in Kent. The Prudoe unit in Newcastle provides an NHS service for adolescents who have a learning disability in addition to offending and mental health problems.

The first of the NHS units in Manchester necessarily had a national remit, having to admit those young people with the most serious problems from across the country. As further units open and develop, it is increasingly possible for them to have more regional and local links, offering admissions for those who live nearby.

The units are also developing outpatient work, which includes consultation and liaison services to other local organisations such as young offender institutions, secure units, youth offending teams and child and adolescent mental health services. Eventually this may allow for regional networks of adolescent forensic mental health, so that all those involved in work with the young people who present the greatest risk can access appropriate advice and services. Currently, though, the funding mechanisms are such that the focus has been on building inpatient units, and adequate community and inreach services remain patchy.

The majority of the young people admitted for inpatient care have serious mental disorders, such as schizophrenic or bipolar illnesses, although those with developing personality disorders or with evidence of autistic or attention deficit disorders or post-traumatic stress disorder may be admitted for assessment, and for treatment where this is possible.

As with adult services, the therapeutic approach includes the full range of psychiatric treatments – such as oral and intra-muscular pharmacotherapy and electroconvulsive therapy (although this is rarely used) – and access to different therapy modalities as appropriate. In addition, all the young people are offered educational programmes according to their ability.

CONCLUSION

Overall, mental health services for detained adolescents have vastly improved since 1999, but significant areas of unmet need remain. An increase in resources is necessary to improve the networks that allow smooth transitions across services for those with complex needs, and to develop services for specific, poorly resourced types of problem, such as learning disability and sexually harmful behaviours. The needs of the mental health workers themselves also have to be addressed, from basic physical safety requirements to the psychological stresses of working in such "alternative" environments.

CHAPTER 9

Women in Prison

Richard Taylor and Jessica Yakeley

GENDER DIFFERENCES IN CRIME

In 2006–2007 in England and Wales, 87,200 women were arrested for violence against another person, compared to 400,900 men (Ministry of Justice 2008d). The ratio of male to female homicide in England and Wales has remained stable at about 10:1 in recent years (Home Office 2006b). Around 80% of all violent offences in the UK are committed by males (Home Office 2004b). However, recent statistics suggest that overall numbers of male and female perpetrators of violent crimes against another person are increasing, compared to other offences (Ministry of Justice 2008d). Also, the proportion of recorded domestic violence incidents in which the offender is female has increased significantly in recent years (Home Office 2004b).

Studies of female homicide show that 80% of victims are close family members, 40–45% of female homicide offenders kill their children, and roughly one third kill their partner (Wykes 1995). The relationships between offender and victim show marked differences according to the gender of the offender – most victims of male violent perpetrators are not known to the offender, whereas the victims of violent women are most often close family members, their partners or children. This can present particular challenges for mental health professionals working with remand prisoners, for example, charged with child cruelty or homicide of a male partner. There may be ongoing criminal proceedings with parallel family court or child protection issues in relation to surviving children. There may be a background of domestic violence, substance abuse, or a new pregnancy and request for admission to a mother and baby unit to deal with, in addition to the ongoing clinical problems of mood disorder, self-harm and personality disorder.

The early criminology literature on gender differences emphasised biological factors. Lombroso & Ferrero (1895) argued that women were, by evolution, less developed and thus able to adapt more easily than men to difficult environments, and so less likely to commit violent crimes as a way of adaptation. Pollack (1950) argued, controversially, that lower offending rates for women were merely an artefact, as women may not necessarily commit fewer crimes than men, but are less likely to be detected. He proposed that the criminal activities of women were more likely to be based on deceit. D'Orban's (1971) review of the literature concluded that gender has an influence on the treatment of female offenders at all stages of the criminal justice system, but that the effects are complex.

Social and learning theorists argued that, for example, girls were more protected whilst growing up and therefore less likely to offend (Sutherland 1947). Hagan, Simpson & Gillis (1979) suggested that informal controls instituted in the home were the strongest factors controlling crime. The feminist criminologists from the late 1960s viewed women as predominantly the victims of violence, committed against them by their partners or fathers within a patriarchal society (Yakeley 2009). Kennedy (1992) has argued, from a legal perspective, that the criminal justice system continues to discriminate against female defendants in the way various aspects of the criminal law are interpreted and in the context of a predominantly male judiciary – for example, in the different ways that the provocation defence operates for male and female defendants in domestic killings. She asserts that "a web of prejudice, privilege and misinformation affects women in all their dealings with the law" (p.235). A psychoanalytically oriented body of literature (Welldon 1988, Motz 2001) has challenged the notions of women as victims of violence, and has explored a psychoanalytic explanation for the patterns of female violence where the victims are partners, children or the woman's own body (see below).

IMPRISONMENT OF WOMEN

Chao & Taylor (2005) describe the UK profile of women prisoners. Twenty per cent of known offenders are women, and they represent 6% of the prison population in England and Wales (HM Inspectorate of Prisons 1997). The average female population in prison rose by 173% between 1992 and 2002, as opposed to 50% for men (Home Office 2003b). The age of women prisoners is also young, with only 16% over 40 years of age in 2002 (Home Office 2003b), and ethnic minorities are over-represented, making up 29% of the female prison population (but only 9% of the total female population in England and Wales). There is a significant issue in relation to drug smuggling and the use of women as mules by drug gangs (see below), and 19% of female prisoners are foreign nationals (Fawcett Society 2003).

Gibbens' (1971) classic study of HMP Holloway surveyed 638 women, representing one in four of all women received to prison during 1967, and concluded that 15%

of sentenced women prisoners had a mental illness, 22% a history of a past suicide attempt and 7% had alcoholism. Maden, Swinton & Gunn (1990) found that 23% of sentenced prisoners were dependent on drugs, and subsequent studies identified high rates of psychosis in the remand population (Maden *et al.* 1996, Singleton *et al.* 1998). Maden argued that, for women in prison, the essential disadvantage was being a mentally disordered offender rather than being a female offender, and that the principal problem was the failure of mental health services to divert mentally disordered offenders to appropriate regional secure psychiatric services. Maden argued that the number of women involved was so small that their transfer from prison to hospital should be an achievable target.

A subsequent study looking at the transfer of female offenders with mental disorder from prison to hospital found that only 62 women from 3,309 receptions at HMP Holloway were transferred to hospital in 1995. The speed of response in these cases was inadequate, particularly for those diagnosed with a personality disorder (Rutherford & Taylor 2004). A further study (Chao & Taylor 2005) examined 119 women referred for transfer from HMP Holloway to specialist forensic mental health services. Fifty per cent of women with a personality disorder and 38% of those with a psychotic illness were rejected for transfer to hospital.

Since the publication of Maden's review in 1996 there have been significant developments in female secure psychiatric services. There has been a policy shift towards the provision of single sex accommodation in both low and medium secure units. However, there has been an overall reduction in the provision of high secure psychiatric services. The concern, notably identified by lobby groups such as WISH (Women in Secure Hospitals), that some female mentally disordered offenders find their way to an inappropriately high level of security, has resulted in the development of specialist alternative services such as enhanced medium security, with improved specialist therapeutic input without unnecessary and excessive perimeter security. Service provision gaps include a shortage of appropriate low and medium secure inpatient psychiatric facilities, particularly for personality disorder, within the NHS, although there have been significant increases in single sex mental illness beds, and NHS outsourcing to the private sector has filled the gap to a certain extent.

Women offenders referred to hospital are commonly labelled as having complex diagnoses, particularly mental illness co-existing with personality disorder and/or substance misuse. These added factors, although common, make them difficult to manage and may contribute to decisions not to divert to a hospital environment. The need to manage and contain psychotic prisoners awaiting transfer, along with depressed prisoners and those self-harming, will be familiar to mental health professionals working in male and female prisons alike. However, in a women's prison setting the refusal by psychiatric services to agree to the transfer of highly distressed prisoners with a complex interplay of personality disorder, mood disorder, psychotic symptoms and self-harm can be particularly challenging for the prison inreach mental health team.

HMP HOLLOWAY

Until recently HMP Holloway was the largest women's remand prison in Western Europe. It became an all women's prison in the early twentieth century. It was rebuilt in the 1970s and 1980s, designed to be run on hospital lines, which contrasts with its function as a remand prison for many disturbed and violent offenders. Until recently HMP Holloway had capacity for 550 inmates, including young offenders, although with the opening of additional facilities in and near London the numbers have reduced significantly. There can be over 5,000 receptions a year. The average stay is 28 days, but some women remain on remand for over a year.

The health care inpatient wing in 2003 contained 30 beds and had a throughput of nearly 400 women a year (Chao & Taylor 2005). The majority were admitted on mental health grounds (88%), a small minority on physical health grounds (8%) and the remainder owing to "management problems" (4%). HMP Holloway has continued to attract publicity, although, since 2001, closer partnership with NHS providers has led to a gradual and sustained improvement. Sir David Ramsbotham, the Chief Inspector of Prisons, highlighted the problems of a large female remand prison (Ramsbotham 2003). A report published in September 2001 concluded that women were being neglected owing to limited resources. The budget per inmate per annum was £40,500, compared with £150,000 or more for secure hospital inpatient psychiatric care. However, some improvements were noted at the unannounced inspection in October 2004 (Owers 2005). Holloway no longer houses sentenced juvenile prisoners, which had been identified as a problem, and special provision has been made for the juvenile remand unit. An innovative "first night in custody" wing has also helped to ameliorate the emotional impact for new remand prisoners.

HMP Bronzefield and HMP Peterborough (new public-private women's prisons in southern England) have now opened, reducing the catchment area for HMP Holloway, with a consequent drop in overall numbers by almost two hundred inmates and a reduction of pressure on resources at Holloway. Holloway is still expected to deal with more disturbed prisoners from elsewhere in the women's prison estate, and staff expertise has gradually accumulated, notably on the lifers' unit and in the greatly improved inpatient health care centre with specialist input from a range of providers including forensic psychiatry, community mental health, drugs and alcohol rehabilitation and improved primary care. General practitioners now hold clinics on the wings where there is a permanent nursing presence, obviating the need for time-consuming escorts of prisoners to an outpatient clinic.

PSYCHIATRIC PRESENTATIONS IN WOMEN

Howard (2006) has argued that schizophrenia in women appears to be a different disorder to that in men. There is evidence that women with schizophrenia have a better outcome compared with men and less evidence of negative symptoms. Women are said to have a better treatment response and to be more likely to have mood symptoms.

Howard also argued that women with schizophrenia may initially be misdiagnosed because of the use of narrow diagnostic criteria that exclude episodes of a brief duration and with affective symptoms. Given the high rates of substance misuse in the prison population, the complication of drug-induced psychosis or dual diagnosis may also add to diagnostic difficulties and management problems.

Travers (1996) has argued that there are a number of gender influences on women in forensic settings, that are often overlooked. These include enduring behavioural disturbance, high rates of violence towards carers, more extensive histories of trauma, serious self-harming, and increased rates of negative countertransference amongst staff. Travers argues that dedicated forensic services for women must provide a safe environment where challenging behaviours can be tolerated. Bland, Mezey & Dolan (1999) have argued that much of the behavioural and psychological disturbances are the result of long-term experiences of trauma, abuse and deprivation. Psychotherapy, although difficult to deliver, is said to be crucial in allowing meaningful connections to be made between current distress and past events.

Assaults on staff are an important issue, particularly in prison health care centres where psychotic women prisoners may wait for many weeks or months for transfer to the NHS. Prison and health care staff have to deal with significant aggression from disturbed prisoners. This can cause tension between health care and prison discipline staff. Prison discipline staff who have worked in health care centres become adept at identifying mentally disordered prisoners, and they share the exasperation of mental health inreach staff when NHS transfer is not available or is delayed. Aiyegbusi (1996) argued that risk assessment research on women in high security showed that staff can accurately predict physical aggression but cannot prevent it. Given that, in prison, antipsychotic medication can only be given under capacity, rather than mental health, legislation in an emergency and in the patient's best interests, the management of acute psychosis during a delayed transfer can be particularly problematic in a women's prison setting.

VIOLENCE AGAINST THE BODY – A PSYCHODYNAMIC APPROACH

Welldon (1988) was the first author to challenge the narrow view that women were solely the victims of violence, but could also be perpetrators. She argued that women tend to direct their aggression against their own bodies or their children, or perhaps more broadly against their own reproductive potential. Self-harm in the form of cutting is an obvious example of violence to the self, which anecdotally is more common in women in both prison and psychiatric settings. Welldon challenged the collective denial about women being capable of abusing their own children. Motz (2001) has further developed Welldon's work to consider the psychology of female violence in general, where the woman's body or creations of her body are unconsciously used for violent and perverse purposes. This psychodynamic approach has been applied to a number of the clinical issues commonly dealt with in women prisoners.

FORENSIC ISSUES OF PARTICULAR RELEVANCE TO WOMEN IN PRISON

Child abuse

In the last 25 years society has become much more aware of the extent of child abuse that occurs within families. The Children Act 1989 establishes the orders available to the courts, and sets out criteria for deciding whether the child reaches the threshold of significant suffering or harm from the parents or caregivers, so that the local authority can institute care proceedings. This Act was revised in 2004 (Department of Health 2004) to highlight the need for inter-agency communication and co-ordination, following the inquiry into the death of Victoria Climbié in 2000 (Laming 2003), the issue recently revisited in relation to Baby P in 2008. Both Welldon (1988) and Motz (2001) draw attention to transgenerational patterns of perverse mothering, and how women who were themselves neglected and abused by their mothers re-enact this destructive behaviour with their own children.

Women charged with child cruelty may find themselves subjected to bullying or abuse from fellow prisoners in much the same way as sex offenders are victimised in the male prison system. However, given the absence of large numbers of sex offenders in female prisons compared to male prisons, the vulnerable prisoner unit system is not available to women in prison and the burden of dealing with the emotional fall-out of the disturbed background of these individuals, coupled with their negative experience of imprisonment, will often fall to prison listeners, voluntary agencies and prison mental health inreach teams. An awareness of child protection issues is important for any professionals working with women in prison, as frequently there will be parallel criminal and family proceedings ongoing. An awareness of the negative (countertransference) reactions provoked by this group of inmates in both prison and health staff is important in order to avoid further inadvertent victimisation.

Factitious illness by proxy (FIP), also known as Munchausen's syndrome by proxy (MSBP), is a form of child abuse in which a child's carer (usually a mother) falsely presents the child to health services as ill. Women who carry out this behaviour often have complex histories of childhood abuse or neglect, including sexual abuse, self-harm, eating disorders and other somatic disorders. A significant proportion of these mothers have also been diagnosed with Munchausen's syndrome themselves, with histories of multiple presentations of unexplained symptoms, hospital admissions and surgical procedures (Rosenberg 1987, Adshead 2001b). Although these women may be viewed by professionals as deliberately fabricating their symptoms or malingering, a more useful explanatory model is that this is a complex form of abnormal illness behaviour on the spectrum between conscious fabrication and unconscious somatisation, often associated with personality disorder and where the issue of secondary gain may be hard to determine. Where a woman caregiver, usually the mother, is remanded in custody charged with criminal offences, the combination of physical health symptoms (real or factitious) and mental disorder can pose a significant challenge to the assessing psychiatrist or mental health professional.

Child abduction and stealing

D'Orban (1972, 1976) has made a significant contribution to the understanding of the relatively rare occurrence of child abduction. In five years of working at Holloway one of us encountered only one case, when the woman was an alleged accomplice to a male abductor. Kidnapping for ransom is rare in the UK, although currently of epidemic proportions in Latin America; however, abduction of a child by a female perpetrator may be commonly associated with mental disorder. D'Orban found that of 24 offenders, 8 had schizophrenia, 6 had learning disability, and the rest had varying degrees of personality disorder. Three offence patterns based on motivation were proposed: comforting, psychotic and manipulative offences. *Comforting* offences tended to be committed by younger women from adverse backgrounds with mild learning difficulties. The offence may be motivated by a sense of emotional deprivation. The women are fond of children and long to have a baby. They may abduct a child known to them. This form of child abduction may be associated with pseudocyesis (false pregnancy). In *psychotic* offences, the diagnosis is schizophrenia. The women may have lost children to childcare proceedings because of earlier illness episodes and may have a delusion that the child is their own. In the *manipulative* group (perhaps an inverse of the Medea syndrome in infanticide (see below), a child may be abducted by a personality disordered, but relatively well socially adjusted, woman who abducts a child in the setting of an insecure relationship with a partner in an attempt to prolong a relationship.

Boudreaux (2000) has reviewed the available American literature on child abduction. In the USA child abduction (broadly defined to include abduction by parents during a custody dispute) is estimated at 160,000–350,000 cases per year. The number of abductions by strangers is 3,200–4,600 per year. Stranger abductions are more commonly sexually motivated. A psychodynamic understanding of non-sexual child abduction offences, where the intention is to keep the child, is through processes of projection and projective identification where offenders unconsciously project their own neglect and sense of abandonment into the child. Child abduction cases can be very high profile in terms of media coverage and this can complicate appropriate psychiatric management, both inside and outside a prison setting.

Infanticide

The Infanticide Act was initially introduced in 1922, and reduced the offence of child murder to infanticide (roughly equivalent to manslaughter) in cases where it was believed that the mother had killed her child because she had not fully recovered from the effect of giving birth, which had caused a disturbance in the balance of her mind. The reduction in offence to infanticide was due to an increasing reluctance to convict mothers of murder, as this would automatically lead to the death penalty. The Act was revised in 1938 to include not having recovered from the effects of lactation (breast-feeding) as well as childbirth, as a further cause of mental disturbance at the time of the killing that could reduce the charge of murder to infanticide. In the UK, an infanticide conviction, like manslaughter, gives judges discretion over sentencing. The mandatory life sentence is avoided. Originally, infanticide was brought in to avoid the death penalty in an era when unwanted and concealed pregnancies and subsequent child destruction was a much more common problem. In practice, community orders, with or without mental health treatment requirements, rather than custodial sentences, are common.

Various researchers (Resnick 1969, Scott 1973, D'Orban 1979) have attempted to classify infanticide based on the motivations of the mother into categories such as an unwanted child, mercy killing, psychosis, battering parent or Medea syndrome (where the woman kills her child as revenge or retaliation against her partner). Motz (2001) critically reviews the Infanticide Act, and suggests that the notion of female hysteria is implicitly woven into its structure. The motivations for infanticide are complex, may not be conscious, and may be influenced by social and cultural factors as well as biological. The management of women remanded in custody and charged with the killing of their own babies under the age of one must include careful psychiatric evaluation and almost certainly a period of observation in a health care centre. Cases of puerperal psychosis or schizophrenia will need to be urgently referred for transfer to the NHS. Evaluation of the contribution of affective disorder and personality disorder will be more complex, and contextual issues such as pre-existing child abuse and the care of surviving siblings will need to be addressed.

Domestic violence and "battered women who kill"

The plight of women abused by their partners has been the subject of much debate in recent years. These women are often seen as the victims of men who control and dominate their partners within the home by coercive and violent means. It is argued that society has tolerated or turned a blind eye to this, owing to male prejudices. It may be difficult for the woman to leave, not only because of her financial dependence upon the husband or partner, but also because of lack of support from the social and legal systems. There may be fear of later retribution, anxiety about alternative accommodation, and worries about the potential for losing contact with children. These fears may be exacerbated in some cultural or ethnic groups – for example, in relation to fear of honour killing.

The model of learned helplessness has been used to explain the abused woman's continued dependence upon her partner. Learned helplessness was first described in laboratory rats, which showed symptoms of apathy, passivity and loss of motivation to respond when repeatedly exposed to painful stimuli with no means of escape (Seligman 1975). It is proposed that the battered woman who sees no means of escape from the abusive relationship responds in the same way, developing feelings of helplessness and hopelessness, lowered self-esteem, passivity and social isolation (Walker 1984). Battered woman syndrome is described as a constellation of behavioural and cognitive patterns seen in women who have been exposed to violence in intimate relationships. The resultant depression and cognitive distortions of powerlessness are said to impair the individual's ability to escape from the abusive situation. The model of learned helplessness, however, has been criticised by Downs (1996) as being too simplistic. Downs argues that the syndrome's logic denies women their reason and will, reinforcing their victimisation, and that women often adopt "heroic means of survival, retaining accurate, reasoned perceptions concerning [their abusers]", and consequently that "to portray battered women as irrational and lacking will undermines otherwise valid self-defence claims and hurts women more generally" (p.12). It also fails to take into account dynamic factors between victim and perpetrator that may also contribute to the process. Motz (2001) argues that the woman's active participation, albeit unconscious, in the violent relationship may be understandable in the context of her inability to leave, despite repeated experiences of abuse.

Roughly one third of all women who commit homicide kill their husband or partner (Wykes 1995), and many of these women have been abused by the man they killed (Kirkpatrick & Humphrey 1986, Foster, Veale & Fogel 1989). In the UK the charge of murder carries a mandatory life sentence, but since the 1957 Homicide Act, if this charge is reduced to manslaughter on the grounds of provocation or diminished responsibility, the sentence is discretionary. In the UK battered women who kill abusive partners have found it difficult to successfully run self-defence, which, if successful, results in acquittal.

The case law relating to the partial defence of provocation has been complex in relation to cases of battered women who kill their partners. The partial defence of provocation requires not only that there were things said or done by the deceased that constitute provocation, but also that the perpetrator must have been subject to a sudden loss of self-control. Attempts were made in various criminal cases in the late 1990s to argue that for an abused woman there may be a form of "slow burn" provocation, which does not fit neatly into the legal definition of sudden loss of self-control. Cases such as R v Ahluwalia and R v Thornton are examples of this. In both cases a male victim who had repeatedly been physically abusive to the female perpetrator was killed whilst asleep. Provocation has been further complicated by subsequent case law developments such as R v Smith and latterly Attorney General for Jersey v Holley. Smith appeared to allow the presentation to the jury of abnormal mental characteristics to modify the partial defence of provocation, whereas the case of Holley may have tightened up this definition. Previously there had been some elision of the boundaries between diminished responsibility and provocation; however, it may now be that mental characteristics can only apply to the woundability of the defendant but not to his or her loss of self-control. Mezey (unpublished) has conducted research on the outcome of murder trials involving battered women. Although murder convictions are common at the first trial, there are frequently re-trials and the final outcome may be manslaughter, usually on the grounds of diminished responsibility as a consequence of battered woman syndrome in combination with depression or personality disorder. The defence more successfully used in such cases to reduce a charge of murder to one of manslaughter has been diminished responsibility, often on the grounds that the woman suffers from battered woman syndrome.

Proposals have been made to change UK murder law regarding cases of domestic violence (Ministry of Justice, Attorney General's Office & Home Office 2008). The defence of provocation will be abolished altogether, and sexual fidelity on the part of the victim will no longer constitute grounds for reducing murder to manslaughter. Two new partial defences will be introduced: "killing in response to a fear of serious violence" and "killing in response to words and conduct which caused the defendant to have a justifiable sense of being seriously wronged". Moreover, the existing common law requirement for loss of self-control in these circumstances to be "sudden" will be removed. These changes may be favourable for the abused woman who kills her abusing partner, but not in the heat of the moment of being physically beaten by him. However, the partial defence of diminished responsibility will become more stringent, in that it will now have to be grounded in a valid medical diagnosis linked to accepted classificatory systems. Battered woman syndrome remains a controversial concept, not currently included in either ICD-10 or DSM-IV.

Future policy regarding the treatment of violent women in both mental health services and the courts should welcome the recognition of cultural and societal influences on female violence, but should not collude in the denial of female agency and aggression. Erin Pizzey (2008), a feminist all her life and founder of the modern women's shelter movement, cautions against accepting a neat division between female victims and male oppressors, reminding us that in many abusive couples both partners are guilty of verbal and physical assault, and that women may choose alternatives to killing their partners in these violent relationships.

Drug mules

Organised drug gangs frequently employ vulnerable women as mules to smuggle illicit drugs into the UK. The penalties for drug smuggling are harsh, with average sentences between five and eight years for a first offence. Large numbers of women, predominantly from West Africa, South America and the Caribbean, are serving lengthy sentences of imprisonment in UK prisons, having been apprehended for drug smuggling. The individual socio-economic circumstances of these women are often tragic. Many of them have dependent children in their home country and may have been subject to various forms of duress or coercion to co-operate with the smuggling operation. This particular problem represents one way in which women, although complicit in the activities, bear the brunt of the penalty for an operation generally organised by male overseers. Managing the mental health and social consequences for this particularly disadvantaged group of women prisoners remains a significant challenge. Charities such as Hibiscus, which works in Ghana, regularly use simple cartoons to demonstrate the severe penalties for anyone getting involved in smuggling. Many of these women are naïve first-time offenders who have left children behind. Frankly mentally ill drug mules are rare.

POLICY AND FUTURE DEVELOPMENTS

Maden's (1996) exhortation to move the mentally ill out of prison and into specialist secure mental health hospital placements remains valid today. New resources have been provided for prison mental health inreach teams, and partnerships via service level agreements and contracts with local NHS health care (primary care trusts) are the norm. There has been some criticism that contracts have been awarded to general adult psychiatric services at the expense of established forensic mental health providers. It could be argued that accumulated experience of the realities and limitations of the practice of prison psychiatry are lost when contracts are awarded to services without long-term experience of the complexities of liaising with the criminal justice system. Conversely, forensic psychiatry services may be accused of failing to capitalise on the opportunity to improve prison psychiatry and to have too rigidly protected secure forensic beds. It is certainly troubling to hear that transfer of mentally ill prisoners to the NHS is not required simply because of the presence of a mental health inreach team in prison.

The majority (71%) of women still serve short sentences of less than 12 months, with the most common offence attracting a custodial sentence being theft and handling, which accounts for 40% of receptions. The female remand population in 2002 was 23%, and of these, 59% were not given custodial sentences (Home Office 2003b). Chao & Taylor (2005) argued that a reduction in the number of custodial sentences for minor offenders, and limiting the number of women remanded into custody, might help to lessen the burden on prisons, and in turn on the mental health services working within the criminal justice system. However, if the female prison population continues to rise, it is likely that further development of female secure units within the NHS will be necessary. The number of high secure beds has been reduced, and although there were previously women in both Broadmoor and Rampton high secure hospitals, at present there are only 50 high secure female beds remaining, all at Rampton.

A further notable gap in services, given developments for men in this area, is the lack of inpatient facilities for the treatment of women with personality disorder. Although single-sex medium secure units have been commissioned, they generally take dual diagnosis only (i.e. psychosis with co-morbid personality disorder). Whereas both high secure and medium secure facilities for men have been developed through the dangerous and severe personality disorder programme, there is clearly a gap between high or enhanced medium security for women (which will treat personality disorder), and community-based projects such as the day hospital programme at Halliwick Day

Unit, St Ann's Hospital in Tottenham, London, a psychotherapeutic service for women with borderline personality disorder. Further investment in these services would clearly be beneficial, both in treating potential offenders and in providing a viable alternative to custody for some. Private sector hospitals (paid by the NHS) provide a significant number of secure beds for female offenders, including those in specialist personality disorder units, and are increasingly providing a wider range of step-down and community-based programmes. Given the low numbers of women versus men offenders, there may be economies of scale in contracting out some of this provision in an increasingly mixed economy health service.

CHAPTER 10

Elderly Prisoners

Seena Fazel and Preeti Chhabra

Increasing attention has been paid to elderly prisoners over the last decade. This interest has been primarily driven by the increasing numbers of elderly prisoners, but also reflects the widespread acceptance of the general principle that the health care needs of elderly persons are different, and that these needs should be met in a manner specific to the elderly. The number of sentenced prisoners aged 60 and above has more than doubled from 454 in 1992 to 1700 in 2004 (Home Office 2005). This partly reflects overall increases in the sentenced population in England and Wales, which rose from 37,000 to 57,000 in the same time period. However, the proportion of those aged over 59 in prison has also doubled in a decade to 2.6% (see Table 10.1).

Table 10.1 Rise in population of men aged 60 and over in prison establishments in England and Wales from 1994 to 1999, expressed as a percentage of males of all ages (Home Office 2000b). For 2000 onwards the proportion is for sentenced prisoners only (Home Office 2005).

Year	1994	1995	1996	1997	1998	1999	2000	2001	2002	2003	2004
% of all ages	1.51	1.59	1.69	1.75	1.80	2.15	2.20	2.30	2.40	2.52	2.62

A similar trend has been observed in America, where the number of prisoners aged 55 and over has increased from 48,000 in 1999 to 71,900 in 2004 (Beck 2000, Harrison & Beck 2005). In Canada, the growth in the population of older offenders in prison is more than ten times the growth of the population of younger offenders (Uzoaba 1998).

The number of receptions of elderly men to prisons in England and Wales has also increased, but not as fast as the numbers inside prison. In 1998, there were 661 receptions of those aged over 59 in prison, compared to 339 in 1993 (Home Office 2003a). This reflects what criminologists call "punitive bifurcation", whereby those in prison are staying in for longer sentences, while the admission rates are growing less quickly.

Women form only a very small proportion (4.8%) of the prison population (Wahadin 2003) and women over 50 represent only 5% of that total. Over a four-year period from 1996 to 2000, numbers of older female inmates (50+ years) rose by 48% (Wahadin 2003).

Minority ethnic groups are over-represented in the prison population, making up 20–25%. Amongst prisoners, this over-representation of minority ethnic groups is more marked in the elderly population compared with younger adult prisoners: in November 2001, 11% of prisoners over 60 in England and Wales belonged to a minority ethnic group, compared to only 2% of people age 60 or older in the general population (Schuman 1999).

WHAT SORT OF CRIME?

Table 10.2 shows the offence categories that attracted sentences of imprisonment for men of all ages in 1999. The large number of sexual offences among the elderly men is notable. Sexual offences as a proportion of all offences committed by a respective age group greatly increases from young to old (Table 10.3). In prison in England and Wales, about half of the elderly sentenced male prisoners are sexual offenders – a proportion that has been increasing over the last decade. In 1993, 43% of the sentenced male prison population of over-59s in England and Wales were sexual offenders, and this has risen in 2004 to 57% (Home Office 2005). Large numbers of incarcerated elderly sexual offenders are also found in other western countries. In Canada, for example, half of the male sentenced prison population of the over-59s are sexual offenders (Uzoaba 1998).

Older women in prison have a different pattern of offending behaviour. The crimes making up the largest proportion of their offences are: violence against the person (30%); drugs offences (17%); fraud and forgery (15%) and theft and handling (15%) (Wahadin 2003).

DEMOGRAPHIC INFORMATION

Demographic information on sentenced adult prisoners can be found in the large study conducted by the Office for National Statistics (Singleton *et al.*1998). This can be compared with Fazel *et al.*'s (2001b) study of 203 prisoners aged 60 and above. In comparison with younger prisoners from the ONS study (average age 25–29), there were similar rates of employment at the time of the offence (40% in elderly prisoners, 44% in the ONS study). However, elderly prisoners were more likely to have no qualifications (66% *vs.*

Table 10.2 Receptions into prison service establishments of men by age and offence in England and Wales 1999 (Home Office 2000b)

	All ages	21–24	25–29	30–39	40–49	50–59	over 60
All offences	63,635	15,905	17,133	20,596	6,772	2,505	724
Violence against the person	8,926	2,159	2,356	3,126	926	293	66
Sexual offences	2,414	139	282	777	538	402	276
Burglary	7,294	2,517	2,352	2,005	336	71	13
Robbery	1,873	667	546	551	90	16	3
Theft and handling	13,813	3,983	4,099	4,261	1,087	308	75
Fraud and forgery	2,449	285	511	888	458	246	61
Drugs offences	5,932	1,163	1,615	2,127	730	241	56
Other offences	19,842	4,774	5,100	6,516	2,442	861	149
No record	1,092	218	272	345	165	67	25

Table 10.3 Proportion of men imprisoned (remand and sentenced) in England and Wales in 1999 for sexual offences, as a percentage of all offences for each respective age group (Home Office 2000b)

All ages	21–24	25–29	30–39	40–49	50–59	60+
3.79	0.87	1.65	3.77	7.94	16.05	38.12

46%), and to live in rented accommodation prior to detention in custody (64% *vs.* 48%). Elderly prisoners were more likely to be on long-term sickness benefit (14%), but less likely to be unemployed. Although elderly prisoners were more likely to have no qualifications, a higher proportion had attained an A-level or higher degree or to have received vocational training (28%). More elderly prisoners owned their own homes (33%). These differences probably reflect age-related cohort effects.

In comparison with community dwelling elderly persons, elderly prisoners were different in relation to marital status. In a 1997 survey of UK males aged 65 and over, 71% were married (in contrast to 31% in the inmate sample), and 4% were divorced (compared to 42% in the elderly prisoners) (Office for National Statistics 1999). The increased divorce rate in elderly prisoners may be a consequence of imprisonment, and may also be a risk factor for offending. The ONS study did not examine whether younger adult prisoners were divorced, but it found that 18% of sentenced male inmates were living alone.

The 1991 census provides information on other demographic variables, such as employment, social class and educational attainment. The main difference appears to be in relation to social class: elderly prisoners were more often in social class 4 and 5 (32%) compared with elderly persons in the community (13%). Eleven per cent of those aged 65 and over and 59% of those aged 55–64 years were employed in the community, compared with 40% in this sample (average age 65). However, the proportion with no educational or vocational qualifications was similar – 57% in the general elderly population and 66% in elderly prisoners (White et al. 1992).

One of the interesting demographic findings in Fazel et al.'s (2001b) survey is that the rate of homelessness in prisoners prior to custody was negligible. This contrasts with Taylor and Parrott's (1988) investigation of elderly remand prisoners, which found that a third were homeless. This difference may reflect the fact that remand prisoners may be detained for more trivial crimes, such as being drunk and disorderly, which are probably more common in the homeless, and that the latter study was based in London. Homeless persons are also more likely to be remanded in custody than bailed.

In summary, a notable demographic finding is that 40% of elderly prisoners were working at the time of their offence. More elderly prisoners were divorced or single at the time of their offence than community elderly persons. This is probably associated with a lifestyle that puts them at risk of committing crimes.

OVERALL MORBIDITY OF ELDERLY PRISONERS

Elderly prisoners suffer poor physical and mental health. A recent survey (Fazel et al. 2001b) found that 85% of elderly prisoners had at least one or more major illnesses reported in their medical records, and 83% reported at least one chronic illness at interview. The most common illnesses were psychiatric, cardiovascular, musculoskeletal and respiratory (Table 10.4).

PSYCHIATRIC MORBIDITY OF ELDERLY PRISONERS

Fazel et al. (2001a) found that one in three elderly prisoners have a potentially treatable mental illness (see Box 10.1). The main findings of this study were that 32% (95% CI: 26–38%) of sentenced elderly prisoners had a diagnosis of psychiatric illness using a standardised semi-structured diagnostic instrument, and 30% (24–36%) had a diagnosis of personality disorder. In total, 53% (46–60%) of the sample had a psychiatric diagnosis.

This is a higher level of treatable psychiatric morbidity than in surveys of adult prisoners that typically find that one in seven prisoners has a potentially treatable mental illness (Fazel & Danesh 2002).

Table 10.4 Morbidity of elderly prisoners

System	Major illnesses recorded in medical records	Self-reported chronic illnesses	Self-reported chronic illnesses	
	No. elderly prisoners (%)	No. elderly prisoners (%)	% prisoners aged 18–49*	% community elderly aged 65–74**
Psychiatric	92 (45)	18 (9)	NA	1
Cardiovascular	71 (35)	72 (36)	3	29
Musculoskeletal	48 (24)	88 (43)	16	25
Respiratory	31 (15)	43 (21)	15	12
Genito-urinary	26 (13)	34 (17)	1	4
Endocrine	21 (10)	18 (9)	2	9
Gastro-intestinal	21 (10)	32 (16)	5	8
CNS	18 (9)	20 (10)	5	4
Dermatological	12 (6)	16 (8)	3	2
Hearing/ eyesight	12 (6)	30 (15)	4	NA
Haematological	6 (3)	2 (1)	0	1
Other	13 (6)	14 (7)	0	4
No illness	31 (15)	34 (17)	NA	NA

* Bridgwood & Malbon (1995)
** Prior (1998)

The rate of depression reported in this study (30% [23–36%]) was higher than previous studies of younger adult prisoners and community studies of the elderly in the UK (Fazel *et al.* 2001a). A meta-analysis of all prison surveys found a typical rate of 10% of depression in male prisoners (Fazel & Danesh 2002), consistent with another investigation of 95 sentenced male prisoners aged 50–72 that found 10.5% with a major depressive episode (Koenig *et al.* 1995). A community study of 468 men aged 65–69 using the Geriatric Mental Status Schedule (GMS) found 6% had a depressive illness: 4.6% with depressive neurosis, and 1.7% with depressive psychosis (Saunders, Copeland, Dewey *et al.* 1993). The relative risk for depression was calculated to explore the quantitative contribution of some of these factors. In the Fazel *et al.* (2001a) sample, depression was increased in prisoners with a past psychiatric history (relative risk 2.1), and those with poor self-reported

---

Box 10.1 Psychiatric morbidity of elderly prisoners

Diagnoses	No. (%) of prisoners
Psychoses	
Depressive	9 (4)
Other	1 (1)
Total	10 (5)
Neuroses	
Depressive	51 (25)
Hypochondriasis	1 (1)
Total	52 (26)
Organic disorders	
Dementia	2 (1)
DSM-IV personality disorder	
Antisocial personality disorder	17 (8)
Any personality disorder	61 (30)
Total	78 (38)
Current substance abuse/dependence	10 (5)
TOTAL*	108 (53)

* Total is less than the sum of individual disorders because some prisoners had more than one disorder.

---

physical health (relative risk 2.2). The ONS survey of younger adult prisoners found that the risk for neurotic disorders was increased in those who were economically inactive at the time of their offence and in those who had spent less time in prison (Singleton *et al.* 1998). In contrast, Fazel *et al.* (2001a) demonstrated no relationship between paid employment and the length of time spent in prison with depression in elderly prisoners. Surveys of younger prisoners have not explored the association between physical illness and depression. However, a large investigation of GMS elderly depressed individuals in the community (Copeland, Chen, Dewey *et al.* 1999) found that physical illness at the time of interview was predictive of depression (as was being widowed, divorced, or separated).

Alcohol and substance abuse

Alcohol abuse and dependence particularly affects older prisoners. In a UK study of remand prisoners, Taylor and Parrott (1988) reported a steady increase with age in the numbers of prisoners experiencing alcohol withdrawal symptoms; such symptoms were observed in one third of prisoners over 65. A large American study (Arndt, Turvey & Flaum 2002) reported that 71% of older inmates reported a substance misuse problem, and found that compared to younger prisoners, older inmates were more likely to abuse alcohol only. Specific interventions such as educational programmes within prisons may have a long-term effect on alcohol use (Crundall & Deacon 1997) and it may be appropriate to target these towards older prisoners.

Sex offenders

As noted earlier, sex offenders make up almost half of the older prison population. There has been much speculation as to why this should be the case. It has been argued that elderly sex offenders have a long-lasting "Achilles heel" normally held in check by compensatory satisfactions or pressures but liable to re-emerge in times of stress, and that old age, ill health and disability may lead to such impulses manifesting themselves (Fazel & Jacoby 2000). Psychodynamic theories have also been proposed. The need to compensate for a "collapse of narcissism" – the loss of outward symbols of masculinity such as work, physical health, sexual activity – could also help to explain why men with previously unblemished records commit sexual offences in old age (Fazel & Jacoby 2000).

Fazel *et al.* (2002) showed that elderly sex offenders and non sex offenders have similar prevalence rates of mental illness. However, elderly sex offenders have increased schizoid, obsessive-compulsive and avoidant personality traits, supporting the view that sex offending in the elderly is associated more with personality factors than with mental illness or organic brain disease.

SERVICE IMPLICATIONS

Five per cent of the elderly prison population represents a large number of psychotic inmates, consistent with the 4% found in the systematic review of all published prison surveys in adults. If this is extrapolated to the total elderly prison population, then the 5% with psychosis represents around 70 elderly sentenced men who would be psychotic at any one time in 2002 in prisons in England and Wales, almost all with a depressive psychosis. Most psychiatrists would wish to see these individuals transferred to a hospital, whether secure or not, for treatment.

Similarly, around 400 elderly inmates would be suffering from a major clinical depression in English and Welsh prisons in 2002. Most of these individuals can be treated within the prison setting. In the sample interviewed, only 14% of the depressed prisoners were being treated with anti-depressants, demonstrating significant unmet treatment needs (Fazel *et al.* 2004). However, three-quarters of the sample were being prescribed other medication, and elderly prisoners were therefore in regular contact with prison doctors for their physical health needs. These contacts should provide ample opportunity for assessment and treatment of psychiatric illness within the prison setting.

The most concerning aspect of research on elderly prisoners is the large number of untreated and under-treated depressed elderly men in custody. The prison service can respond by making improvements in the identification of depression in the elderly. This could include increased general awareness among all prison staff of the increased risk of depression in the elderly prisoner. Prison officers should be encouraged to refer those elderly prisoners who appear withdrawn, isolated and depressed to the prison medical staff. A similar increased awareness among prison medical staff, and the transfer of commissioning responsibility for prison health services to the National Health Service, should improve the situation (Smith 1999). A screening questionnaire for depression at prison reception for those aged 59 and above may be helpful. The 15-item version of the Geriatric Depression Scale would be well suited to the prison environment, as it is simple to administer, designed for community samples, and only takes a few minutes to complete (Shiekh & Yesavage 1986). Prisoners could be identified at reception, by referral from prison officers, or when seen for physical problems, and referred to a prison medical officer or visiting psychiatrist. Those prisoners with chronic physical problems and a past psychiatric history are at particular risk of depression. In addition, training and recruitment of prison medical staff remain important challenges (Bluglass 1990), and seminars on the special needs of elderly prisoners could be considered for prison health care managers and senior medical officers.

Such educational interventions, though, are not sufficient. The Hampshire Depression Project, a randomised controlled trial of an educational intervention for the detection and treatment of depression in primary care in the UK, did not find that an educational programme based on clinical practice guidelines improved the recognition or outcome of depression in a community setting (Thompson et al. 2000). In contrast, the Seattle group found that a "multi-faceted" intervention in primary care that involved increased intensity and frequency of outpatient follow-up by both primary care physicians and consulting psychiatrists was effective in treating those with major depression (Katon et al. 1995). The evidence, therefore, suggests that prison psychiatrists should collaborate with prison medical officers to target and treat depression effectively in custody. A primary care survey (Fazel et al. 2004) found that only 18% of inmates with recorded psychiatric morbidity were being prescribed psychotropic medication. Even regular review of prisoners' medical records, with a view to aligning medication regimes with identified illnesses, would be a simple but effective intervention.

In the longer term, there may be a need to consider specialised prisons for the elderly. Older prisoners differ from younger inmates not only in their need for medical care, but also in their psychosocial needs (Aday 1994). Older inmates are often unable to cope with the fast pace and noise of a regular facility (Anderson & Morton 1989). They report feeling unsafe and vulnerable to attack by younger inmates, and expressed a preference for rooming with people their own age (Krajick 1979, Walsh 1989, Aday & Rosefield

1992). Vega and Silverman (1988) also reported that abrasive relationships with other inmates occurred daily for 55% of their respondents, and these were highly disturbing and stressful for them. The physical condition and structure of the prison, designed for young, active inmates, can create significant problems for older, frailer inmates, and particularly for those with limited mobility.

Another area of consideration is sentencing policy for the elderly. Much debate has been generated over the policies of successive UK governments and the ineffectiveness of incarcerating persons who pose little risk to the public. According to the US Parole Commission, age is one of the most significant factors that predicts whether an inmate will return to crime in the event that he or she is released. The older the inmate is upon release, the lower the rate of recidivism (Beck & Shipley 1997). It should not be assumed that the detention of the elderly prisoner is necessarily in the best interests of society, and individual and community-based punishments may often be more appropriate.

CHAPTER 11

People with Intellectual Disabilities in Prison

Kiriakos Xenitidis, Maria Fotiadou and Glynis Murphy

TERMINOLOGY AND CLASSIFICATION

Intellectual disabilities

Intellectual disabilities, or learning disabilities (LD), is the term currently used in the United Kingdom to describe a condition of significant impairment of intellectual functioning (originating during the developmental period), associated with significant impairment of adaptive skills and resulting in a reduced overall level of functioning of the individual. Mental retardation is the term used in the two major classification systems of mental disorders, DSM-IV (American Psychiatric Association 1994) and ICD-10 (World Health Organisation 1992). Both classification systems allow for the sub-classification of mental retardation into four categories using intelligence quotient (IQ) as the main, though not the only, criterion. The general population has a mean IQ of 100 (s.d. 15) and intellectual disabilities are considered to be present when IQ is below 70 (i.e. more than 2 s.d. below the mean), provided adaptive behaviour is also significantly impaired. The four sub-categories for intellectual disabilities in ICD-10 are mild (IQ between 50 & 69), moderate (IQ between 35 & 49), severe (IQ between 20 & 34) and profound (IQ<19) mental retardation. Very few people with severe or profound intellectual disabilities ever become involved in the criminal justice system (CJS). However, they may at times show challenging behaviour, such as aggression, which could be considered similar to behaviour classed as criminal, but their cognitive impairments mean that while *actus reus* could be proved, *mens rea* could not.

In defining intellectual disabilities three elements are necessary: the intellectual deficit, the social impairment and the onset early in life. Intelligence has been described as "the aggregate or global capacity of the individual to act purposefully, to think rationally and to deal effectively with the environment" (Wechsler 1944, p.3). Although modern IQ tests provide a quantitative measure of a person's intellectual capacity, the reliance on IQ alone to define learning disability is discouraged. The person's global level of functioning in terms of the degree of acquisition of a number of adaptive skills, as measured by standardised tests, is considered equally important. The consideration of the origin of the impairment during the developmental period (usually regarded as up to the age of 18 years) is essential in distinguishing between intellectual disabilities and cognitive deficits resulting from accidents or a disease process later in life (e.g. head injury or dementia).

Mental health problems

In recent years a consensus has emerged that intellectual disabilities and mental illness are distinct concepts which can co-exist, and that people with intellectual disabilities can develop a wide range of mental health problems (Reiss 1988, 1994) including mental illness (Sovner & Hurley 1983), personality disorders (Reid & Ballinger 1987) and behavioural disorders (Xenitidis, Henry, Russell *et al.* 1999). Moreover, the increased risk of people with intellectual disabilities developing mental health problems, compared to the general population, has been consistently demonstrated (Eaton & Menolascino 1982, Russell 1997).

EPIDEMIOLOGY

Prevalence of intellectual disabilities and mental health problems

There is considerable variation in the findings of epidemiological studies of intellectual disabilities, mainly because of variation in case identification criteria and terminology (Haveman 1996). Moreover, "true prevalence" rates are difficult to obtain because comprehensive surveys based on whole population screening tend to be very resource-intensive. Thus, the majority of studies rely on identification of cases through records of service agencies and estimate the "administrative prevalence" of the condition, ignoring those who are not in contact with services. Clearly, an administrative prevalence approximation to a true prevalence depends on the comprehensiveness of the service, available resources and local arrangements with regards to eligibility criteria for gaining access into the service.

Keeping these limitations in mind, the true prevalence of mild intellectual disabilities is estimated to be 3–4% of the general population, and the true prevalence of moderate to profound intellectual disabilities is estimated to be 3–4 per 1,000 of the general population (McLaren & Bryson 1987). Administrative prevalence figures are much lower, of the order of 1%, particularly in adulthood, as people with mild intellectual disabilities often do not seek services after leaving school (Richardson & Koller 1985). There are reports of increasing prevalence (at least administrative) of intellectual disabilities over the years (McGrother *et al.* 1996) despite prenatal screening and other preventative techniques. This is likely to be partly due to an increase in case recognition and availability of service provision. Other factors may contribute; for example, in the case of Down's syndrome, increase in life expectancy has increased prevalence by more than preventive measures have reduced it. Interesting moral arguments against increasing availability of measures for the prevention of Down's syndrome have been put forward (Gillam 1999) which may influence both true and administrative prevalence rates. A number of factors affect the distribution of intellectual disabilities in a population. Differential mortality rates within the intellectual disabilities population result in fewer people with more severe intellectual disabilities surviving into old age. The distribution of mild intellectual disabilities is strongly skewed in relation to social class, the poorer classes being affected considerably more. At the severe end of intellectual disabilities, most commonly associated with biological abnormalities, the pattern of distribution is much more even in relation to social class.

Corbett's classic epidemiological study in Camberwell in South London showed that 37% of adults with severe and profound intellectual disabilities living at home met the criteria for a psychiatric disorder (Corbett 1979). A similar prevalence rate of 39% was found in an American study in a day centre setting (Reiss 1990). As far as specific psychiatric syndromes are concerned, Crews, Bonaventura & Rowe (1994) studied a sample of people with intellectual disabilities living in a residential setting. They reported total prevalence of 15.55%, with the following prevalences for the major diagnostic categories: schizophrenia 0.63%, affective disorders 8.88%, other psychoses 2.36%, organic mental disorders 55%, anxiety disorders 0.63% and personality disorders 0.86%. However, reports on the prevalence of mental health problems in people with intellectual disabilities generally vary from 14% to more than 80% with a modal prevalence of 45% (Borthwick-Duffy 1994). The main reasons for this wide discrepancy in prevalence rates are the different criteria applied in defining "intellectual disabilities" and "mental health problems", and the diversity of settings and sampling methods used, with very few studies using unselected samples. In addition a number of factors have been identified to account for the difficulties in diagnosing psychiatric disorders in the learning disabled. Sovner (1986) described a number of processes that interfere with accurate psychiatric diagnosis in people with intellectual disabilities. These are:

1. *intellectual distortion*: difficulties in abstract thinking and communication make collecting data relevant for a psychiatric diagnosis problematic

2. *psychosocial masking*: the potential for misdiagnosis due to poverty of "real life experiences" of people with intellectual disabilities

3. *cognitive disintegration*: deterioration of intellectual functioning in response to emotional stress, leading to potential for misdiagnosis due to atypical presentation of symptoms

4. *baseline exaggeration*: increase in severity of pre-existing maladaptive patterns of behaviour due to emotional stress.

The phenomenon of *diagnostic overshadowing* has also been described and refers to the tendency not to make a psychiatric diagnosis, due to attribution of behaviour to the learning disability itself rather than co-existing specific psychopathology (White, Nichols, Cook *et al.* 1995).

Numerous studies have found very high rates of mental health needs in people with intellectual disabilities in the CJS (Day 1988, White & Wood 1988, Murphy *et al.* 1991, Lindsay *et al.* 2002, O'Brien 2002, Lindsay *et al.* 2004b).

OFFENDING BEHAVIOUR IN PEOPLE WITH INTELLECTUAL DISABILITIES

Most prisoners have an IQ that is lower than average (HM Inspectorate of Prisons 2007a) and many have numeracy and literacy problems. However, systematic information on the prevalence of LD in prisons is scarce. Most studies focus on the prevalence of mental disorder in prisoners. IQ therefore is rarely assessed using validated instruments, but may be evaluated indirectly with instruments such as the Mini Mental State Examination or past diagnosis (Faulk 1976) – see Table 11.1. The relevance of offending behaviour in people with intellectual disabilities has been increasingly recognised (Hollins *et al.* 1997a, 1997b).

It used to be thought, especially in the eugenics era, that people with intellectual disabilities were disproportionately responsible for crimes, and a very large number of studies of the association between crime and intellectual disabilities took place, especially in the USA. By 1930, for example, Woodward (1955) commented that there had been over 300 studies. She found that early studies reported much higher percentages of prisoners to have intellectual disabilities than later studies. Similar trends have been reported ever since, and a summary of classic studies in the US and UK is shown in Table 11.1. The variation in figures over the years appears to have been largely due to poor methodology in the early studies (McBrien 2003), including the use of selected samples (e.g. only testing those referred), group tests (instead of individual ones) and literacy tests or quick screening tests (instead of full IQ tests), insensitivity to issues of ethnic origin and language, and a number of other factors.

It appears now that in the USA the true prevalence of intellectual disabilities in prisons is about 3% (i.e. the same as it is in the general population). In other countries it may be higher. In the UK, on the other hand, perhaps as a result of government policy and the increased options of diversion from custody, the prevalence in prison seems to be under 1%, only one study (Singleton *et al.* 1998) finding a higher figure. In the UK it may

Table 11.1 Prevalence of offenders with intellectual disabilities in US & UK prisons

Author & year of study	Location of study	Number of participants	Test(s) used	% of prisoners with LD
Brown & Courtless (1971)	Inmates in USA prisons	90,000 (80% of prison population)	Large variety	9.5%
MacEachron (1979)	Inmates in 2 USA prisons	436 of the 3,938 combined prison population	Variety	1.5%–5.6% (depending on how measured)
Denkowski & Denkowski (1985)	20 prisons in USA*	19,1133	WAIS-R	0.2%–5.3% (state-to-state variations)
Coid (1988)	1 prison in England	Retrospective study, 10,000	None specified	0.34%
Gunn, Maden & Swinton (1991)	UK, 16 prisons, 9 YOIs	404 youths 1,365 men	None specified	0.4%
Murphy, Harnett & Holland (1995)	1 London prison (remand)	157 men	WAIS-R	0% < IQ70 5.7% < IQ75
Birmingham, Mason & Grubin (1996)	1 prison, northern UK (remand)	569 men	None specified	1%
Brooke et al. (1996)	13 Prisons & 3 YOIs in UK	750 youths and men	Quick test	1%
Singleton, Meltzer & Gatward (1998)	1 in 34 of all UK male prisoners; 1 in 8 of all UK male remand prisoners; 1 in 3 UK women prisoners	3,142 prisoners in total – i.e. 1,437 remand & 1,705 sentenced prisoners (2,371 male, 771 female)	Quick test	People with scores in bottom 5% of the population: 5% to 11% of prisoners

* Denkowski & Denkowski also look at IQ scores on group tests in 16 other institutions. These have been omitted.

also be that proportionately more of the people with intellectual disabilities convicted of crimes are given community sentences than prison sentences (compared to the USA). Mason & Murphy (2002a, 2002b), for example, found that 4–6% of people on probation had intellectual disabilities, suggesting that probation may be the preferred form of sentence where people with intellectual disabilities are convicted of crimes (and where probation is legally possible).

A recent systematic review involving ten relevant surveys from four different countries with a total of approximately 12,000 prisoners indicated that typically 0.5–1.5% of prisoners were diagnosed with intellectual disabilities, with a range of 0–2.8% across studies (Fazel *et al.* 2008).

In most jurisdictions, prison is a late stage in the CJS, preceded by questioning at the police station, being charged with a specific crime, appearing in court and, if convicted, sentencing. The prevalence of people with intellectual disabilities at earlier stages of the criminal justice system appears to be higher than it is in prisons, at least in the UK. Two studies have shown that between 5% and 9% of people arrested by the police have a learning disability (see Table 11.2). Several studies in Australia have shown high rates of people with intellectual disabilities in court, while one study in the UK showed a much lower figure (see Table 11.2). There have also been some investigations of the numbers of people on probation in the UK (see Table 11.2). These studies need to be interpreted carefully, particularly in the light of the jurisdiction where the study took place and the types of tests used. Many suffer from similar methodological difficulties to prison studies (McBrien 2003).

Table 11.2 People with intellectual disabilities at other stages of the CJS

Author & year of study	Location of study	Test(s) used	% of prisoners with LD
Gudjonsson *et al.* (1993)	Two South London police stations	Short WAIS-R	9% had an IQ<70 34% had an IQ<75
Lyall *et al.* (1995b)	Cambridge police stations	None (screening questions only)	5% had attended special schools for people with LD; 10% had attended other types of special schools
Hayes (1993)	Two urban and two rural courts, NSW, Australia		14%
Hayes (1996)	Two rural courts in NSW, Australia		21%
French, Brigden & Noble (1995)	Two magistrates courts, Berkshire	Self-report	<2%
Mason & Murphy (2002a)	One area probation service in Kent	Screening questions, VABS & WAIS-R	6%
Mason & Murphy (2002b)	Probation services throughout Kent	Quick test, clock drawing test, VABS	4%

There have been some researchers who have attempted to examine the general propensity of people with intellectual disabilities to commit crimes, as compared to other people, using retrospective studies of large cohorts. For example, Hodgins (1992) examined convictions for a Swedish birth cohort of 15,117 people born in Stockholm in 1953, who were followed up for 30 years. Evidence of LD was taken from registers of the children who were placed in special classes at school because of LD (this included 1.5% of the men and 1.1% of the women). Hodgins reported that the likelihood of conviction for a man with LD was three times higher than for those without disabilities. For women with LD the likelihood was nearly four times higher than for women without disabilities. The odds ratios were even more extreme for violent offences (five times higher for men with LD and 25 times higher for women).

A further study by Hodgins *et al.* (1996) of a total population of over 300,000 people in Denmark, born between 1944 and 1947, followed up at age 43 years, gave similar results: people with LD (excluding those with serious mental illness) who had had admissions to psychiatric wards had an increased risk of committing offences of various kinds compared to people who had never been admitted (risk ratios were 5.5 and 6.9 for women and men respectively, for crimes entered onto the computerised criminal record system which came into operation in Denmark in 1978). There was no particular pattern to the crimes, according to the researchers.

It is difficult to interpret these retrospective cohort figures. They cannot really be considered to throw much light on the question of the relative proportions of people with and without intellectual disabilities who commit crimes, since there are a large number of filters that operate differentially for the two groups, between being labelled as having a learning disability and not being so labelled, and between committing potentially criminal behaviour and entering the various levels of the criminal justice system. For example:

- People who have been labelled as having a learning disability in childhood may be more likely to retain that label if they show antisocial behaviour, whereas people whose behaviour is acceptable may "disappear" from the service system (Richardson & Koller 1985). Thus, administrative samples of adults with LD may be very biased samples of the total population.

- Whether a crime is reported to the police by the victim is very variable. Numerous crimes are under-reported, particularly sexual crimes, as victim surveys demonstrate. Crimes against other people with intellectual disabilities (many of which are committed by perpetrators with intellectual disabilities) are particularly likely to be under-reported by the victims if they have limited verbal skills (Murphy 2007).

- Whether a crime is reported to the police by witnesses who are members of the public is also variable. In the case of criminal behaviour taking place in public, witnesses may be reluctant to report it if the alleged perpetrator is someone with intellectual disabilities.

- A crime may not be reported to the police by staff in services. There is evidence from intellectual disabilities services that staff are reluctant to report to the police potential crimes that occur in the service setting (Lyall, Holland & Collins 1995a, McBrien & Murphy 2007). Reasons include fear of scandal in services and beliefs that the person with intellectual disabilities will not benefit from CJS involvement.

- On the other hand, once informed of a crime, if the perpetrator is not on the spot at the time, the police may be disproportionately likely to find people with intellectual disabilities, since their evasion skills are likely to be limited, compared to non-disabled people.

- Once arrested for questioning, people with intellectual disabilities may be particularly likely to be charged and convicted because of their vulnerabilities in the CJS, including not understanding their rights, being suggestible on interview, having difficulty withstanding cross-examination, and making unwise decisions while in custody (see below for details).

In the UK, some community-based studies have been undertaken focusing on people receiving LD services in particular geographical areas and asking how many show behaviour that has come to the attention of the CJS, regardless of whether they were convicted (Lyall *et al.* 1995a, McNulty, Kissi-Deborah & Newsom-Davies 1995, McBrien, Hodgetts & Gregory 2003). In the largest and most methodologically robust of these, McBrien *et al.* (2003), based in a city with a general population of almost 200,000, examined the numbers of convictions and contacts (as suspects) with the criminal justice service, for all 1,326 adults known to LD services. It transpired that:

- 0.8% of the 1,326 were serving a current sentence

- 3% had a conviction of some kind (current or past)

- a further 7% had had contact with the CJS as a suspect, but without conviction

- an additional 17% had challenging behaviour that was "risky", in the sense that it could have been construed as offending.

This study suggests that about 10% of the people in touch with LD services will have had contact with the CJS at some time in their lives, as suspects. Similarly, Vaughan, Pullen & Kelly (2000), in a study of mentally disordered offenders and community teams in Wessex (total population 1.8 million), found 13% of the people known to LD teams fitted a definition of "mentally disordered offender". (A larger percentage showed challenging behaviour.)

In all probability, these kinds of community-based studies may be more helpful for service planning and less helpful for arguments about the extent to which intellectual disabilities put someone at risk of criminal behaviour. Community-based studies, because they consider only people who are known to services, probably overestimate the true proportion of people with LD at risk of offending, since many adults with mild disabilities who are not at risk of offending lose touch with services when they leave school, and are therefore not counted in the denominator (Richardson & Koller 1985).

PEOPLE WITH INTELLECTUAL DISABILITIES IN THE CRIMINAL JUSTICE SYSTEM

Characteristics and vulnerabilities

Prisoners with LD are commonly male and often have chaotic family backgrounds, a history of physical and/or sexual abuse, unemployment, homelessness, poverty and deprivation. However, such backgrounds are also common features of prisoners without intellectual disabilities, to the extent that MacEachron (1979) could find very little difference between disabled and non-disabled prisoners in her study in Maine and Massachusetts, USA. There was also no significant difference between the two groups in the severity of the most recent offence, the length of current sentence, the degree of recidivism, participation in rehabilitation programmes, recommendations for parole, the degree to which parole had ever been revoked and the use of probation as a juvenile. The only significant distinction found in types of crime was that those with disabilities had fewer violent incidents in prison than the comparison group.

Similar characteristics have been reported regarding people with intellectual disabilities in other parts of the CJS. Thus the background of people with LD who have been involved in the CJS as a suspect or offender is very often characterised by social deprivation and family breakdown or disorder in childhood (e.g. Day 1988, Winter, Holland & Collins 1997, Barron, Hassiotis & Banes 2004), long histories of antisocial or "challenging behaviour" (e.g. Day 1988, Winter *et al.* 1997), high rates of adult unemployment (Murphy *et al.* 1995, Barron, Hassiotis & Banes 2004) and a raised incidence of abuse in their own histories (Lindsay *et al.* 2001, Barron *et al.* 2004, Lindsay *et al.* 2004a). People from ethnic minorities often seem to be over-represented and this may be in part due to the use of tests which may not be culture-fair (Noble & Conley 1992, Hayes 1993, 1996).

Much of the research literature refers to male offenders only. This is partly because relatively few offenders are female, both in the disabled and non-disabled populations. For example, over 90% of violent offences and over 95% of sexual offences are committed by men. Female offenders show educational underachievement and lower than average intelligence scores. In a sample of 1,272 randomly selected female offenders awaiting trial, severe cognitive impairment was found in only five women i.e. in 0.4% of the women (Teplin, Abram & McClelland 1996).

People with intellectual disabilities have a number of vulnerabilities in the CJS. First, when arrested by the police, in most jurisdictions, people have a number of rights.

However, it has been shown in both the UK and the USA that people with intellectual disabilities do not usually understand these rights, for example their (limited) right to remain silent, to have a person informed of their arrest and to consult a lawyer (Clare & Gudjonsson 1993, Fulero & Everington 1995, Clare, Gudjonsson & Harari 1998). They have also been shown to be more suggestible and acquiescent, on average, than people without such disabilities, when questioned (Heal & Sigelman 1995, Finlay & Lyons 2001), and this may make them especially vulnerable, when questioned by the police, to making self-incriminating statements and/or false confessions (Perske 1991, Gudjonsson 1992, Clare and Gudjonsson 1993, Cardone & Dent 1996, Everington & Fulero 1999). This tendency to false confessions may be exacerbated by the fact that many people with LD misunderstand legal terms which are basic to the legal process: Smith (1993), for example, found that about 20% of the people referred for pre-trial competency assessments in South Carolina did not understand the terms "guilty" and "not guilty", to the extent that some actually had the meanings of the terms reversed. Some people with LD may also misunderstand the likely events in the criminal justice process, thinking, for example, that if they make a false confession, even to a serious crime, in the police station, they will still be allowed to go home and will be able to correct their false confession later in court (Clare and Gudjonsson 1995).

In some jurisdictions, in recognition of the difficulties people with intellectual disabilities have in understanding their rights, being interviewed and making decisions in the CJS, provision has been made to try to support them (and other vulnerable adults). For example, in England and Wales, since 1984, people with intellectual disabilities have to have an appropriate adult (AA) with them in the police station when interviewed, and all police interviews with them must be audio-taped. (Similar provisions were also made in Australia (Baroff, Gunn & Hayes 2004).) The AA's role in the police station was to protect vulnerable suspects from their tendency to "provide information which is unreliable, misleading or self-incriminating" (Home Office 1995b, p.403). However, it appeared there were two main problems with the appropriate adult scheme: first, it was difficult for the police to be sure when someone had a learning disability, so that many people who were entitled to an AA were not provided with one (Bean & Nemitz 1994, Medford, Gudjonsson & Pearse 2000); and second, AAs, who could be parents, carers, or social workers, often did not speak during the police interview and seemed unclear about their role (Pearse & Gudjonsson 1996). Clearly for such provision to be effective there needs to be both a training scheme in place for AAs and a system for identifying people with LD when they arrive at the police station. Such information could then usefully follow the suspect through the CJS, to ensure that their vulnerabilities are recognised in court, on probation and/or in prison too.

Specific conditions

AUTISM

Approximately three quarters of people with autism also have intellectual disabilities (Bradley, Summers, Wood *et al.* 2004). The three main characteristics of autism (including Asperger's syndrome) are delayed and abnormal language, social communication impairment and restricted and/or repetitive interests. Some of these characteristics may make people with autism more likely to break the law. For example, they may have difficulty understanding the social basis of laws. They may also have difficulty understanding their own and others' emotions, such that they may have a reduced ability to empathise. As empathic sensibilities may be an inhibitory factor in crimes, especially against a person (but see Joliffe & Farrington (2004) for a review of empathy and offending), autism may make a person more likely to be aggressive. Evidence exists showing that people with autism are more susceptible to displaying challenging behaviour (Murphy *et al.* 2005). In addition, people with autism may be so set on following their restricted interests (such as checking bus timetables) that they may be liable to break the law in ways that people without autism would not understand (for example, hitting bus drivers who run late). On the other hand, the fact that people with autism tend to be dogmatic and inflexible may make them rigidly follow the letter of the law, which could be a protective factor. The relationship between autism and offending is not yet clear, but a number of individuals with autism do commit offences.

ADHD (ATTENTION DEFICIT HYPERACTIVITY DISORDER)

This disorder is characterised by overactivity, impulsivity and poor attention and concentration. It is often associated with behavioural problems on the one hand, and intellectual disabilities on the other. Although it is a condition typically manifested in childhood and tends to disappear by late teenage years, sometimes it persists into adulthood. One of the characteristics of ADHD is poor impulse control, which is a risk factor for offences. Childhood ADHD is linked to childhood conduct disorder, which in turn is associated with adult personality disorder and criminality (Mannuzza *et al.* 1991). ADHD is often missed as a diagnosis in individuals with intellectual disabilities, although symptoms of ADHD are more common in people with intellectual disabilities.

SUBSTANCE MISUSE

The association between crime and substance misuse has been well established, both in the general population and in mentally disordered offenders in particular. Although alcohol and drug misuse are less common in people with intellectual disabilities, in general it is an important variable to keep in mind where offenders with intellectual disabilities are concerned. A recent study showed that over a quarter of offenders with intellectual disabilities had a history of alcohol or illicit drug misuse (Barron *et al.* 2004).

EPILEPSY

People with intellectual disabilities are at higher risk of developing epilepsy compared to the general population. Epilepsy has been linked with offending behaviour on rare occasions. This can happen either as a result of "automatic" behaviour during an epileptic seizure, or before or after a seizure. Some of the impairments associated with organic brain syndrome are also experienced by people with LD. Early starters show a more global, persistent and stable pattern of offending than late starters.

Specific offences

There has been considerable debate about whether people with intellectual disabilities are disproportionately likely to commit particular crimes. Most studies have shown a range of crimes amongst samples of people with intellectual disabilities who are at the police station and/or remanded in prison and/or convicted (see pp.115–116, under Characteristics and vulnerabilities). Nevertheless it is sometimes asserted that they are especially likely to commit arson or sexual offences. Such assertions seem to rest on misinterpretations of data from Walker and McCabe's (1973) English study of people detained under the Mental Health Act in a particular year. They found that a disproportionate number of the sexual offences and arson offences in their sample had been committed by the people in it who had intellectual disabilities. Of course, this does not in any way prove that people with intellectual disabilities are particularly likely to commit sex offences or arson offences because:

- only a minority of all sexual offenders and arsonists are detained under the Mental Health Act (and people with intellectual disabilities may be disproportionately so detained)

- most sexual offences are never reported to the police, so no conclusion can be drawn about who are the likeliest offenders

- most malicious arson is motivated by insurance fraud, something people with intellectual disabilities are very unlikely to be party to (since they generally own very little property and do not normally insure it).

Suffice it to say that most studies show a range of crimes in samples of people with intellectual disabilities in the CJS (MacEachron 1979, Hodgins *et al.* 1996, Glaser & Deane 1999, Barron *et al.* 2004). It is likely that those who commit the most serious crimes are more often to be found in the secure or prison services than in the community, though there is no hard evidence of this and most practitioners would assert that whether people with intellectual disabilities are diverted out of the CJS or not seems to be very arbitrary.

ASSESSMENT OF PEOPLE WITH INTELLECTUAL DISABILITIES IN THE CJS

Assessments of people with intellectual disabilities may be requested at a variety of points in the CJS, for a number of purposes. For example:

- the police may request an assessment of someone they are holding for questioning. This may be very important for suspects, especially as there are a number of provisions (e.g. an AA) that they are entitled to at the police station stage

- if the police charge the person with a crime, his or her solicitor may request an assessment of the person, before he or she appears in court. One of the issues at this stage is whether the person is fit to plead (see below)

- if the person is remanded to prison or to hospital, the court may request an assessment (usually by the local psychiatrist) and advice as to where the person should be sent by the court, if convicted

- finally, there are likely to be assessments needed when the legal process is over, wherever the person is sent, in order to help him or her not to re-offend.

Whenever possible, assessments should be broad and multidisciplinary, and should lead to the development of a person-centred plan, with a view to improving the person's skills. (Realistically this kind of broad assessment is likely to be possible only after the legal process is completed.) The content of the assessment will vary with the purpose, but the following provides a general outline:

1. Determine the presence of learning disability according to the criteria already described.

2. Clarify the survival skills of the individual, in which way they are limited and how they can be improved. The survival skills to be assessed include:

   - orientation (for example, the patient may be intermittently confused because of epilepsy or a coexisting infection)

   - physical independence and mobility

   - daytime occupation

   - education

   - economic self-sufficiency (entitlement to benefits and employment).

3. Consider the presence or absence of mental health needs, including conditions such as autistic spectrum disorder, and substance misuse.

4. Assess fitness to plead, according to the Pritchard criteria (see Box 16.2 on p.179 and see Murphy & Clare (2003) for a review). This is likely to be raised when the person is mute, unresponsive or presents with impairment in communication due to disordered mood, thought process or cognition. As a general rule, a severely handicapped person will probably not meet criteria for fitness to plead.

5. Assess fitness to stand trial. Fitness to stand trial has no legal definition but unfitness arises in physical illness and in situations where the patient suffers or is considered to suffer from an acute mental illness that would normally require inpatient assessment or treatment.

6. Assess the social support system available to the patient in order to define how this can be mobilised to the patient's maximum benefit.

7. If possible, a functional analysis should be completed, so as to understand the links between the person's past history, living environment (at the time of the offence), relationships (and social supports), skills, disabilities and mental health needs, and offending behaviour. Such assessments may take some time (i.e. weeks, rather than hours), as they depend in part on information from the person him/herself but also need to be complemented by information from others. A number of specific offence-related assessment tools exist that can assist with this process – for example, for aggression (Benson & Ivins 1992, Walker & Cheseldine 1997, Taylor *et al.* 2004a), arson (Murphy & Clare 1996, Taylor, Thorne & Slavkin 2004b) and sexually abusive behaviour (Lindsay *et al.* 2004a).

8. In some cases, courts may ask for advice on "disposal". This will include, for example, the possibilities of pre-trial transfer to hospital for assessment under relevant sections of the Mental Health Act 1983 (as amended by the Mental Health Act 2007), contact with the local community team, or a community order with or without a mental health treatment requirement.

A key question in the process of court proceedings is the concept of fitness to plead and stand trial (see Chapter 16, pp.179–180). Fitness to plead requires that the defendant is able to plead (i.e. make a plea of guilty or not guilty), comprehend the proceedings of the court and the evidence, instruct a solicitor, and challenge a juror. Fitness to plead is decided by the court, and solicitors may ask for an assessment by a psychologist or psychiatrist to advise the court. If the defendant is unfit to plead, the court proceeds with a trial of facts, which determines if the defendant committed the offence, but not if he or she is guilty. If the court finds the act was committed, it can make three disposals: a hospital order, a supervision order, or an absolute discharge (see Box 16.3, p.180).

TREATMENT OPTIONS

General issues

In prisons, a limited number of treatment options for prisoners are available by reason of resource availability and staffing. Such treatments need to be modified for prisoners with LD and often special training and expertise is required to deliver them. Treatment may be made available under a legal framework, either in hospital (under the Mental Health Act 1983), in custody (prison-based therapeutic programmes), or in the community (community order with mental health treatment requirement).

Notwithstanding being in prison (or in other parts of the CJS), people with intellectual disabilities should always be asked to give their consent to assessments and treatments. The vast majority of those who become enmeshed in the CJS have only mild disabilities and can understand assessments and treatments, their risks, benefits and alternatives, if these are simply explained (Arscott, Dagman & Kroese 1999).

Specific treatments

DRUG TREATMENTS

Drug treatments should only be used to treat an underlying mental health problem – for example, the treatment of depression in a woman who shoplifts – and only with the person's informed consent. It is important to include systematic assessment of the person's mental state before medication and after it has begun, to ensure that it is helpful, particularly since many psychotropic medications have serious side effects and are rarely well validated for people with intellectual disabilities.

Anti-libidinal medication may be used in the treatment of sex offenders, aiming at a reduction of their sex drive. Such treatment, of course, involves ethical issues, since the medication may lead to side effects, such as feminisation, and consent of the man in question needs to be very carefully sought. It should never be the treatment of first resort but may occasionally be appropriate where other treatments have failed.

PSYCHOLOGICAL TREATMENT FOR OFFENDERS WITH INTELLECTUAL DISABILITIES

Psychological assessment and treatment packages for mentally disordered offenders have been adapted for use with offenders who have a learning disability (Clare & Murphy 1998). Very few of the studies investigating the effectiveness of cognitive-behavioural therapy (CBT) in reducing offending-type behaviour for people with intellectual disabilities, however, have involved control or comparison groups of any kind (Benson, Johnson Rice & Miranti 1986, Lindsay & Smith 1998, Rose, West & Clifford 2000, Taylor *et al.* 2002a, Taylor *et al.* 2002b). Even fewer have involved randomised controlled trials (RCT), as noted by Barron *et al.* (2002), Lindsay (2002) and Taylor (2002), although one small RCT has appeared that examined the effectiveness of anger management training (Willner *et al.* 2002).

Examples of specific CBT packages are given below. Aside from these comprehensive treatment packages, clinical psychologists would also provide other treatment, which would not necessarily be associated directly with a specific offence, but which may reduce the risk of re-offending by treating, for example, underlying depression or anxiety. Furthermore, other skills deficits which are thought to contribute to the likelihood of offending can also be addressed through training packages for social skills and problem-solving skills.

1. Sex offences

Ten years ago, the majority of sex offender treatments for people with intellectual disabilities were behavioural (rather than cognitive-behavioural) and of limited efficacy. Nowadays, cognitive-behavioural therapy programmes are being offered to all sex offenders, including those with intellectual disabilities (see Chapter 13). There may be advantages to group treatment, since peer challenge seems to be an important component in reducing cognitive distortions. (See Lindsay *et al.* (2004a) for a review.) Research studies have suggested that treatment can reduce re-offending (e.g. Lindsay & Smith 1998, Lindsay *et al.* 1998a, 1998b, 1998c) and that following treatment offenders are able to have increased community access (Xenitidis *et al.* 1999). Studies also report a reduction in attitudes consistent with sexual offending and reductions in minimisation and denial of offences (Lindsay & Smith 1998, Lindsay *et al.* 1998a, 1998b, 1998c, Rose *et al.* 2002).

In England and Wales, the main programme offered in prisons is the Adapted Sex Offender Treatment Programme (SOTP). This programme is highly structured and modularised but it does not run in every prison. It is Home Office funded and accredited, but as yet no data on its effectiveness have been published. In the community, a variety of other similar programmes run, such as that provided by Lindsay's group in Scotland, which has been well evaluated (Lindsay *et al.* 1998a, 1998b, 1998c), and the Sex Offender Treatment Services Collaborative programme, SOTSEC-ID, which has also shown positive results (Murphy *et al.* 2004).

2. Arson

CBT for arson may also be administered in an individual or group setting. Treatment components include functional analysis of fire-setting, education about the dangers of fire, interpersonal skills (social skills, assertiveness), emotion recognition and management (e.g. anger management), and relapse prevention. There is a dearth of studies regarding the outcome of treatment for adult arson offenders with intellectual disabilities. A recent study found that following group treatment for fire-setting, offenders showed a small reduction in fire interest and attitudes associated with fire-setting, improved anger disposition and increases in self-esteem (Taylor *et al.* 2002a).

3. Anger and aggression

Behavioural approaches, without cognitive components, used to be the only available treatment for people with intellectual disabilities and aggressive behaviour. These methods have demonstrated good outcome in terms of a reduction of aggression (Whitaker 2001), but once the intervention ceases, there is a strong likelihood that the aggression will reappear, since behavioural approaches do not focus on helping individuals to self-regulate behaviour. Individual or group cognitive-behavioural treatments for anger and aggression are therefore likely to be more effective, provided the person is motivated to change his or her behaviour. CBT for anger and aggression tends to include training in the recognition of emotions, arousal reduction, cognitive-restructuring and self-instruction, problem-solving and stress-inoculation. Individual case studies of cognitive-behavioural treatment for anger with individuals with intellectual disabilities and seriously aggressive behaviour have shown good outcome in terms of reduction of aggression (Murphy & Clare 1991, Black & Novaco 1993), and a number of studies have now demonstrated that group anger management training is effective in reducing self-rated anger (Benson *et al.* 1986, Rose *et al.* 2000, Whitaker 2001, Taylor *et al.* 2002b, Willner *et al.* 2002, Taylor *et al.* 2004a).

Risk assessment and risk management

As Halstead (1997) and Johnston (2002) have commented, many services for people with LD only employ structured clinical judgements of risk. While this method of risk assessment may have some face validity, there have been criticisms that such methods are not as good as actuarial methods in predicting risk, at least in the non-disabled population (Grove 2000, Monahan 2002).

For non-disabled offenders, risk is increasingly predicted using measures that combine actuarial historical variables (such as age, gender, numbers of previous offences) with clinical variables (such as diagnoses, psychopathy scores). A number of large-scale studies have found that these instruments do predict risk well and that the instruments often do not differ systematically in their predictive ability for non-disabled offenders (Sjostedt & Langstrom 2002, Harris *et al.* 2003). Nevertheless, research into the use of these instruments is only just beginning in relation to people with LD at risk of offending (Lindsay & Beail 2004): for example, Harris & Tough (2004) have found that the Rapid Risk Assessment of Sexual Offence Recidivism did predict sexual offending amongst men with LD and sexually abusive behaviour, while Quinsey *et al.* (1998) reported that the Violence Risk Appraisal Guide was a good predictor of violent and sexual behaviours in people with LD transferred from institutions to community settings. However, McMillan, Hastings & Coldwell (2004) noted that clinical prediction was as good as actuarial prediction of violent incidents within a forensic institution.

Increasingly, there have been attempts to improve prediction of re-offending by non-disabled offenders, by including dynamic factors (such as mood) in the risk measure, to supplement the normally static actuarial and clinical factors. Attempts to do this for people with LD are just beginning (Boer, Tough & Haaven 2004), and some measures have shown some initial success. Lindsay *et al.* (2004a), for example, have developed a measure called Dynamic Risk Assessment and Management System (DRAMS), which is showing promise as a predictor of aggressive incidents in residential settings.

CONCLUSION

People with intellectual disabilities are sometimes at risk of offending. The ethics of imprisoning people with intellectual disabilities has been questioned. The issues of mental capacity and moral responsibility have been raised, most dramatically in the case of the execution of people with intellectual disabilities in countries with capital punishment.

The response of staff and the CJS to offending behaviour, as exhibited by adults with intellectual disabilities, is variable and often arbitrary. Such behaviour is sometimes disregarded, although at other times people with intellectual disabilities may find themselves involved in the CJS, including prison. Once there, they may not understand their rights and may be significantly disadvantaged, owing to a number of factors outlined in this chapter. There is a need for increasing awareness and identification of intellectual disabilities and associated conditions within populations of suspects and offenders in a variety of settings. Then structures need to be in place for the appropriate treatment options to be made available to them, in order to prevent further offending.

CHAPTER 12

Black and Minority Ethnic Prisoners

David Ndegwa and Dominic Johnson

This chapter looks at the representation of black and minority ethnic persons in the UK prison system, and the prevalence of mental disorders in this group. It also looks at the current government response to identifying people with mental health problems within prison and managing them either within prison or outside prisons, set within the context of the government's "Delivering Race Equality" programme, which seeks to reduce ethnic disparities in the prison population. From a review of current literature, research priorities are highlighted. Suggestions for interventions that might reduce the number of persons who are vulnerable to entry into the criminal justice system are made.

EPIDEMIOLOGY

Despite the absence of evidence that offending patterns differ among ethnic groups, people of black and mixed race backgrounds are more likely to be stopped and searched, arrested, remanded without bail and imprisoned than their white counterparts (Reza & McGill 2006). The total black and minority ethnic (BME) population in prisons is 25% (Prison Reform Trust 2006, 2007). However, the total national population (i.e. BME prisoners who are British nationals) is 17%. Of that group, 10% are black, and 4% Asian (compared to community norms of 2.8% and 4% respectively). Ethnicity recording in the prisons is patchy (HM Inspectorate of Prisons 2007b), making it difficult to generate evidence-based policy for these groups. The BME national group seem to be generally similar to their white counterparts, in terms of age, socio-economic class and offence type; they are over-represented among robbery and fraud offences and under-represented among drug and sexual offenders (Home Office 2006a).

IMPLICATIONS

Overall, there is over-representation of the BME population (mainly persons of African and African-Caribbean descent) in prisons, compared to the general population. However, in general, these are are not migrants but British-born second- or third-generation descendants of migrants. The over-representation of black people at every stage of the criminal justice process, despite the absence of any convincing evidence that there are significant differences in offending between groups, suggests that covert and structural racism may be operating in the criminal justice systems. There is an over-representation of BME groups among those serving long sentences, which includes foreign national females serving prison sentences for drug-related offences and men sentenced to the new, indefinite public protection orders because of the nature, seriousness and repeat history of their offending. What is less widely publicised is that BME groups are also over-represented among victims of crime (Sharp & Budd 2005).

PSYCHIATRIC MORBIDITY

The Office for National Statistics' (ONS) study of psychiatric morbidity in remand and sentenced prisoners in England found no statistically significantly differences in the prevalence of psychosis or antisocial personality disorder between black and white men and women (Singleton *et al.* 1998). No relationship was apparent between the prevalence of neurotic symptoms and ethnicity.

A more recent review of mental health needs in prisons by HM Inspectorate of Prisons (2007a) suggests that there is little difference in the level of mental distress between BME nationals and white nationals. BME nationals were less well known to mental health services prior to imprisonment and were less often referred to substance misuse services or mental health inreach within prison. Of particular concern is that young offenders are twice as likely to be black or of mixed race, compared to white, but they receive less mental health input.

MENTALLY DISORDERED OFFENDERS FROM BME GROUPS

As a result of improvements in the identification in prison of prisoners with mental illness, and their early diversion to the NHS, there was a major increase in the numbers of people, both black and white, admitted from prison to secure units from 2002 to 2006 (see Figure 5.2). This increase in numbers displaced from prison to hospital, as would be expected, also led to an increase in the number of black people who were detained in hospital. Prior to that, large numbers of mentally ill black people were to be found particularly in the remand prison population.

There was a change also in the type of section which was used to divert such persons. Most people were diverted using Home Office Transfer Warrants (Sections 47 and

48 of the Mental Health Act 1983). These prisoner-patients were largely all also subject to Restriction Orders (under Section 49 of the Mental Health Act 1983).

Diversion schemes set up to divert mentally disordered offenders from the criminal justice system have not been particularly sensitive to the needs of BME arrestees and re-mandees. The focus has been on those who are obviously mentally ill or already known to services – which may not apply to BME offenders. Diversion is usually to hospital inpatient services rather than community services (outpatients, assertive outreach services or home treatment services).

It is well established that BME groups are over-represented among patients admitted to secure units, and at every stage of the formal psychiatric detention process (Cope 1990, Cope & Ndegwa 1990, Morgan *et al.* 2004). Concerns about the sensitivity of mental health services to the needs of BME patients, and the perpetuation of perjorative ethnic stereotypes by mental health professionals, have been raised by published inquiries into the deaths of Orville Blackwood (Special Hospitals Service Authority 1993), Daksha Emson (North East London Strategic Health Authority 2003) and David Bennett (Norfolk, Suffolk and Cambridgeshire Strategic Health Authority 2003).

PERSONALITY DISORDER, RISK AND ETHNICITY

A review of mentally disordered offenders in 1994 raised the question of the relative absence of personality disorder diagnoses in black mentally disordered offenders (Reed, DoH & Home Office 1994). In 1999 the British government published proposals for managing people whose severe personality disorder caused them to be dangerous to others. In 2000 the dangerous and severe personality disorder (DSPD) (see Chapter 19) programme was established jointly between the then Home Office and the Department of Health, and by 2004 an additional 140 new secure places and 75 specialist rehabilitation hostel places were to be provided for this group.

The number of black and ethnic minority patients admitted to these programmes is currently very small, particularly in the high secure estate (maximum secure hospitals and prisons). The numbers in medium security are increasing; in particular in those pilot services where persons with co-morbid mental illness are admitted. In an unpublished review within South London & Maudsley NHS services, looking at those persons currently within the prison service who would meet the criteria for admission to inpatient medium secure services, specialist hostel accommodation or specialist community personality disorder service, from two inner city areas with high psychiatric morbidity and risk of violent crime, it was found that out of about 800 prisoners examined, about 50% were black, and met the admission criteria. These prisoners had been identified from the case records held by the Prolific Offender Team, the Public Protection Team and the Resettlement Team. These were offenders where case note information indicated they had a severe personality disorder which was linked to their risk of serious violence.

BME FOREIGN NATIONALS IN UK PRISONS

There is increasing concern about the proportion of foreign BME nationals in the prison system. Between 1997 and 2007 there has been a 152% increase in the number of foreign nationals, half of whom come from just six countries: Jamaica, Nigeria, Pakistan, India, Turkey and the Republic of Ireland (Prison Reform Trust 2007). They are over-represented amongst drug-related offenders. Twenty per cent of female prisoners are foreign nationals, most of whom have been convicted of drug trafficking.

It may be useful to compare evidence from international studies of the prevalence of mental disorder in prisons. Two studies of Nigerian prisoners suggest that they have high levels of mental illness, but low levels of substance misuse and personality disorder, compared to developed countries (Adesanya *et al.* 1997, Agbahowe *et al.* 1998). The authors postulate that this difference is related to the cost and difficulty of obtaining heroin and cocaine in Nigeria at the time of the study. A further Nigerian study found high rates of mental health problems in prisoners, though the majority of the sample reported no history of mental illness prior to their incarceration. The study identified a significant association between cases of mental illness and awaiting trial, and reports of poor prison accommodation (Fatoye *et al.* 2006). None of these studies raises the issue of self-harm.

In terms of specific offences, Mafullul, Ogunlesi & Sijuwola (2001) studied 118 homicide offenders. There was evidence of a psychotic motive in 9% of the sample referred for pre-trial psychiatric assessment. However, 25 offenders had had contact with traditional healers for treatment of psychiatric disorders, 13 of whom may have had psychotic motives in the offence. As in industrialised countries, a significant proportion of the sample were intoxicated with alcohol at the time of the offence. A recent Kenyan study looked at psychiatric morbidity in convicted male sex offenders (Kanyanya, Othieno & Ndetei 2007). This study highlighted high rates of substance misuse and personality disorder and low rates of mental illness amongst sex offenders, similar to findings from European nations (Fazel *et al.* 2007).

SERVICE PROVISION IN DEVELOPING NATIONS

Information on this area is scarce. One study described how one doctor provided outpatient clinics for a prison housing some 608 inmates. The facility had occasional visits from a local psychiatric hospital for disturbed inmates (Agbahowe *et al.* 1998). One prison was reported to have a staffed health clinic, but access to medication was dependent on relatives procuring it, as clinic supplies were chronically short. This study also highlighted poor accommodation and food, factors which correlated with poorer mental health (Fatoye *et al.* 2006). All studies report large numbers of prisoners on remand awaiting trial.

WHAT IS NEEDED?

In January 2005 the Department of Health (2005a) published *Delivering Race Equality in Mental Health Care* (DRE). It is a five-year action plan for tackling discrimination in the NHS and local authority mental health services. The DRE programme, if successful, hopes that by 2010 there will be a reduction in the ethnic disparities found in prison populations. This is an ambitious objective in the sense that it aims to reduce the number of prisoners from ethnic minorities in prison at the same time as reducing the number of those with mental health problems within prison. The main objective relevant to prisons in the programme is going to be difficult to achieve, and in particular it will be difficult to demonstrate that any moves towards that objective are attributable to the existence of the DRE programme, and not changes that would have happened anyway as a result of other government initiatives.

What is needed is first and foremost to reduce the number of black people who offend. There is also a need to reduce the number who are sentenced to prison terms and who receive indeterminate sentences, and the number of those who re-offend after release. The Commission for Racial Equality (1999) suggests that reduction of the BME prison population will require the country to address the under-achievement of BMEs in the poor schools they attend, to reduce inequalities like discrimination in the workplace, reduce the use of the stereotypes of dangerousness, and address poverty. The problems of black people who are caught up in the criminal justice system often begin from childhood. In order to understand and prevent the movement from normal childhood (at home and school) to the criminal justice system, a detailed examination of parenting and school experiences is required. The following is an attempt to illustrate the sort of questions that one needs to ask in the light of the poor outcomes that black children, particularly boys, have in schools.

- What interventions exist in primary and secondary schools to reduce school exclusion?

- What is happening to the BME children who are excluded from school?

- How many of them get back to mainstream normal schools?

- How many of them go to other "specialist" facilities and what outcomes do they have?

- What interventions exist in secondary schools to improve the performance of BMEs (particularly children of African/African Caribbean and Bangladeshi descent)?

- What remedial services exist for those who do not do well in GCSE exams and want to repeat or continue with further education to improve their performance at these crucial gate-keeping exams?

- What interventions exist to address the needs of BME individuals with special needs, where the families are unhappy with what is on offer in state education?

- For each of the above, how many BMEs would benefit from any good evidence-based interventions but are not currently benefiting?

To understand the experience of black men in the work environment, the following questions would need to be addressed.

- What interventions exist to remove discrimination in the workplace, at all stages of the process, including adverts, shortlisting, interview, induction, training, experience and promotion?

- What evidence is there that the paper policies mean anything on the ground?

- If BMEs do not have the necessary skills, e.g. to enter into the professions, what interventions exist for addressing the education and skills deficits so as to make them attractive to employers?

- What interventions exist to assist those who do not want employment but want to be self-employed, e.g. set up their own businesses?

The state is a major parent of black children and the outcomes of this parenting are poor. To understand this phenomenon, the following questions would need to be addressed.

- What interventions exist to assist the particular group of looked after children?

- BMEs are over-represented in this vulnerable group. How good is the parenting these children receive from the state? Are the cut-offs for intervention at age 16–18 appropriate, given the vulnerabilities of the children?

- How good is the education these children receive?

- Is the state a reliable parent that is there beyond their teen years? (Most non-looked-after young adults maintain contact with family/parents beyond their 20s, and they continue to receive guidance, emotional and sometimes financial support from family and parents in their 20s and 30s.)

- What happens to children who have frequent changes of carers, and/or end up in secure establishments run by the child care system because they are difficult to manage?

RESEARCH

There is an urgent need to take a more culturally competent approach to research. It is now well established that an early history of any childhood conduct disorder and/or child maltreatment increases the risk of adolescent offending and later adult offending; but how has this been applied in practice to BME groups? Like their white counterparts, black offenders often have childhood histories of antisocial conduct. Black children are over-represented among children diagnosed with conduct disorder (Meltzer *et al.* 2000), however black prisoners are more likely to have a history of adolescent-onset conduct disorder, which is usually associated with social rather than family factors (McCabe *et al.* 2001, Coid *et al.* 2002). It would be helpful to study the delinquency trajectories in BME and white youth.

Similarly, although substance misuse is common generally in offender populations, black people are over-represented in those who use illicit drugs, particularly cannabis and crack cocaine. Cannabis is associated with early onset of psychosis in those who are vulnerable, and may explain the large numbers of black people who develop psychosis (Arsenault 2004, Arendt *et al.* 2005). Cannabis and crack cocaine use are associated with poor response to medical treatment for psychosis, and with poor engagement, discontinuation of treatment and relapse in those who have developed psychosis already (Kessler *et al.* 1996). Cannabis use is associated with conduct disorder, and illicit drug use generally is associated with an increased risk of violence. Understanding illicit drug use in different parts of the BME community might assist in prevention of offending and reconviction.

There are now interventions which can reduce the incidence of childhood disorders associated with the later development of delinquency and antisocial behaviour, including offending (Scott *et al.* 2001, Scott 2002, Matthew & Scott 2005, Olds 2006). However, such interventions have not been offered to BME groups; nor has their acceptability been explored, despite there being good theoretical evidence that such interventions can reduce antisocial behaviours in the mentally ill and change the nature and frequency of contact with psychiatric services and criminal justice systems after the first episode of psychosis (Hodgins & Müller-Isberner 2004).

There are also a number of interventions offered in prison that address offending behaviour in prisons. However, there is a lack of data about the uptake by prisoners from BME groups. Better ethnicity data recording might make it more obvious where interventions are not being offered. This is a particular issue given the levels of reconviction in BME groups.

Research should focus on areas identified in the expert paper commissioned by the NHS Research and Development Programme in Forensic Mental Health (Ndegwa 2003), i.e. in particular understanding the genesis of those offences prevalent in BME groups (e.g. black-on-black violence, robbery, assaults, drug offences). Issues that may explain the vulnerabilities of BMEs to engagement in particular criminal activity, e.g. identity, drug use, lifestyle, self-esteem, family dynamics – themes developed in America in social sciences and psychology literature – could greatly assist this exploration.

CHAPTER 13

Sex Offenders and Vulnerable Prisoners

Rebecca Milner

INTRODUCTION

The current male sentenced prison population in England and Wales is 63,683 (Ministry of Justice 2008c). Of these, 7,739 are men sentenced for one or more sexual offences (12.2%). There are currently 3,247 female sentenced prisoners in HM Prison Service, and 47 of these women are convicted of one or more sexual offences (1.4%).

HOUSING SEX OFFENDERS AND OTHER VULNERABLE PRISONERS

Male prisoners

Sex offenders and other vulnerable prisoners are often housed in prison under Prison Rule 45 Own Protection (49 for Young Offenders). There are two parts to this rule, Good Order (to maintain the good order or discipline of the establishment, GOOD) and Own Protection (segregation for own protection, OP). Prison service guidance (PSO 1700) on this rule states:

> Governors must ensure that the restrictions on prisoners segregated under Prison Rule 45 (YOI 49) are no more than necessary to protect the prisoner concerned or to maintain the good order and discipline of the establishment.

Prisoners under Rule 45 OP are usually housed in a segregation unit or a vulnerable prisoners unit (VPU). Prisoners in a VPU will associate, exercise and work together, whereas those held in a segregation unit will only associate together on exercise. Very high profile or volatile prisoners will exercise on their own. The regime for segregated prisoners (under Prison Rule 45 (YOI 49)) should be as full as possible, and only those activities that involve associating with mainstream prisoners should be curtailed. Certain regime elements, e.g. TV, radio, CD player, association within the segregation unit, PE, gym access, can be used as incentives/rewards for prisoners that comply with the targets set by the Segregation Review Boards.

Prisoners placed on Rule 45 OP can be sexual offenders, but include other vulnerable prisoners such as those who are being bullied, are in debt, high profile cases, or those who cannot cope with life on a main residential wing.

At most local prisons and lower category prisons (e.g. Category C), prisoners can apply to go on Rule 45 OP when they are received into reception. This would normally be in consultation with the duty governor. A prisoner can be initially segregated for 72 hours by the authority of a governor. After the initial 72 hours a review board is held to decide whether to segregate further. If the prisoner is to be held on continued segregation, a Rule 45 GOOD Board has to be held every 14 days with a medical officer present. In a local prison a sex offender will not routinely be placed on Rule 45 OP and segregated, if he feels secure and comfortable living on the main residential wings. If, however, at any point in his sentence he feels vulnerable and wishes to be segregated for his own protection, he can make that choice and be segregated. This application can be made via a request/complaint form or wing application form. Alternatively the prisoner can express his concerns to his personal officer, or indeed any member of staff, who can then take it forward. The process is the same for any vulnerable prisoner.

At other prisons, including the high security estate, the emphasis is on integrating sex offenders onto the main residential wings rather than segregating them. This is particularly the case in prisons that house many sex offenders. There is no time limit on being segregated. In general (and where possible) prisoners will be encouraged to return to normal location. If this is not possible, then every effort is made to move them to another prison.

Women prisoners

Women prisoners can also request Rule 45 Own Protection, and the same guidance applies as for men. Female sexual offenders apply for Rule 45, along with women who have harmed children, or who see themselves as vulnerable. Due to the small number of female sexual offenders, and generally the small numbers of women in prison, women's prisons do not have separate wings or units purely for this use. Women who apply for Rule 45 OP may spend a short time in the segregation unit. The policy is that they are supported to reintegrate with the rest of the prison as soon as possible. If this is not possible, then they will be transferred out to another prison with the intention that they be re-housed on normal location there. Notorious female offenders who may be vulnerable may also be housed in health care centres, which tend to be small and supportive units. Again, the policy is that they reintegrate onto the main prison wings as soon as possible, and are supported in doing so.

Interventions for sex offenders

Following a number of serious prison riots in which vulnerable prisoners and sexual offenders were targeted, the Woolf Report (Home Office 1991a) and the Criminal Justice Act 1991 made specific recommendations about the management and treatment of male incarcerated sexual offenders. The Core Sex Offender Treatment Programme (SOTP) was designed and developed, based on research evidence regarding treatment efficacy with male sexual offenders, and was introduced nationally in 1992. This has now been expanded and consists of a group of six sex offender programmes. The SOTP programmes are based on a cognitive behavioural approach, known to be the most effective for treating sexual offenders (Hall 1995, Lösel & Schmucker 2005). SOTP is modelled on the risk–need–responsivity principles (Andrews & Bonta 1998). Initially outlined for general offending behaviour programmes, these state that treatment should match risk, focus on (criminogenic) needs and be responsive to offenders' learning needs. The programme is supported by a long-term evaluation strategy, and results of the first evaluations are reported within this chapter.

In 2008 the HM Prison Service merged with the National Probation Directorate to become the National Offender Management Service (NOMS). The aim is to streamline sentences, managing assessment, treatment and aftercare from sentencing, through prison and back into the community. A central team, the Interventions and Substance Misuse Group, provides support to approximately 25 sites delivering the SOTP programme to convicted male sexual offenders, and three community male sex offender programmes spread across three geographical areas in England and Wales. The long-term vision is to provide effective, continuous treatment for men convicted of sexual offences.

DYNAMIC RISK FACTORS

1. Offence-related sexual interests

Hanson & Morton-Bourgon (2005) found that "any deviant sexual interest" and "sexual preoccupations" were both major predictors of sexual recidivism (see also Hanson & Harris 2000). Ward & Siegert (2002) theorised that offence-related sexual interests are a result of a combination of the problems in the other three domains. In essence, sexual self-regulation difficulties are a result of distorted sexual scripts interacting with dysfunctional relationship schemas. Men may have experienced sexual abuse as children, leading to premature sexualisation, and believe that intimacy can only be achieved by sexual contact (Marshall, Anderson & Fernandez 1999).

2. Underlying distorted thinking patterns

Hanson & Morton-Bourgon (2005) found that the general category of sexual attitudes was significantly related to sexual recidivism, but the effect was small. Some propose that sexual offender treatment should focus on addressing offence-supportive attitudes such as the belief that children enjoy sex and are unharmed by it (Ward & Keenan 1999, Mann et al. 2007). Other key areas of offence-supportive cognition to be addressed in treatment include entitlement thinking (Hanson, Gizzarelli & Scott 1994), hostile grievance thinking (Mann & Hollin 2007) and suspiciousness of women (Malamuth & Brown 1994).

3. Intimacy skills/interpersonal functioning

Sexual offenders are often deficient in the skills required to develop and maintain successful adult relationships (Cortoni & Marshall 2001). Hanson & Morton-Bourgon (2005) found that the general category of intimacy deficits showed a small but significant relationship to sexual recidivism. There is a link between emotional loneliness and sexual offending (Seidman et al. 1994), and unskilled attempts to rectify this could result in sexual offending. Attachment styles of sexual offenders have been widely researched, with sexual offenders typically showing insecure attachment styles (Smallbone & Dadds 1998). Low self-esteem is a core issue in insecure attachment. Some meta-analytic studies (Hanson & Bussière 1996, Hanson & Morton-Bourgon 2005) have found no relationship between low self-esteem and recidivism risk, whereas some recent individual studies have found a link (Thornton, Beech & Marshall 2004, Webster et al. 2007).

4. Self/emotional regulation

Poor self-regulation is a fundamental issue for general criminality, and has also been found to be relevant in sexual offenders (e.g. Polaschek et al. 2001). Thornton (2002) divided self-regulation problems into three areas: lifestyle impulsiveness, poor problem-solving and a lack of emotional regulation. Hanson & Morton-Bourgon (2005) found general self-regulation problems to be a major predictor of sexual recidivism. Whilst research does not link chronic emotional difficulties or mood disorder with increased risk of sexual offending (e.g. Hanson & Bussière 1998), some studies have identified acute, negative emotional states as a precursor to sexual offending or offence-related sexual fantasy (McKibben, Proulx & Lusignan 1994).

To be successful a treatment programme, or family of programmes, would need to be broad enough to address each domain, and also be specific enough to modify these driving mechanisms and assist with the acquisition of functional alternatives (Beech & Ward 2004). In addition, group work must be responsive to the needs of its participants. The SOTP family of programmes has developed over the years to include programmes and modules to cover each of these four research-based domains. It has also considered responsivity and provides programmes for those who have particular learning needs.

THE SEX OFFENDER TREATMENT PROGRAMME (SOTP)

The SOTP consists of five group work programmes – the Core, Extended, Adapted, Rolling, and Better Lives Booster – and one individual programme, the Healthy Sexual Functioning programme. All the programmes use methods such as discussion, role-play and skills practice to help offenders understand and change their thinking, develop new skills and prepare for an offence-free and personally fulfilling life. The Healthy Sexual Functioning programme also uses behaviour modification strategies to help men manage offence-related sexual fantasy.

Core

The Core programme is for medium to high risk sexual offenders. The programme is designed to help offenders:

- develop an understanding of how and why sexual offences were committed

- learn about patterns in sexual offending

- understand and rethink any excuses used to justify offending

- collaboratively identify their treatment needs

- undertake exercises which help to outline the victim's perspective

- develop personally satisfying and meaningful life goals that are inconsistent with sexual offending, and lead the individual to live a more fulfilling life without sexually offending.

Extended

The Extended programme is for high and very high risk offenders who have met the treatment targets of the Core programme. The programme targets socio-affective functioning, specifically distorted thinking (schemas), poor emotional regulation and intimacy skills. There is also a focus on relapse prevention.

Adapted

This is the equivalent of the Core programme and is available for sexual offenders who might learn less quickly than others or who might have difficulty with the language or literacy requirements of the Core programme. The programme tends to use more active learning methods, using pictures and symbols rather than words. It is designed to increase sexual knowledge, modify offence-justifying thinking, develop ability to recognise feelings in self and others, to gain an understanding of victim harm, and develop relapse prevention skills.

Rolling

The Rolling programme is for low and medium risk sexual offenders and also provides treatment for men who have committed internet sexual offences. It is a continuously running course, with offenders leaving when they are judged to have met the targets that are personally relevant for them. Treatment areas covered are similar to those of the Core programme, but with a focus on relationship skills and attachment deficits.

Better Lives Booster

The SOTP Better Lives Booster programme is for sexual offenders who have met the treatment targets of one or more of the initial SOTP programmes, including Core, Extended or Adapted programmes. The aim of the programme is to refresh, maintain and enhance learning from these primary programmes. Outstanding individual treatment needs are targeted and the ethos of the programme is based on the Good Lives Model (Ward & Gannon 2006), ensuring a focus on offenders' planning for offence-free and personally fulfilling lives. There are adapted versions of the programme available, and a version of the programme is being rolled out in the community.

THE HEALTHY SEXUAL FUNCTIONING (HSF) PROGRAMME

The best predictor of sexual recidivism is a deviant sexual interest (Hanson & Bussière 1998, Hanson & Morton 2003), and so treatment in this area is essential. The HSF programme is for men who are currently experiencing offence-related fantasy and is delivered on an individual basis. The treatment goals are to:

- modify distorted attitudes that are supportive of sexual interests
- manage the antecedents to offence-related fantasy and promote triggers to healthy sexual interests
- reduce offence-related interest by removing positive consequences and introducing aversive ones
- promote healthy sexual interest by reinforcing healthy fantasies
- develop skills to manage offence-related sexual interests.

Sexual offenders may undertake one or more of these programmes in prison before being released into the community, where they may do top-up work or attend a Booster programme. The treatment pathway for sexual offenders in prison is determined by a tool known as the Structured Assessment of Risk and Need (SARN).

STRUCTURED ASSESSMENT OF RISK AND NEED (SARN)

SARN assesses risk and need in male sexual offenders. It involves both actuarial prediction of risk, based on historical factors, and empirically guided clinical judgement. It seeks to identify the long-term psychological risk factors or treatment needs relevant to an individual sexual offender. It determines allocation to treatment as well as collaborative treatment planning and evaluation of progress and risk.

The first stage involves a static risk assessment using an algorithm known as Risk Matrix 2000 (Thornton *et al.* 2003). Static risk algorithms are widely used for assessing risk of recidivism in criminal populations and the Risk Matrix 2000 is the most applicable to British sex offenders, and is used by the police and in the community as well as by the Prison Service. It has been validated for use in England and Wales (Craig, Beech & Browne 2006) and Scotland (Grubin 2008). Work is currently under way to conduct further validation of the Risk Matrix 2000 using HM Prison Service data.

The second stage involves an assessment of dynamic risk factors, also known as treatment needs (Treatment Need Analysis). In this stage 15 factors known to be relevant to risk of sexual recidivism are examined to see which are relevant to a given offender. These factors are introduced into first stage treatment during the Core programme, and collaborative working between facilitators, supervisor and offender assesses the presence or absence of needs. Further examination of case records, psychometric testing, interview data and information from previous programmes is made by the (nationally trained) writer of the report, and the information is drawn together in a process of structured clinical judgement. The results of this assessment are used to set treatment targets for the individual offender and these are worked on during the SOTP.

The 15 dynamic risk factors have a research base in the literature and are divided into the four domains already discussed above: sexual interests, distorted attitudes, relationship management and self-management (Table 13.1).

The third stage of the SARN is a risk report. This report reviews the four domains and comments on any progress the offender has made in addressing his individual treatment needs and risk factors. It incorporates information from pre- and post-psychometrics, interview with the offender, group work products and facilitator reports. It comments on possible protective factors for the offender, consults with the offender manager in the community about recommendations/release, and makes a clear and defensible statement about current risk level. These reports are written by trained professionals (usually prison psychologists) and supervised by a trained, experienced chartered psychologist who has achieved a standard level of inter-rater reliability.

Table 13.1 The 15 dynamic risk factors of the SARN

Sexual interests	Distorted attitudes
• sexual preoccupation	• adversarial sexual beliefs
• sexual preference for children	• sexual entitlement beliefs
• sexualised violence preference	• child abuse supportive beliefs
• other offence-related sexual interest	• view of women as deceitful
Management of relationships	**Self-management**
• inadequacy	• lifestyle impulsiveness
• distorted intimacy balance	• poor problem-solving
• grievance thinking	• poor management of emotions
• lack of emotional intimacy with adults	

TREATMENT ALLOCATION

In terms of allocating men to the programmes, HM Prison Service has relied on British research with sexual offenders, which has examined the relationship to reconviction of both static and dynamic risk factors. Beech *et al.* (2001) followed up men who had undergone community-based treatment in the UK. Reconviction was predicted by static and historical factors and by dynamic risk factors, both making independent contributions to predicting sexual recidivism. As such these distinctions between risk levels have influenced placement onto treatment programmes in the UK. Beech, Fisher & Beckett (1999) found that high deviancy child abusers needed twice as many treatment hours compared to low deviancy child abusers in order to show a "treatment effect". They also found that a shorter version of the Core SOTP worked equally well with low deviance/ low risk offenders as the longer version.

Bearing these results in mind, HM Prison Service allocates offenders to treatment based on risk level as measured by the RM2000 (first stage of the SARN) and treatment need (second stage SARN). In prisons, essentially those scoring as high risk/high treatment need are allocated to longer treatment, Core/Extended/Booster, whilst those at a lower risk/treatment need complete the shorter Rolling programme and complete Booster work in the community. This is illustrated in Table 13.2 below.

Table 13.2 Who does what programme?

		Static Risk (RM2000)			
		Low	**Medium**	**High**	**Very High**
Treatment Need	**Low**	Rolling (Booster work in the community)	Rolling (Booster work in the community)	Core and Booster	Core, Extended and Booster
	Medium	Rolling (Booster work in the community)	Core and Booster	Core, Extended and Booster	Core, Extended and Booster
	High	Rolling/Core and Booster	Core, Extended and Booster	Core, Extended and Booster	Core, Extended and Booster

PROGRAMME DELIVERY AND TREATMENT STYLE

The programmes, except Healthy Sexual Functioning (HSF), are delivered as group work, with up to nine convicted male sexual offenders in one group. Men of different offence types work together in the same group. The programmes are delivered by a multidisciplinary team of three facilitators, which may include prison psychologists, prison officers, probation, education and chaplain staff. The HSF is delivered by a trained and experienced psychologist on a one-to-one basis. Programme integrity is key, so all sessions are videotaped and the group is allocated a supervisor, usually a qualified psychologist, who, in addition to clinical supervision, monitors the videotapes to ensure the programme is being delivered as per the treatment manual. Facilitators undertake a two-week assessed national training course to deliver the Core programme, and can then specialise in the other programmes by undertaking further training. Caring for staff health is essential and facilitators undertake mandatory counselling, as well as clinical supervision, whilst delivering SOTP. In addition experienced facilitators undertake the Staying Strong training, designed to aid coping, promote psychological health and identify burnout.

Establishing group cohesion and a warm, non-punitive therapeutic style are also key aspects of the SOTP, as the literature suggests that these two factors are an important feature of effective treatment for sexual offenders. Beech, Fisher and Beckett (1999), using the Group Environment Scale (Moos 1986) and SOTP group data, measured the clinical success of groups in terms of the abandonment of pro-offending attitudes. They found a clear correlation between the therapeutic climate and clinical success, with cohesion identified as the most important attribute of the group for successful treatment effect.

Research on treatment style using data from the SOTP was conducted by Fernandez (1999). In this study, videotapes of sex offender groups were studied and rating scales were developed to measure therapist techniques and therapist style. Ratings were then related to clinical change measured by pre- and post-treatment psychometric testing, and also to in-session behaviours by the group members. The therapist techniques measured were centred around three core skills: encouraging active participation, non-confrontational challenge, and use of open questions. Aspects of therapist style that were measured included warmth, empathy, genuineness, hostility, coldness and deception. Fernandez found that taking responsibility by clients was linked to warm, empathic and genuine behaviours by therapists. Group participation increased when therapists actively encouraged participation, used open questions, and challenged in a non-confrontational way. Improvements in perspective-taking were related to encouragement by therapists to participate and sincerity on the part of therapists. Acceptance of future risk was related to non-confrontational challenge and warmth/empathy/genuineness. Last, improvements in coping skills were related to the use of open questions by therapists. There was no relationship between changes in self-esteem and therapist behaviour.

National training, on-site clinical supervision and video monitoring, and external video monitoring by National Offender Management's Interventions and Substance Misuse Group (ISMG) are in place to monitor and help develop group cohesion processes and a warm and non-punitive therapeutic style in facilitators.

ASSESSMENT

All sex offenders completing SOTP programmes complete a series of psychometric questionnaires and semi-structured interviews pre- and post-treatment. This test battery has been designed to map onto the dynamic risk factors covered by the SARN, as shown above (Offending Behaviour Programmes Unit 2004). Following treatment, each offender's pre- and post-psychometric scores are profiled onto a graph which indicates an individual's pre-treatment needs, progress during treatment, and outstanding treatment needs, as compared to a comparison group of sexual offenders treated by HM Prison Service. These profile graphs are interpreted by prison psychologists and incorporated into the SARN reports to help, along with clinical interviews and information from group sessions, to assess progress in treatment.

Friendship, Mann & Beech (2003) have conducted an evaluation of the prison-based Core SOTP. The study relates to the Core SOTP prior to 1996, and before an accreditation policy to formalise systems was introduced. Two-year reconviction rates were compared between a group of prisoners who had participated in the programme and a retrospectively selected sample of sexual offenders who shared the same broad characteristics as the treatment group but had not participated in SOTP. The treatment group consisted of 647 convicted male adult sexual offenders serving a custodial sentence of four years or more and who had voluntarily participated in Core SOTP. The comparison group consisted of 1,910 adult male offenders who were serving a custodial sentence of four years or more for a sexual offence but had not participated in Core SOTP.

Two-year sexual and violent reconviction rates were calculated for the treatment and comparison groups. The two-year rates of sexual reconviction were low in both the comparison groups, although the rate was higher for high risk offenders, as measured by the Static 99 (Hanson & Thornton 1999, 2000). The issue of the low reoffending base rate is one that has been discussed by researchers evaluating treatment programmes. Friendship & Thornton (2001) have suggested that as the rate of sexual reconviction is already low (less than 5% within two years of release) for untreated sexual offenders, then any reduction in this rate as a result of treatment would be very small and likely to be statistically insignificant. Any small differences between treatment groups should therefore be seen as a positive. Certainly in the area of reducing sexual offending, any small gains are significant to society, even if not statistically so.

There were no significant differences in the sexual reconviction rates between the two groups, however the issue of the low base of reoffending should be observed here. When the sexual and violent reconviction rates were combined there were overall significant differences ($p<0.01$) between the treatment and comparison groups in the rate of reconviction (see Table 13.3).

Table 13.3 Two-year combined sexual and reconviction rates for the treatment and comparison groups (Friendship *et al.* 2003)

Risk category	Treatment group		Comparison group	
	Number	%	Number	%
Low	5	1.9	25	2.6
Medium-low	6	2.7	83	12.7
Medium-high	6	5.5	31	13.5
High	13	26.0	16	28.1
Overall	30	4.6	155	8.1

In terms of risk level, significant differences were found in the medium-low ($p<0.01$) and medium-high ($p<0.05$) offender groups. For low and high risk offender groups there was a trend in the desired direction, with the treatment group showing a slightly lower level of reconviction. This would indicate that higher risk offenders need additional intervention, in line with the risk–need–responsivity principles.

In conclusion the Core SOTP has a significant impact on sexual and violent reconviction for medium risk offenders and is also successful at reducing reconviction for low risk offenders. However, higher risk offenders need additional treatment. It is important to recognise that sexual offenders are reconvicted at a very low rate and that future studies should supplement reconviction data with other non-official data.

The adapted programme evaluation (Williams, Wakeling & Webster 2007) explored treatment change in sex offenders attending a programme specifically designed for men with cognitive and social functioning deficits. Two hundred and eleven men who had undertaken the adapted programme between 1997 and 2003 were included in the study. Six psychometric assessment measures targeting the goals of the programme were adapted for use with this population, and the first phase of the study established reasonable psychometric properties as determined by internal consistency and factor analyses. The second phase of the study showed significant pre- to post-change on five out of the six measures, indicating treatment change. The link between treatment change on self-report measures and recidivism needs to be explored, and future evaluation will focus on recidivism data.

CONCLUSIONS AND THE FUTURE

HM Prison Service runs the largest national sex offender treatment programme in the world, delivering six manualised programmes across approximately 25 sites in England and Wales. A recent merge with community programmes will present the opportunity for continuous treatment for sexual offenders. Evaluation shows that the programme is having an impact on reconvictions for sexual and violent offences. Developments have included a standardised assessment battery and a tool for assessing risk and need and reporting on progress (the SARN).

Knowledge about sex offenders and effective sex offender treatment continues to develop across the world, and a recent large-scale meta-analysis conducted on controlled outcome evaluations showed treatment to be beneficial (Lösel & Schmucker 2005). Treated offenders showed 37% less sexual recidivism than controls. HM Prison Service, now as part of NOMS, will continue to add to this growing pool of knowledge and understanding. It is encouraging that research to date indicates a positive impact in terms of a) reduction in offending and b) desired change on treatment targets, as measured by psychometric assessment. Programmes that help reduce reoffending are beneficial both in terms of limiting the financial cost to society of apprehending, prosecuting and imprisoning perpetrators and also, and arguably more importantly, in preventing further victims whose lives will be affected by sexual trauma. Finally, effective treatment programmes potentially benefit perpetrators themselves, in that it is hoped they will go on to live more personally fulfilled and offence-free lives.

CHAPTER 14

Consent to Treatment, the Mental Health Act, and the Mental Capacity Act[1]

Simon Wilson and Raj Dhar

INTRODUCTION

Although many prisons in the UK have "hospital wings" or "health care centres", these are not equivalent to NHS hospitals (Wilson 2004), and psychiatric patients cannot be given treatment under the Mental Health Act within prison. However, it is clear that there are many prisoners suffering from acute and severe mental illnesses, requiring urgent medical treatment, who are awaiting transfer to NHS hospitals.

TRANSFER FROM PRISON TO HOSPITAL AND THE MENTAL HEALTH ACT 1983 (AMENDED 2007), ENGLAND AND WALES

When individuals are suffering from a mental illness of a nature or degree that warrants medical treatment in a hospital, for their own health or safety or for the protection of other persons, they can be taken to hospital and treated against their wishes under the Mental Health Act 1983. The prisoner suffering from a mental illness cannot be treated

---

1   Some of the content of this chapter has featured in a previous publication in the *Journal of Forensic Psychiatry* (Wilson & Forrester 2002). The publishers have given permission for use of this material.

in this fashion within a prison, as prisons are not recognised as hospitals under the National Health Service Act 1977. There has been consistent resistance to attempts to consider statutory treatment in prison, presumably for fear of abuse or simply because of the ideology that prisons are not for the sick. The possibility of including prison within the scope of mental health legislation was raised during meetings in the Review of the Mental Health Act 1959 (Department of Health and Social Security *et al.* 1978) and dismissed out of hand (Bowden 2002). Similarly, the most recent Mental Health Act 2007 amendments to the 1983 Act make no changes to the status quo, other than the continuance of community treatment orders (which will have little power of compulsion) already started prior to imprisonment.

The Government's policy for prison health is enshrined in the principle of "equivalence of care" (Home Office 1990b, 1991b, HM Prison Service & NHS Executive 1999). Prisoners should receive the same level of health care as they would were they not in prison – equivalent in terms of policy, standards and delivery (Health Advisory Committee for the Prison Service 1997). The prison population is conceptualised as a community and the health care provided within prison should be equivalent to primary care in the NHS, including specialist outpatient services. Any prisoner requiring more than primary care is to be transferred from prison to hospital to receive it. For those with mental disorder this can be done under Part 3 of the Mental Health Act 1983, and indeed this is recommended best practice: "[p]rison is unsuitable for a person coming within the scope of the Mental Health Act" (Department of Health & Home Office 1992). There are a variety of mechanisms for achieving such transfer under the English and Welsh Mental Health Act 1983 (as amended by the Mental Health Act 2007), and these are listed in Table 14.1.

In acute cases, however, usually the quickest and most appropriate means of effecting a transfer will be via a Home Office warrant, following reports from two doctors, under Sections 48 (for unsentenced prisoners) or 47 (for sentenced prisoners) of the Mental Health Act 1983. Section 48 is reserved for those needing "urgent" treatment, and this "should be applied where a doctor would recommend in-patient treatment if a person were seen as an out-patient in the community" (Department of Health & Home Office 1992, para. 9.6). Such transfers are not uncommon, given the high rates of mental disorder in prisons (Gunn *et al.* 1991, Brooke *et al.* 1996, Singleton *et al.* 1998), and there were 668 Home Office transfers made in 2000 (Home Office 2004a). These are supposed to happen in a "timely" fashion in accordance with Standard 5 of the Government's National Service Framework for Mental Health (Department of Health 1999a). Unfortunately, in practice, prisoners wait a considerable length of time before such transfer is possible (Robertson *et al.* 1994, Reed & Lyne 2000). In these circumstances, the prisoner may be very ill, and may be denied treatment because of the lack of any statutory framework for treatment against his or her wishes.

Table 14.1 Brief overview of sections of Part 3 of the Mental Health Act 1983 which are relevant to prisoners. (All sections include, of course, some criteria in relation to the person being considered as having some form of mental disorder requiring hospital admission.)

Section of Mental Health Act 1983	Applies to	Recommended by	Order made by
35 (Remand to hospital for medical report)	Unsentenced defendant where offence might result in imprisonment	One doctor	Court
36 (Remand to hospital for treatment)	Unsentenced prisoner where offence might result in imprisonment	Two doctors (one from hospital where patient is going)	Crown Court
37 (Hospital Order)	Convicted person where offence might result in imprisonment	Two doctors	Court
38 (Interim Hospital Order)	Convicted person where offence might result in imprisonment	Two doctors (one from hospital where patient is going)	Court
45A (Hospital & Limitation Direction)	Convicted person	Two doctors (one from hospital where patient is going)	Crown Court
47 (Ministry of Justice Transfer)	Sentenced prisoner	Two doctors	Ministry of Justice
48 (Ministry of Justice Transfer)	Unsentenced prisoner needing urgent treatment	Two doctors	Ministry of Justice

A typical case might be of an inmate with an active psychotic illness including florid delusions and hallucinations. If refusing treatment with antipsychotic medication, he would almost certainly not be given this treatment unless or until he became very disturbed, perhaps smearing faeces on the walls, or attempting to harm himself or another inmate, for example. Medical treatment can, however, be given under common law within prison. Reed and Lyne (2000) state: "treatment without consent [in prison] is possible only in emergencies under common law." (p.1031).

TREATMENT WITHIN THE PRISON AND THE MENTAL CAPACITY ACT 2005

Treatment decisions in prison

Although prisons contain high levels of physical and psychiatric morbidity, clinicians working in such environments have to adapt, clinically and ethically, to a regime that focuses primarily on discipline and order. Although such a culture may seem incompatible with a treatment decision-making model based on autonomy and best interests, the clinician is legally bound to respect the prisoner's right to consent to or refuse treatment. Prisoners have no fewer rights in this regard than non-prisoners, and treatment given without proper informed consent would be an unlawful interference and could amount to an offence of assault or battery. Although assault and battery are terms used loosely legally, the former means the apprehension of immediate unlawful force, and the latter actual unlawful force. The degree of force entailed is so minimal that even touching, in the context of giving treatment, would suffice.

In order for treatment to be lawful on the basis of consent, the consent received must be valid. To achieve this, consent must be given whilst in an "informed" state of mind, and must be made "voluntarily", free of any coercion or duress. Although some have tried to argue that a requirement of voluntariness may make it impossible for a prisoner living in a coercive environment to give informed consent, it has been held that being a prisoner, *per se*, does not prevent the giving of informed consent (Freeman v Home Office). The existence of coercive forces in prison will, however, require greater care on the part of the clinician to ensure that such influences do not materially interfere with the consent-to-treatment process.

Although it is always the right to decide that is sacred, and consequently it is irrelevant whether one refuses or consents to treatment, it is usually the refusing patient that causes most clinical concern. Again the common law has made it clear that all persons have the right to make an unwise or irrational treatment decision, even if clearly not in their best interests (Re M.B.).

Mental capacity and treatment decisions

Although the rights described above are fundamental, they are not absolute, and rely on a presumption of capacity – that is, that the individual has the ability to make a given decision. It is crucial to distinguish the *decision made* from the *ability to make* a decision. The decision made may be blatantly wrong, but that, in itself, is not evidence enough to conclude that there is an "impairment in ability". There must be direct evidence of impaired decision-making that has had an impact on the specific treatment decision. The prisoner who has capacity to decide on treatment remains autonomous in respect of any treatment offered in prison, irrespective of whether he or she has a physical or mental disorder.

Treatment without consent

There are circumstances when treatment may be given without consent. First, treatment that is in the patient's best interest can be given without consent from the patient in an emergency situation, under the defence of necessity. Although necessity is relatively straightforward in legal meaning and widely applicable in a range of situations, if challenged it is not an easy defence to plead successfully. It is truly a "weighing up" defence, the court deciding whether the course taken by the defendant on the facts known to him or her at the time was the better of the evils. For the defence to be relied upon, there has to be an element of seriousness and emergency about the situation. For treatment decisions in a prison setting, most clinicians would probably rely on this defence only for genuinely life-threatening situations.

As described above, the right to refuse or consent to treatment is based on a presumption of capacity. Thus, if that presumption is rebutted by evidence that the person deciding on treatment lacks the capacity to make that decision (Re T., Re M.B.), then, provided the treatment is in his or her best interests, it may be given without consent. Considering first the evidence of lack of capacity, the test comes from the landmark case of Re C. The "C test" as it became known was later affirmed by Lady Butler Sloss in the Court of Appeal in Re M.B. and also held to apply more specifically to the treatment decisions in a prison context in Re W. The "C test" is as follows: "first comprehending and retaining information, secondly, believing it and thirdly, weighing it in the balance to arrive at a choice" (Re C., p36).

Re C. also established that capacity was decision-specific, and therefore logically any assessment of capacity should be "functional" rather than based on "status" or "outcome". The degree of capacity required will vary according to the gravity of the decision at issue (Re T.). It was further held in Re M.B. that capacity can be temporarily impaired, as it was in that particular case, the material facts of the case being that a needle phobia had rendered the patient in labour incapacitous and unable to accept anaesthesia necessary for a caesarean section. Other causes of temporary incapacity that were cited included pain, fear and anxiety.

The case law involving capacity has recently been codified into statute in the form of the Mental Capacity Act 2005 (hereafter referred to as the MCA). Many of the principles that emerged out of case law have been enshrined in the statute, and the treatment of an individual who is not or cannot consent will now require application of the decision-making framework as set out in the MCA.

Consequently, for the prisoner who lacks capacity, the treatment of physical disorders will be governed by the MCA. Furthermore, as described above, the absence of provisions within the Mental Health Act (MHA) 1983 to allow for treatment of a mental disorder in prison would mean that the MCA could also apply to the treatment of mental disorder in the prison population. It is perhaps ironic that, of all citizens, it is the capacitous prisoner who retains this autonomy in respect of the treatment of mental as well as physical conditions; a position that was strongly advocated by the Richardson Committee (in their review of the MHA 1983) when they recommended that the treatment of mental disorder under the MHA should be based on incapacity (Department of Health 1999b, Eastman & Dhar 2000).

Staff need to have a basic understanding of the safeguards in place to protect individuals, including prisoners, who lack decision-making capacity.

The framework of decision- making within the MCA 2005

The MCA 2005 essentially provides a framework for decision-making on behalf of those who lack the capacity to make decisions for themselves. This framework applies to a variety of decisions, including treatment decisions. It does not give those who decide on behalf of an incapacitous person any additional rights or powers beyond that which the individual would have had, had he or she retained capacity, so that any legal rights or powers that were not available to the capacitous prisoner or those providing treatment prior to loss of capacity will remain unavailable. Thus in respect of the prisoner, although various decision-making rights may be lost due to incarceration, the right to decide on treatment is preserved, and those acting on behalf of the incapacitous prisoner can uphold the right to refuse treatment on the prisoner's behalf if it is deemed not to be in his or her best interests.

According to the framework laid out in the Act, the first step in determining whether treatment can be given to the prisoner who cannot or will not give consent is to establish whether he or she meets the "diagnostic threshold" by adducing some evidence of disability of mind. This requirement serves to ensure that irrational decision-making alone is insufficient. It must be caused by some disability of mind. The next step is to establish that factually there is a loss of capacity arising from the mental disability. This will require application of the capacity test, as defined within the Act, to the relevant treatment decision.

Under MCA Section 3 the presence of capacity requires the individual:

a) to understand the information relevant to the decision (under subsection 4, meaning the reasonably foreseeable consequences of deciding one way or another, or failing to make the decision)

b) to retain that information (this need only be for long enough to make the decision (Section 3))

c) to use or weigh that information as part of the process of making the decision

d) to communicate his decision (whether by talking, using sign language or any other means).

To safeguard against biases Section 2 (3) states that a lack of capacity cannot be established merely by reference to:

a) a person's age or appearance; or

b) a condition of his, or an aspect of his behaviour, which might lead others to make unjustified assumptions about his capacity.

Evidentially the MCA places the burden of proof on those alleging incapacity (in the context, the treatment provider) and applies the civil standard: on the balance of probabilities. Capacity can fluctuate depending on the cause of incapacity, and so capacity assessment ought to be repeated before any final judgement is made.

If the individual fails on any of the limbs, then he or she fails the test. If the individual is indeed found to lack capacity according to the test, then a further principle stated in the MCA is that reasonable steps should be taken to restore capacity and to assist the individual in making the decision before finally concluding that he or she lacks capacity. If lack of capacity is the final outcome, then the next issue is whether treatment can be given, and if so, who can make the decision on behalf of the patient. The MCA introduced a new hierarchy of decision-making in the event of an individual lacking capacity. This hierarchy means that if any of the following exist, then the decision to treat will be made through that mechanism, rather than by those proposing treatment:

- advance directives

- lasting Power of Attorney

- deputy appointed by the Court of Protection.

Of the three mechanisms listed, the advance directive is the most powerful and significant. It is a statement of refusal of treatment made by the patient him- or herself in advance of the treatment being offered. If there is a valid and applicable advance directive, then it cannot be overridden, even if the individual lacks capacity and the treatment is in his or her best interests. In order for the directive to be valid it must have been made when the individual had capacity, and must specifically direct that a certain treatment is to be refused. For treatments other than those that are life-sustaining there are no formalities, and the advance directive can be made orally to another person without witnesses. Life-sustaining treatments can also be refused in advance, but the directive must be in writing, must have been witnessed and must include an express statement that it would apply even if a risk to life. If such a directive exists, then the treatment that is the subject of the directive cannot, under any circumstances, be given, irrespective of whether it is in the best interests of the patient.

If no such directive exists, then the treatment may be given, provided it is considered in the best interests of the patient in accordance with Section 4 of the Act:

1. In determining for the purposes of this Act what is in a person's best interests, the person making the determination must not make it merely on the basis of:

   a. the person's age or appearance, or

   b. a condition of his, or an aspect of his behaviour, which might lead others to make unjustified assumptions about what might be in his best interests.

2. The person making the determination must consider all the relevant circumstances and, in particular, take the following steps.

3. He must consider:

    a. whether it is likely that the person will at some time have capacity in relation to the matter in question, and

    b. if it appears likely that he will, when that is likely to be.

4. He must, so far as reasonably practicable, permit and encourage the person to participate, or to improve his ability to participate, as fully as possible in any act done for him and any decision affecting him.

5. Where the determination relates to life-sustaining treatment he must not, in considering whether the treatment is in the best interests of the person concerned, be motivated by a desire to bring about his death.

6. He must consider, so far as is reasonably ascertainable:

    a. the person's past and present wishes and feelings (and, in particular, any relevant written statement made by him when he had capacity),

    b. the beliefs and values that would be likely to influence his decision if he had capacity, and

    c. the other factors that he would be likely to consider if he were able to do so.

7. He must take into account, if it is practicable and appropriate to consult them, the views of:

    a. anyone named by the person as someone to be consulted on the matter in question or on matters of that kind,

    b. anyone engaged in caring for the person or interested in his welfare,

    c. any donee of a lasting power of attorney granted by the person, and

    d. any deputy appointed for the person by the court,

as to what would be in the person's best interests and, in particular, as to the matters mentioned in subsection (6).

Case law prior to the MCA has established that treatment in the patient's "best interests" will include that necessary to save life or prevent a deterioration or ensure an improvement in the patient's physical or mental health (Re F.), as well as a broader range of interventions. "Best interests" is often misinterpreted in very narrow fashion when applied to prisoners, to mean that treatment can only be given when the prisoner's life is in danger, or serious harm is likely, or the prisoner is faced with irreversible deterioration.

The test of "best interests" at common law is broader than this, however, including, for example, donating bone marrow (Re Y.), and undergoing diagnostic procedures (Re H.). Furthermore, in Re F. Lord Brandon held that "In many cases…it will not only be lawful for doctors on the ground of necessity, to operate on or give other medical treatment to adult patients disabled from giving their consent: it will be their common law duty to do so."

These legal tests apply equally to prisoners refusing medical treatment. They can, then, be treated in the face of a refusal, without such treatment constituting an assault, provided that they are incapacitated; and, if there is no advance directive, lasting power of attorney, or deputy from the Court of Protection, provided that the treatment is in their best interests. However, doctors working in prison have generally been reluctant to administer treatment under these circumstances, waiting instead until an emergency supervenes. The reasons for this are likely to be complex, but might include faulty legal advice previously given by the Prison Service (see Wilson & Forrester 2002 for detailed review); an unacknowledged need for the patient to get more unwell so as to expedite hospital transfer; anxiety that any hospital transfer will be cancelled altogether if the patient improves (Earthrowl, O'Grady & Birmingham 2003), and perhaps a concern about historical abuses of medication in prisons (the more widespread use of the "chemical cosh" historically[2]).

What standard of assessment of capacity and best interests is required?

The MCA was designed to remain informal in its application so as to be as accessible and universal as possible. Reflecting this informality is the general defence, under Section 5:

> before doing the act, D takes reasonable steps to establish whether P lacks capacity in relation to the matter in question, and b) when doing the act, D reasonably believes – i) that P lacks capacity in relation to the matter and ii) that it would be in P's best interests for the act to be done.

This is essentially a Bolam test based on reasonableness.[3] The defence does not apply to the treatment itself, only to the decision to give the treatment.

---

2   The "chemical cosh" refers to the abuse of sedating medication to control disturbed behaviour with no need for there to be any underlying medical condition.

3   The Bolam test is the standard legal test of medical negligence. Did the person act in accordance with a practice accepted as proper by a responsible body of medical opinion?

Further provisions relevant to those who lack capacity

Further provisions and safeguards for those with long-term incapacity (the Bournewood scenario[4]) will be available when "bolt-on" legislation to the MHA 2007 comes into force in April 2009. Although the situation of the long-term incapacitous prisoner may *prima facie* appear similar to the facts of the case of L. v Bournewood, the obvious difference is that in Bournewood the individual was not legally detained but *de facto* detained. The issue was then whether his rights could be adequately protected without the safeguards provided under the MHA. In the prisoner's case there is no such option for detention under the MHA, and in any event he or she is already detained in prison. The Bournewood bolt-on safeguards may provide some guiding principles (rather than direction) on how best to safeguard the rights of the long-term incapacitous prisoner detained in prison.

CONCLUSIONS

Medical treatment can be administered to prisoners with mental illness when they lack capacity to consent, and when such treatment is in their "best interests" and does not conflict with a valid advance directive, lasting power of attorney, or deputy from the Court of Protection. Treatment with anti-psychotic medication is in their best interests, in that it would ensure an improvement in their mental health in both the short and long term. One might suggest that this is likely to result in many mentally ill prisoners being treated at an earlier stage and as frequently as necessary – an improvement on the present situation. However, hospital treatment will provide a good deal more than compulsory medication, and the prospect that some prisoners may miss out on this if their mental state improves as a result of forcible medication in prison while they are waiting for a hospital bed, may well be another relevant factor to consider in making judgements about "best interests". All mentally ill prisoners refusing treatment should have their capacity to consent assessed by their treating doctor, in consultation if necessary with a doctor experienced in these matters (probably a psychiatrist), and the results of these assessments should be fully recorded in the Inmate Medical Record. When the prisoner is incapacitated, serious consideration should be given to administering medical treatment in prison without having to wait for a hospital bed to become available, although, being mindful of the breadth of the "best interests" test, considerations about the realities of cancellations of hospital transfers should perhaps also be included in any decisions about administering treatment in prison.

In many respects it is not surprising that the amendments to the Mental Health Act 1983 exclude any provision that might allow compulsory treatment in prison under the Act. Such a change would have placed the mentally disordered offender in a fundamentally different position to that which existed before. The proposal that compulsory treatment in prison should be authorised under the Mental Health Act has been met

---

4   This case refers to the detention of an incapable but non-protesting adult without using the Mental Health Act.

with forceful objection from some. There is an understandable concern that such a move would go too far in a direction away from proper hospital care, the prisoner being at risk of being deprived of a truly "equivalent" level of treatment. The lack of provision within the Mental Health Act does, however, create two interesting issues. First, some incapacitous prisoners could be treated for their mental disorders under the Mental Capacity Act in prison, without the protections afforded by the Mental Health Act (such as regular inspection by the Mental Health Act Commission). Second, the prisoner who retains capacity remains autonomous in relation to the treatment of physical or mental disorder, something that would not be the case were he or she living outside of prison, capacity being largely irrelevant to the Mental Health Act. A large number of key organisations and bodies with an interest in the care of mentally disordered individuals supported the notion that the Mental Health Act 1983 should be amended so that involuntary detention and treatment depended on a capacity test; thereby making no distinction between mental and physical disorders when it comes to compulsory treatment (Department of Health 1999b). Those proposals were not adopted, and so, in fact, it is only the prisoner group that benefits from this legal position. However, in clinical terms there are disadvantages to the prisoner. The prisoner who, through lack of capacity or insight, does not consent to treatment for a mental disorder may remain untreated for many months whilst awaiting transfer out of prison to hospital. As a result, those prisoners who are acutely unwell but not necessarily in need of emergency treatment for a life-threatening situation may remain untreated because of the lack of a clear legal power authorising treatment. Capacity case law, and now legislation, makes it clear that individuals who lack capacity can be treated against their will, provided the treatment is in their best interest. The codification of this case law now means that there is a proper framework in existence to protect the rights of those who lack capacity. This includes, for example, giving a statutory footing to the advance directive. Ultimately these safeguards will allow the prisoner lacking capacity and in need of treatment for mental or physical disorder an improved level of protection, although probably not the same level of protection were the MHA to apply. Prison medical authorities may thus feel legally more secure when proceeding with treatment that would previously have fallen within the common law framework, and this may be relevant to those individuals who are clinically stuck in that period of time between the onset of symptoms of illness and transfer to hospital.

CHAPTER 15

Hunger Strike and Food Refusal

Danny Sullivan and Crystal Romilly

HISTORY

> Fasting is an institution as old as Adam. It has been resorted to for self-purification
> or for some ends noble as well as ignoble. Buddha, Jesus and Mohammed fasted so
> as to see God face to face… In my fast, I have but followed these great examples,
> no doubt for ends much less noble than theirs. (Gandhi 1944, p.67)

Gandhi cited three reasons for fasting which were, first, to overcome bestial passions;
second, to rest the overworked stomach; and third, to reform individuals and society. In 1924, when Hindus and Muslims were killing each other, he undertook a 21-
day fast as a plea for tolerance. When Ramsay MacDonald planned to make Harijans
(Untouchables) a separate electorate, Gandhi threatened to fast "unto death". In 1933
he also carried out a 21-day fast in the cause of the Harijans. He wrote, "All fasting
and penance must as far as possible be secret. But my fasting is both a penance and a
punishment, and a punishment has to be public – punishment of those I try to save. The
only way love punishes is by suffering." (Gandhi 1944, p.11)

In Britain the use of hunger striking as a political tool dates from the years leading
up to the First World War, when suffragettes and Irish nationalists refused solid food in
prison. From 1912 onwards the suffragettes campaigning for votes for women became
more militant and engaged in criminal damage and arson. The first such woman to
engage in hunger striking was Miss Wallace Dunlop on 2 August 1908, as a protest
against not being treated as a political prisoner: "'Release or death' was her motto.
From that day…the hunger strike was the greatest weapon we possessed against the

government" (Kenney 1924). Miss Dunlop was released. However, subsequent suffragette hunger strikers were force-fed.

Emmeline Pankhurst endured ten hunger strikes in prison in 18 months. Her sister, Mary Clarke, was force-fed in Holloway in 1910, and died soon afterwards at home. No women died in prison, but several, such as Lady Constance Lytton, were thought to have had their health ruined by the experience of hunger striking and force-feeding. The hunger striking tactic was followed by the far more dangerous and unpleasant hunger and thirst strike, which both Mrs Pankhurst and her second daughter, Sylvia, endured. The Government did not want to create martyrs, so when there was danger of death they released the prisoners. Once the Government had passed into law the Prisoners' Temporary Discharge for Ill Health Act in April 1913 (widely known as the "Cat and Mouse Act"), the release was only temporary. Even opponents of women's suffrage were appalled by force-feeding. Keir Hardie (1909) wrote, "Women worn and weak by hunger are seized upon, held down by brute force, gagged, a tube inserted down the throat, and food poured or pumped into the stomach. Let British men think over the spectacle."

Hunger striking was first taken up by Irish Nationalists in 1912. It was a weapon also used by Sinn Feiners in 1920, and Terence MacSwiney, Lord Mayor of Cork, died in a London prison after a fast of 74 days. An account by Frank Gallagher (1929) from a diary he kept while on hunger strike at Mountjoy Jail in Dublin in 1920, from Easter Monday for ten days, gives a vivid picture of the emotional toll and near delirium experienced by the hunger strikers. Following MacSwiney's death in 1920, hunger striking was banned by Sinn Fein until the 1970s and 1980s, when it was again taken up by the IRA. Several Irish prisoners in English prisons starved themselves in the 1970s, and as late as 1974 Irish prisoners at Brixton prison were force-fed.

American women suffragettes adopted the hunger strike in the period 1918–1920, as did conscientious objectors who did not want to fight in the First World War. It was used again during protests against the Vietnam War in 1969. Inmates at Soledad prison in California also used it as a protest against prison conditions in the 1970s. It has since been used in prisons in South Africa, Turkey and elsewhere as a protest against detention and prison conditions, often by members of political movements. Many detainees at Guantanamo Bay detention camp have engaged in food refusal since this US facility has been used to detain people suspected of terrorism-related offences. The legal status of these detainees has been subject to remarkable debate, and reports in medical journals describe force-feeding, with concern that the debate over the legal status of detainees has obscured the use of force-feeding as an aversive procedure or as a form of torture, and contrary to existing international instruments (Annas 2006).

Hunger striking has been described as a communication, a protest by the powerless, intended to wrest moral authority from the state. The intention of the hunger striker is not to die; he or she may be prepared to die if necessary, but it is not the aim. Most hunger strikes end before there is any risk of serious medical consequences. The history of hunger striking for political aims indicates that this has frequently been an effective strategy in bringing about changes in prison management regimes and in realising broader political goals.

Force-feeding and hunger striking prisoners

Until fairly late in the twentieth century, the policy for managing hunger-striking prisoners in the UK was described as "brusque force-feeding". In the 1909 suffragette case Leigh v Gladstone, it was held that the Home Office has a duty to preserve the health of prisoners, so that hunger-striking prisoners must be force-fed. Similarly, prison rules bound the prison medical officer to care for the mental and physical health of the prisoner. Nothing in the prison rules specifically justified force-feeding, but the Home Office Standing Orders, Rule 17 (1) Prison Rules 1964: SI No. 388, specified the advisability of admitting the person to the prison hospital for assessment of the need for compulsory feeding. In practice, prison medical officers seem to have thought they were obliged to force-feed. The Suicide Act of 1961 changed the law so that suicide was no longer illegal; however, aiding and abetting suicide remained a criminal offence. This may have encouraged prison medical staff to believe they had a duty to force-feed when a prisoner appeared to be set on starving himself to death. However, without making any change in either statute law or prison regulations, there was a significant change in policy when Roy Jenkins, the Home Secretary at the time, made this decisive statement in the House of Commons on 17 July 1974 (Jenkins 1974) in relation to the Price sisters (IRA prisoners at Brixton):

> The doctor's obligation is to the ethics of his profession and to his duty at common law; he is not required as a matter of prison practice to feed a prisoner artificially against the prisoner's will.

This statement by the Home Secretary marked a decisive change in the way hunger striking was managed in prison, and it has remained the attitude of successive governments ever since. The British Medical Association published the following policy statement on force-feeding (Anon 1974a, p.52):

> The final decision must be for the [prison medical officer] to make, and it is not for any outside person to seek to override the clinical judgment of the doctor by imposing his own decision upon the case in question.

The issue was the subject of intensive debate within the medical profession, both internationally and in the United Kingdom. The World Medical Association at Tokyo in 1975 declared that artificial feeding should not be forced on capacitous patients.

In practice, major political hunger strikes in the UK have been managed ever since in a manner consistent with the Declaration of Tokyo. This includes the hunger strike in Long Kesh Prison ("The Maze") in Northern Ireland in 1981, in which ten Irish Republican prisoners died, the first and most famous being Bobby Sands. They died after fasting for between 45 and 61 days, but no case descriptions or results have ever been published.

CONTEXTS

There are no studies of hunger strikers which reflect demographic or personal characteristics, although some have, in selected samples, referred to factors which increase likelihood. In custodial settings, remanded prisoners and those immediately post-sentencing are particularly at increased risk of hunger strike (Larkin 1991). There may be associations with personality disorder, especially paranoid, antisocial and borderline types (Larkin 1991).

In those without apparent mental disorder, the unifying theme with hunger striking is motive. Those who perceive their detention as political, or who are denied rights they believe due to them, appear more likely to be involved in strikes. Prudence is warranted owing to the difficulties in quantifying the prevalence of hunger strikes. The numerator is defined by effectiveness at obtaining publicity, the denominator is ill-defined due to difficulties in defining what constitutes a hunger strike.

In populations detained by reason of immigration status – illegal immigrants, asylum-seekers, imminent deportees – hunger strikes are not uncommon. They are often associated with other protest actions: sewing up lips and eyes, sieges, firesetting, rooftop protests, attempts to escape, and other gestures which demonstrate resistance. An association with mental disorder is not clearly apparent. Rather, it is the hopelessness and desperation of the protester's situation, and the lack of perceived alternative recourses available, that usually underlie such actions. It may be appropriate in such contexts to speak of demoralisation rather than depression (Clarke & Kissane 2002).

In dealing with hunger strikes in such situations, it is important to be aware of structural impediments to effective management. In many situations detention centres are the location of these protests, and often the management of these centres has been contracted out to private providers. Treating psychiatrists may have a different contractual relationship with these organisations. It is crucial that doctors working in custodial institutions are keenly aware of the rules under which they practise in specific environments. Confidentiality between detainees and doctors may be compromised. In some cases the local peer body for psychiatry may have recommended against participation in work in detention centres. Any psychiatrist reviewing these situations should be mindful of his or her loyalties and ensure that duties to patients can be maintained without significant compromise. The consequences of involvement as a treating psychiatrist may be professionally catastrophic and there are indications that, in privately run facilities, psychiatrists may be politically exploited to justify force-feeding or absolve the contractors of responsibility for consequences.

In some situations, psychiatrists may feel it politic to withdraw service. This is an awkward situation which may cause distress. However, when a doctor feels compromised by his or her employer – expected to act in ways contrary to his or her own sense of good practice, his or her ethical principles or the guidelines of professional bodies – it may be necessary to cease service provision. Such an action conflicts with the duty to provide care for patients, but when the ability to provide unimpeded care is significantly compromised, a doctor acting in good faith is likely to be supported. Recourse to professional bodies, registration boards and indemnity organisations would be strongly recommended in such situations. There may be a case for whistleblowing if constraints upon patient care are particularly severe.

FORMAL GUIDELINES FOR MANAGING HUNGER STRIKERS

There are two main documents applying to hunger strikers, although other international instruments and local law may be relevant. The first is the anti-torture statement known as the Declaration of Tokyo (World Medical Association 1975). Article 6 of the Declaration refers specifically to hunger striking in prison:

> Where a prisoner refuses nourishment and is considered by the physician as capable of forming an unimpaired and rational judgment concerning the consequences of such a voluntary refusal of nourishment, he or she shall not be fed artificially. The decision as to the capacity of the prisoner to form such a judgment should be confirmed by at least one other independent physician. The consequences of the refusal of nourishment shall be explained by the physician to the prisoner.

Subsequently the World Medical Association (1992) approved a specific declaration on hunger strikers in Malta in 1991. In their preamble, they state:

> Hunger strikes occur in various contexts but they mainly give rise to dilemmas in settings where people are detained (prisons, jails and immigration detention centres). They are often a form of protest by people who lack other ways of making their demands known. In refusing nutrition for a significant period, they usually hope to obtain certain goals by inflicting negative publicity on the authorities. Short-term or feigned food refusals rarely raise ethical problems. Genuine and prolonged fasting risks death or permanent damage for hunger strikers and can create a conflict of values for physicians. Hunger strikers usually do not wish to die but some may be prepared to do so to achieve their aims. Physicians need to ascertain the individual's true intention, especially in collective strikes or situations where peer pressure may be a factor. An ethical dilemma arises when hunger strikers who have apparently issued clear instructions not to be resuscitated reach a stage of cognitive impairment. The principle of beneficence urges physicians to resuscitate them but respect for individual autonomy restrains physicians from intervening when a valid and informed refusal has been made. An added difficulty arises in custodial settings because it is not always clear whether the hunger striker's advance instructions were made voluntarily and with appropriate information about the consequences. These guidelines and the background paper address such difficult situations.

The World Medical Association declaration offers helpful advice on the management of hunger strikers. First, physicians must assess individuals' mental capacity. This involves verifying that an individual intending to fast does not have a mental impairment that would seriously undermine the person's ability to make health care decisions. Second, the hunger striker needs to be informed of the likely consequences of his or her decision. Third, the doctor needs to maintain a private therapeutic relationship with the striker, so that he or she allows regular examination, and the possibility of interventions such as saline drips is retained.

Of 24 deaths in 2001 classified as self-inflicted by the Safer Custody Group (within HM Prison Service) but not receiving a coroner's verdict of suicide, one was attributed to fluid refusal. In the 12 years from 1991 to 2003, three prisoners died as a result of food refusal. Thus it is not a particularly common problem in prisons in England and Wales, but when it occurs it may be difficult and upsetting for health care and other prison staff. It is important for health care staff in particular to know the legal position, and to have guidelines for managing the patient in a professional way.

The European Committee for the Prevention of Torture discusses the central importance of the doctor's professional independence when working within a prison where the duty to care may enter into conflict with considerations of management and security, stating that "a prison doctor acts as a patient's personal doctor" (Committee for the Prevention of Torture 1993, para. f73). Once a doctor has begun to attend on a hunger-striking prisoner, all the responsibilities which are part of that relationship apply, such as respecting confidentiality.

In South Africa, medical practitioners during the apartheid regime faced these ethical dilemmas, and a position paper adopted by the Faculty of Medicine of the University of Witwatersrand on 20 March 1989, and published in the *South African Medical Journal* on 2 September 1989, set out the principles to follow very clearly. The doctor should establish the mental competence of the patient, explain the consequences of refusal of nourishment, including the uncertainties and complications, continue to monitor the mental and physical state of the patient, alleviate distress (the refusal to accept intervention should not prejudice any other aspect of health care), and show fidelity to the will of the patient. Of course, anyone who persists with a hunger strike will reach a stage of delirium and altered consciousness when they no longer have the capacity to make or express the decision to continue to refuse nourishment. The position paper stated that a conscious person's refusal of treatment must be respected in a period of unconsciousness. However, it also stated that unless there are written instructions to the contrary, the patient should be resuscitated when necessary. It is therefore important to discuss this situation with the patient so that he can make an advance directive stating what he wishes to happen in this eventuality. It is preferable that this is done in writing and documented in the prisoner's inmate medical record, if possible in front of a witness. If the patient reaches this stage and the factor which drove him to the hunger strike in the first place no longer applies, then the doctor should resuscitate the patient so that he can re-consider his position in the new circumstances.

A "dear doctor letter" (Wool 1996) on *Food Refusal, Advance Directives, and Mental Capacity* was sent in January 1996 to all doctors working in UK prisons by the Director of Health Care for the Prison Service, spelling out how to assess capacity and explaining advance directives. To have capacity the doctor must be satisfied that the patient is able to comprehend and retain the information as to the treatment offered, to believe it, and to weigh the information balancing risks against needs. The letter also restated the Instruction to Governors 39/1994 specifying when a doctor should inform the Directorate of Health Care about a prisoner refusing food (and fluid). This advice followed the case of Secretary of State for the Home Department v Robb. In August 1994 a prisoner, Derek Robb, indicated that he no longer wished to eat or drink and that he wished to die. Proceedings were issued by the Home Office seeking declarations of the legal position, in the interests of protecting health care staff. The judgement was delivered by Thorpe J on 4 October 1994, declaring that food and fluid refusal is not attempted suicide, therefore it is not aiding or abetting suicide for health care staff not to institute treatment. He noted that health care staff may lawfully observe and abide by the refusal of the defendant to receive nutrition, and may lawfully abstain from providing hydration and nutrition to the defendant whether by artificial means or otherwise, for as long as the individual retains the capacity to refuse this.

The other salient recent case in the UK is that of Ian Brady (R (Brady) v Ashworth Hospital Authority [2000]). In response to a hunger strike apparently precipitated by his forcible restraint and transfer within a secure hospital, a judicial review was sought of the legality of force-feeding him. Mr Justice Kay ruled that not only was force-feeding justified as treatment for Brady's mental disorder (severe personality disorder), but he was also incompetent and thus could be fed in his best interests (Dyer 2000).

Despite recent judicial support for the considered decisions of medical practitioners in these cases, and the clear statements of relevant international instruments, there remain many countries in which attitudes and local law may unfortunately differ.

The current HM Prison Service guidance on managing hunger-striking prisoners is contained in Prison Service Instruction 38/2002, *Guidance on Consent to Medical Treatment* (Department of Health, HM Prison Service 2002).

FOOD REFUSAL AND MENTAL DISORDERS

It has already been noted that hunger strikes do not generally arise from mental disorders, excepting adjustment disorders. Nevertheless, a proportion will exhibit overt psychiatric illness, diagnosable by the vigilant clinician. A list of differential diagnoses in hunger strikes includes:

- dementia – Alzheimer's type

    – fronto-temporal

- organic cause – cerebral tumour, metabolic, endocrine, gastrointestinal conditions

- psychotic disorder

- mood disorder

- adjustment disorder

- specific phobia

- obsessive-compulsive disorder

- post-traumatic stress disorder

- factitious disorder

- eating disorder

- personality disorder

- mental retardation

- autism spectrum disorders.

In addition, the core skills of psychiatrists are of value in understanding and managing human distress, and in identifying and resolving systemic issues impacting on management.

Larkin (1991) selected known cases of food refusal from a dispersal prison and noted only three cases over an eight-year period, none diagnosed as mentally disordered. However, in a nearby remand prison there were 49 hunger strikes in 39 prisoners over the same period, of which 29 files were accessible to review. Larkin's conclusions, acknowledging methodological limitations, were that those likely to be experiencing serious mental illness tended to refuse both food *and* fluids, and were more likely to be unable to provide a reason for food refusal.

O'Connor & Johnson-Sabine (1988) described 12 cases from different settings without stated selection criteria; they noted the same likelihood of fluid refusal but could not otherwise discern differences in duration of strike or weight loss. One case had a history of anorexia nervosa, but none went on to develop it. The link with eating disorder is pertinent. There may be an increased prevalence of offending in a sub-population of eating-disordered patients (Vandereycken & van Houdenhove 1996). Some patients with anorexia nervosa also have personality disorders and abuse illicit substances, and thus may be incarcerated. One of the Price sisters, on hunger strike as an IRA political prisoner in the early 1970s (Anon 1974b) reportedly went on to develop anorexia nervosa (Anon 2000). There are numbers of other anecdotal reports of hunger strikers subsequently exhibiting eating disordered behaviour, both anorexic and bulimic. These accounts are in accord with descriptions of subsequent abnormal attitudes to food in those detained as prisoners of war by the Japanese in World War II (Polivy *et al.* 1994). An anthropologist has postulated that starvation might impede competence early in the course of a hunger strike (Fessler 2003), but there is still no empirical evidence that voluntary fasting can lead to the development of eating disorder.

Depression, possibly with substantial adjustment features, but also potentially linked to offending, may precede food refusal. Kalk *et al.* (1993) suggested that depression was a feature in 77% of their sample of political hunger strikers. Assessment seeking other features of depressive illness is mandatory. Collateral history may add weight to the diagnosis. Treatment with antidepressant medication is warranted, but careful assessment of decision-making competence is mandatory at regular intervals, and consideration should be given at an early stage to transfer to a psychiatric or medical hospital. For those depressed patients refusing treatment and in a life-threatening condition, treatment with electroconvulsive therapy may be life-saving and justified. The distinction between depression and adjustment disorders should rely not only upon current symptoms, but also on past history and response to environmental interventions such as visits or privileges. In the presence of overt and significant depressive symptoms, one should be cautious to assume that a hunger strike is based upon competent adjudication of the situation.

In detention centres, a history of torture or of post-traumatic stress disorder (PTSD) is not unusual. Incarceration may lead to acute decompensation, retraumatisation and possible hunger strike. In particular, demoralisation, hopelessness and isolation from social supports may be salient in the genesis of hunger strikes, and offer possible avenues to address the concerns which may lead to food refusal.

The prevalence of psychosis in prison populations is greatly increased. Fears of adulteration of food and other persecutory phenomena may lead to food refusal. Some delusional patients may improve with food provided in sealed containers which they can open themselves; however, the underlying psychotic disorder warrants treatment and, without medication, is likely to deteriorate even with such interventions.

Food refusal in the elderly prisoner may represent dementia, possibly mediated through paranoid beliefs about food, or alternatively, in those with more advanced disease, reflecting inanition. It must be remembered that fronto-temporal dementias in younger people may present with offending behaviours because of disinhibition and impaired executive function, thus leading to imprisonment. Should this have not become apparent, it may be that psychiatrists are called to review such patients, although the more typical presentation is one of overeating, dietary change and carbohydrate craving. Huntington's disease should also be considered, given that presentations may include weight loss, offending and persecutory ideas, as well as movement disorder and dementia.

In elderly people refusing food, consideration should primarily be given to personality and situational variables. Food refusal may represent protest (Duggal & Lawrence 2001) or serve as an instrumental means to influence another party, such as a relative. The elderly prisoner may be stricken by hopelessness, expectation that he or she will never see freedom again, or other problems in adjusting to incarceration. The presence of depressive symptoms or physical illness may further confuse the situation. Attention paid to interpersonal dynamics, the social context and communication may be of help to treating clinicians. Clear communication of the limits of powers of health care providers may be of help, but in some cases intransigence may be insurmountable. It is also worth noting that elderly people may evoke a sympathetic countertransference and that the attitudes of staff as well as the clinician may involve significant feelings of guilt.

Those with mental retardation may refuse food on reception into prison, or subsequently. Some people with mild retardation – or even the higher functioning, moderately mentally retarded – may not *appear* to be disabled. Nevertheless, bewilderment, fear, misunderstanding and poor adjustment may lead to food refusal. Those with mental retardation may be subject to bullying or be otherwise vulnerable in a custodial environment. Cognitive rigidity and limited verbal or negotiating skills may result in an inability to shift an attitude of intransigence. Diagnoses of mental retardation should always be considered. These may not be exclusive, and incarceration may lead to marked decompensation and the development of affective or psychotic illness in the mentally retarded prisoner. If the correctional system offers specialised units for the management of prisoners with mental retardation, these may provide an environment which is more amenable.

More unusual diagnoses should be entertained. Unusual attitudes to food may be features of neurotic disorders or autism spectrum disorders; factitious disorders are frequently associated with antisocial traits or behaviours; and organic causes should always be excluded. As with psychosis, where reasons for food refusal are not apparent, a careful and thorough history may reveal occult causes for "hunger strike". The role of the psychiatrist is to cast a critical eye over situations of food refusal and to ensure that treatable conditions have not been overlooked due to the "patient" being a "prisoner".

ASSESSMENT

The psychiatrist, in assessing the hunger striker, must always remember his or her duty to the patient. Navigating the conflicting responsibilities of a prison doctor requires consideration of multiple duties and roles, paramount among which is duty to the patient, notwithstanding that the patient may be a prisoner. We contend that doctors must preserve their independent decision-making capacities and pay heed to local constraints, but also recognise that international human rights instruments have laid down a clear ethical foundation for practice (World Medical Association 1975, 1992). Despite this, in a number of countries the practice may remain one of force-feeding prisoners despite competent refusal.

Furthermore, the psychiatrist is but one element in the multidisciplinary team. It remains important to be aware of the impact of a hunger strike upon other staff members. Various staff will exhibit signs of distress, or display punitive attitudes towards the hunger striker. The psychiatrist is well placed to recognise and manage these reactions. Hunger strikes evoke responses in staff which may compromise appropriate management, and should be anticipated and discussed openly in team meetings. The interface with correctional staff may require clarification, and psychiatrists should make explicit to other staff – within the bounds of confidentiality – their ethical and legal obligations, and reasoning for their stance in the management of food refusal.

It is also true that other team members may provide valuable input. Some hunger strikers will eat surreptitiously or give their food to others; others will discuss their situation with trusted nurses or correctional staff; and the accounts of correctional staff are frequently crucial to diagnose occult psychosis, confirm that depressive symptoms are sustained and not intermittent, and describe interactions with others and the patient's self-care. Collateral history is important both within correctional institutions and outside, and the psychiatrist should assess all hunger strikers with careful reference to as many other sources of information as possible.

A number of authors have noted that assessment may be compromised by the presence of institutional staff (Kalk *et al.* 1993, Silove *et al.* 1996). The traditional impediments to good psychiatric practice in prisons may well be magnified, and psychiatrists must be firm in their boundaries. Where confidentiality and the doctor–patient relationship are compromised by institutional situations, the health service manager and the prison governor should promptly be notified. If the conditions of treatment imposed by the institution are impossible, one must – preferably in consultation with colleagues – discuss whether to withdraw from the treating role or whether to continue despite impediments to ethical practice. The issue of legal liability warrants discussion with one's indemnity organisation in these situations. Doctors are frequently in a remarkably powerful position to gather public support for a principled stance when frustrated by authorities. Indeed, much of the literature on hunger strikes has originated from doctors placed in awkward positions.

The first step in managing a prisoner who is refusing food is to determine if the patient has the capacity to make the decision to refuse food. If the food refusal is judged to be part of a mental disorder (see above) then it may be appropriate to transfer the patient to a psychiatric hospital under mental health legislation for further assessment and treatment, which could include artificial feeding. If he lacks capacity owing to physical disorder, then he should be transferred to a medical ward in a general hospital.

However, if the person is competent, he is entitled to refuse food and indeed any other treatment or intervention. If mental disorder has been excluded, one should consider alternative motives of the hunger striker (Reyes 1998). These may include:

- expressions of helplessness, powerlessness and frustration

- attention-seeking gestures – to publicise a cause or highlight distress

- bargaining through the threat of death by starvation

- attempts at suicide, rational or irrational

- protest at injustice or the perception of wrongful conviction or treatment.

The hunger striker should be advised that he will continue to receive medical supervision and be offered food. He must be informed that the authorities do not require the prison doctor to force-feed, so that medical intervention will only occur at the patient's request. It is important for the doctor to remain supportive, to assess the patient regularly and to maintain a dialogue. The patient should be able to cease voluntary total starvation if he chooses, without loss of face.

A sympathetic and thorough examination of the subjective situation of the hunger striker will aid in management. Solutions may exist which can be realised by the psychiatrist as intermediary, mediator or simply clarifier of the situation. The point is well made that solutions which save face may be missed in the oppositional environment of a custodial institution (Brockman 1999), and that psychiatrists may be perceived by prisoners and staff as outside these structures (Hinshelwood 1993). Doctors should, however, be clear on their position of advocacy and should be wary of being drawn in to a partisan position, rather than looking after the health interests of the prisoner.

It is important to clarify at an early stage the intentions of the hunger striker. Some will accept intravenous fluids, while others will reject all intervention from medical staff. Clarifying the exact nature and objective of the protest offers an opportunity for non-judgemental assessment and, in some cases, the building of rapport. The provision of value-neutral information about the consequences of various levels of food refusal may deter some hunger strikers and aid others to reduce the likelihood of permanent sequelae should they later cease food refusal.

In some group hunger strikes it may become apparent that individuals have varying degrees of commitment to the ends. Those who may seem coerced or swayed by the influence of their comrades warrant particular attention. Moving people to alternative locations in the ostensible interests of their health care may provide an opportunity for a more frank assessment uncompromised by the dynamics of a collective action, in which some participants may not be so keen on the consequences of a hunger strike but feel unable to disagree with the group (Oguz & Miles 2005).

Early assessment of hunger strikers is most crucial. Silove *et al.* (1996) pointed out that their experience (with Cambodian women in an Australian immigration detention centre) was made difficult by the strikers' fluctuating mental states, the need for interpreters, cultural differences and administrative confusion, as well as interference and bullying from officials linked to the immigration authorities. Forming an early understanding of the motives and attitudes of hunger strikers may pre-empt and prevent these added complications.

MANAGEMENT

The management of a hunger strike demands flexibility and daily review. It involves dealing not only with the striker but also with other staff, prison management and possibly the media and other professionals. Professional boundaries and an understanding of the ethical problems (confidentiality, split roles, etc.) faced in managing a hunger strike are crucial. Early planning, and the counsel of other psychiatrists, are likely to reduce the conflicts and anguish of this task. Comprehensive and contemporaneous documentation is, of course, crucial. It has been recommended that letters be written to the patient to clarify communications, and copies filed in the notes. Speaking to relatives, when possible, is also appropriate.

Physical complications of hunger strikes

The course of a hunger strike will be determined by the pre-existing physical status of the patient, as well as the nature of the strike. Refusing fluids is immediately hazardous to the prisoner and leads to rapid physical decline, as described by Emmeline Pankhurst of her experiences in 1913: "thirst strike…is from beginning to end simple and unmitigated torture" (Johannes Weir Foundation for Health and Human Rights 1995, p.16).

Sensations of thirst may be lost in hunger strikers, leading to rapid dehydration. Oral rehydration solution may be preferable to water in resuscitation, but electrolyte monitoring is strongly advised. Unbalanced glucose or sodium intake may lead to hypokalaemia with consequent metabolic complications.

Review of the literature suggests a mean of 63 days to death, with variation between 42 and 79 days (Johannes Weir Foundation for Health and Human Rights 1995). Other studies have suggested longer survivals, although these would appear to have been in prisoners with some limited nutritional intake. Weight loss is approximately 10kg per month, although it would appear that this loss depends upon the degree and nature of fluid intake. Lean patients will lose weight more rapidly than obese ones (Scobie 1987)! Fat loss is markedly greater than diminution in body mass index (BMI) might suggest. The metabolic effects of starvation are important to understand, particularly given the need to monitor competence. Immediate glucose supplies are exhausted within the first week, and alternative metabolic pathways become active, including gluconeogenesis (creating glucose from fat); relative hypoglycaemia (reflecting conservation of extracerebral glucose use); water and nitrogen retention renally; and ketone bodies increasingly being utilised by the brain. Once fat stores are exhausted, protein is catabolised for energy (Peel 1997). Post mortem findings in people who have died on hunger strike demonstrate effects on multiple organs and include tissue loss and depletion of fat stores (Altun *et al.* 2004).

The reported phases of hunger strikes are as follows (Miller 1986, Johannes Weir Foundation for Health and Human Rights 1995).

- First week: well tolerated, hunger subsides after some days, blood glucose drops.

- First month: orthostatic hypotension and bradycardia become apparent, along with fatigue, muscle pain and reduced mental alertness, and mild hypothermia.

- Approximately day 40: malaise, neurological signs, gastrointestinal complaints, extreme fatigue, bedridden.

- Moribund: euphoria or emotional lability, delirium, coma and death, often very rapid in progression (hours).

In those whose course is reversed, residual symptoms and marked disability may continue for months or irreversible sequelae may occur. Other complications, particularly decubitus ulcers, renal failure and Wernicke-Korsakoff Syndrome, have been noted. Recent evidence suggests that even in those complying with thiamine supplementation, neurological damage occurs: in one study of 41 prisoners on hunger strike for at least four months, all subjects demonstrated features of Wernicke-Korsakoff Syndrome despite taking 200–600mg of thiamine for substantial portions of the fast (Basoglu *et al.* 2006). Case studies describe other neurological complications, such as myelinololysis related to hypernatraemia (van der Helm-van Mil *et al.* 2005).

The risk of refeeding syndrome warrants sound nutritional advice when commencing feeding after prolonged fasting (Crook, Hally & Panteli 2001, Catani & Howells 2007). Wernicke's encephalopathy can also be precipitated by administering glucose and then thiamine: intravenous thiamine must be administered *prior* to oral or intravenous glucose. Kalk *et al.* (1993) report successful initial use of diluted lactose-free balanced feeding. One must also be cautious of fluid overload and the precipitation of heart failure with relatively small amounts of intravenous fluid. QTc prolongation, ventricular tachycardia and other arrhythmias have also been described (Peel 1997). Electrolyte disturbance is frequent and may occur one to two weeks after cessation of hunger strike. When David Blaine conducted a 44-day public fast as performance art in London, his refeeding was carefully conducted under endocrine and nutritional advice. He was noted to exhibit metabolic disturbance consistent with refeeding syndrome (hypophosphataemia and oedema) and his clinical supervisors documented carefully Blaine's metabolic and endocrine parameters (Korbonits *et al.* 2007).

Hunger strikers report subjective and distressing headache, faintness and dizziness; objectively, bradycardia and orthostatic hypotension account for these symptoms in clinical studies (Kalk *et al.* 1993). Abdominal pain was described in a majority of South African hunger strikers followed closely (Kalk *et al.* 1993). Weakness and cold sensations have been linked to impaired thyroid function due to reduced T3 and increased reverse T3 during fasting (Walsh 2001).

The physical management of hunger strikers involves regular blood tests to monitor renal function and electrolytes, and regular urinalysis. Consent should be sought in advance for this monitoring. One recommendation is that monitoring should commence after weight loss of 10%, after ten days, or with a BMI of under 16.5 kg/m². The same author noted that major problems arise after weight loss of about 18% (Peel 1997). Those with pre-existing medical problems may be prone to earlier complications. Other authors caution that serious complications may occur with even less weight loss, particularly in women.

Measurements and recording of daily weight, blood pressure, temperature and pulse rate are necessary. Tissue turgor is useful clinically to monitor the situation, and urinalysis may provide evidence of ketosis and of dehydration. Serum creatinine, urea and electrolytes may aid in appreciating the severity of the hunger striker's state. These results should be communicated to hunger strikers. It is important that they be provided with non-judgemental and clear advice on the consequences for their health, and with an opportunity to discuss their health with a doctor who can give clear advice. Complications should be communicated to the hunger striker and recommendations made for treatment. The competent hunger striker may refuse these suggestions and should accordingly be advised of future consequences should such refusal be maintained.

Mental status

An initial assessment should be thorough and explicitly address competence. The legal test in currency in many common law countries is the test of Re C., although other tests may operate in different jurisdictions or in the future. Most such tests require some determination of understanding, the ability to consider facts appropriately and to express a consistent choice.

The assessment of competence is dynamic and task-oriented. It should be reconsidered frequently, and second opinions routinely sought. Most important of all, while someone is competent there exists the opportunity to assess his or her preferences for future management. Rather than drawing up a binding document, the most crucial goal is to develop an understanding of the hunger striker and his or her situation. The key is not so much in a knowledge of psychopathology, but rather a capacity for rapport and empathy. It should also be noted that integral to assessment of competence is the provision of appropriate information. For hunger strikers, this involves a clear explanation of the potential consequences of hunger strike. In those unwilling to listen to such an explanation, it might be argued that the threshold for assessment of competence is reduced without proof of good understanding.

Mentally disordered patients can be managed, in most jurisdictions, by transfer to hospital and involuntary treatment under mental health legislation. The risk of deterioration in physical state renders these patients high priority. If mental health beds are not promptly available, general hospital beds should be accessed and the risks of delay made explicit. Repeated assessment should ensure that physical deterioration is pre-empted, and in all but the most extreme situations, security issues can be dealt with when transferring out to hospital; early liaison with prison management might prevent bureaucratic hurdles.

Alternatively, if incompetent but not falling under mental health legislation, guardianship or mental capacity legislation may enable treatment, often by appointment of a substitute decision-maker empowered to act in the person's best interests. In situations involving such decisions, legal advice should be sought urgently.

Management

The hunger striker will inevitably at some stage lose competence. The available options then alter, as the doctor is then entrusted with the care of an incompetent patient whose prior wishes become crucial, as do legal precedents in the doctor's jurisdiction. It is worth anticipating these issues from an early stage. Indeed, the Johannes Weir Foundation (1995) has provided significant direction in the practical negotiation of these issues.

One option is to appoint an independent "physician of confidence" with no links to the institution. This may preserve communication and ensure that staff do not feel compromised in managing hunger strikes. The chosen physician should have appropriate seniority and be perceived as independent by prisoner, staff and the public. They should be accepted as such by the hunger striker. They should be willing to take on such an awkward role. In some political environments, such a physician might not be available or their appointment may be resisted. Nevertheless, such a course of action is sensible.

Another option, proposed by Silove *et al.* (1996), is that of an advisory committee: the benefits they note are in the breadth of experience offered (including representation from appropriate cultural or political groupings), and in the gradual accumulation of expertise over time; but at the same time they note the limitations of such a response and point out that such a move may further complicate an already fraught situation.

The early negotiation of an advance directive (AD) may be most useful. An advance directive has, in different jurisdictions, some force at law. It can only be made by a competent person and its development should include an explicit, contemporaneous assessment of competence. How binding is such a decree, is related to the detail expressed. It relies upon the judgement of the interpreter, be they doctor or court, to determine whether the conditions anticipated in an AD are those encountered in reality; for the imagination of the maker may not encompass various situations. Kalk *et al.* (1993) raise the situation of a hypothetical hunger striker whose AD specifies no resuscitation, who then lapses into coma, before a subsequent general amnesty is announced. In such cases a condition not considered may render an AD invalid. Similarly, if one did not witness the drawing up of an AD, there should be a higher threshold to consider it valid. It is, however, clear that, at least in the UK, an AD is seen as quite binding (Re W.).

The doctor must also recognise that the advance directive, a confidential document, may be subject to great media and management interest in an advanced hunger strike. It is worth anticipating and discussing these issues openly with a hunger striker early on, in order to pre-empt the problems which may arise when the striker subsequently becomes incompetent.

Those hunger strikers who are first seen late in their strike, are incompetent, and have not previously been assessed, pose a difficult group. Unless there is clear and incontrovertible evidence of their competence and determination, it may be best to treat them in order to restore them to competence. There is a positive but rebuttable assumption at common law that doctors will act beneficently to their patients. It can also be argued that those wrongly treated and restored to competence may later resume their hunger strikes with added safeguards, should their resolve and inclination be unchanged.

If feeding is warranted, and considered necessary and medico-legally defensible, it should be undertaken safely. This requires cautious insertion of access (nasogastric, intravenous or, rarely, percutaneous entero-gastrostomy (PEG) and provision of appropriate alimentation. Both a nutritionist and physician knowledgeable of refeeding should be consulted. The risks are significant and feeding against a patient's will should not be undertaken lightly. There is a substantial body of literature and case law referring to such situations in patients with eating disorders, but little relating to prisoners (Dresser & Boisaubin 1986).

In some cases the hunger striker will be reluctant but caught up in a group protest. It is important that a doctor managing such a hunger striker be resolute in his or her duty to the patient, which may involve seeing the patient without witnesses in order to obtain true understanding of his or her resolve, and providing options for cessation. In other cases it may be necessary to separate the hunger striker from his or her colleagues so as to reduce the influence of others on a vulnerable or uncertain participant in a group action. The guiding principle should always be the doctor's duty to individual patients.

Overall, the keys to effective management of a hunger strike appear to lie in communication and good faith. Whatever efforts are necessary to establish communication are likely to be beneficial. Doctors who preserve their independence and act in the best interests of their patients are least likely to be compromised or to find themselves a pawn in the greater struggles of food refusal. Consultation with colleagues may provide support in difficult situations. Finally, an understanding of local law and of international instruments provides a solid bedrock for good practice and a defence against inevitable suggestions that management should have proceeded otherwise.

CHAPTER 16

Psychiatric Reports

Huw Stone

OVERVIEW

The majority of psychiatric medico-legal reports are prepared on individuals who have been charged with criminal offences. A significant number of these individuals will be held on remand in prison when the report is prepared. However, these are not the only type of reports undertaken by psychiatrists in prisons. The reports required of psychiatrists will vary depending on the type of prison. For example, in a remand prison the majority of reports will be needed for court proceedings, whereas in a lifer's prison they will be required for parole board reviews. The types of psychiatric reports that may be requested include the following.

1. *Pre-trial court reports*, which address legal issues such as fitness to plead, legal insanity and, in the case of charges of murder, diminished responsibility and provocation.

2. *Sentencing reports for court.* Most are requested by magistrates courts which believe that the defendant may have a mental disorder and want some information about his or her mental health to inform their decision on disposal. This often necessitates a lengthy period on remand in prison. The Crown courts usually require reports to address detention under the Mental Health Act or to assist the judge in deciding whether a longer than normal sentence is appropriate.

3. *Parole board/discretionary lifer reports.* Whilst it is not mandatory to have a psychiatric report for each Parole Board or Discretionary Lifer Panel hearing, they are often provided.

4. *Reports for review of Category A status of prisoners.* Prison rules state that the review of a prisoner's Category A status can include a psychiatric report. This should address principally the effect on the prisoner's mental health of continuing as a Category A prisoner. It should not make recommendations for the continuation of his or her Category A status.

5. *Medical reports* are required for adjudications within prison, usually carried out by the Governor or one of his or her deputies. Occasionally such reports might include psychiatric factors. The purpose of these reports is to assess fitness to be punished. This clearly raises a number of important ethical issues, not least the involvement of doctors in prison discipline.

6. *Reports in relation to detention under the Mental Health Act 1983 (amended 2007).* These are statutorily required reports for assessment under Section 35, 36 and 38, and sentencing under Section 37 of the Mental Health Act. In addition, psychiatric reports are required by the Mental Health Unit of the Home Office in relation to transfer to psychiatric hospitals, under Section 48 for unsentenced prisoners and Section 47 for sentenced prisoners. Over the past 15 years there has been a significant increase in reporting under these sections of the Mental Health Act and the total number of transfers from prison under both sections has increased from 218 in 1989 to 968 in 2007 (Ministry of Justice 2009).

7. *The primary care service in the prison* will often refer prisoners for a psychiatric assessment to ask for advice on their treatment needs in prison.

8. *Reports for coroner's court.* Psychiatric reports may be required by the coroner in cases of suspected suicide, where the prisoner may have had contact with psychiatrists during their prison sentence.

As the above list indicates, the psychiatrist undertaking reports on prisoners in prison can have several different roles, and all of these can lead to potential conflicts of interests. Reports prepared by psychiatrists who work as part of a mental health inreach team in prisons can cause a conflict of interest where the psychiatrist is providing both treatment within prison and reports to the court and/or Parole Board. Other issues which challenge the ethical framework within which all psychiatrists are expected to work include the provision of risk assessments on prisoners who do not suffer from mental disorder, but such assessments are required by statute when the court is considering passing a longer than normal sentence.

There is often a conflict between the psychiatrist's duty to the patient, which includes those prisoners referred for assessment only, versus his or her duty to the courts or Parole Board or Prison Service. Any psychiatrist working in a prison will frequently come across examples of this conflict, including the attempted use of psychiatric assessments and reports to allow a prison to transfer a prisoner to another prison because they feel that they cannot manage that individual. Such a transfer may not be necessarily in the patient's own interests and it is crucial that the psychiatrist makes clear his or her opinion of what is in the best interests of the patient. However, this conflict between duty to the patient and duty to the body commissioning the report can also lead to problems with partiality of reports, where psychiatrists are often forced into the position of either the defence or the prosecution's expert and therefore are expected to support either side's particular legal strategy.

It is also important to remember that the adversarial legal system that exists within the criminal courts also extends to the Parole Board and Discretionary Lifer Panels. Last, a slightly less common but nevertheless important area of conflict of interest is one where psychiatrists assess prisoners who deny their offences and may be possible victims of miscarriages of justice. Although the Parole Board has stated that prisoners who deny their offence cannot be refused parole solely because of that denial, it is extremely difficult for a psychiatrist to comment on a prisoner's risk of re-offending when the prisoner denies that he or she has committed the offence, which may be the only evidence of risk to others.

QUALITIES OF A GOOD REPORT

Despite the number of reviews and book chapters (Bluglass 1995, Grounds 2000, Stone *et al.* 2000) concerned with preparing reports for the psychiatric courts, these have paid scant attention to the quality of the reports, with one exception (Bowden 1990). While the issue of admissibility of expert evidence is often an issue in the criminal courts, judgements are not made concerning the quality of an individual report, or indeed the quality of the expert preparing the report. Before considering the qualities of a medico-legal report, it is instructive to consider what would constitute a good expert report from any field, not just medicine.

The key stages in the preparation of any report are:

- research
- planning
- writing
- revision.

If the quality of any one of these stages is poor, then the whole report will suffer.

Research

Any report will only be as good as the actual material on which it is based. It therefore follows that all information contained within the report should be validated or, if this is not possible, this should be clearly stated. When preparing reports for the criminal courts, reading the original witness statements in full is essential, rather than reading only a case summary prepared by a police officer or solicitor. All relevant documentation should be obtained before interviewing the subject, which will comprise, as a minimum, the depositions, including the indictment, witness statements, transcripts of interviews and the unused material. If relevant, past psychiatric records, reports and general practice records must be obtained, in addition to probation and/or social services records. However, the most important part of the research for a medico-legal report is the interview with the patient. The setting and timing of the interview is crucial, as is the allowing of sufficient time for the interview, while taking into account the availability of the subject, particularly when he or she is in prison. It may be necessary also to interview an informant, to confirm the patient's background history and provide additional information.

Planning

Before writing the report it is important to draw up a plan. This should include the fact that all relevant information has been collected and reviewed. The report will obviously have to address the reason why it was requested and the stated purpose of the report. As noted earlier, there are many reasons why a psychiatric court report is requested. Therefore, in all medico-legal reports it is essential to obtain a detailed letter of instruction from the person who is requesting the report. This should include:

- the issues to be addressed
- the location of the patient
- time scale for preparing the report
- who will read the report.

Writing

A suggested format for ensuring the quality of any type of expert report is the "ABC" system: **A**ccuracy, **B**revity and **C**larity.

ACCURACY

The facts relied on in the report that lead to the opinion must be correct. All relevant facts should be included, not only those that support the writer's opinion.

BREVITY

Include only the necessary and relevant facts. Do not repeat sections of the report or repeat verbatim parts of the depositions and other papers which are available to all those concerned in the case. Keep language to that which is brief and to the point, using short sentences and short paragraphs. Remember any report is a summary, and therefore a distillation of the facts and an opinion. It is not a verbatim account of the whole case, so it is not necessary to quote large sections of material. The simple fact is that long reports are not read and they suggest that the writer has been unable to synthesise the information and come to a succinct opinion.

CLARITY

Avoid making subjective comments, for example, "he claimed that…" As Bowden (1990) notes, technical words should be avoided or, if this is impossible, then definitions should also be given. He goes on to say "clichés should be avoided as should extraneous and sometimes flippant or derogatory information, which is not relevant to the gist of the report" (Bowden 1990, p.187).

Revision

Checking and proof reading is one of the most important stages of preparing a psychiatric court report. This is because both the quality and the credibility of the report (and its writer) are affected by obvious typographical errors.

Format

A variety of different formats for reports have been suggested (Bowden 1990, Bluglass 1995, Grounds 2000, Stone et al. 2000). While there is no one agreed format for medico-legal psychiatric reports, a number of principles appear to be accepted (Box 16.1). It is good practice to use headings to break up the text of the report. Some writers suggest 1.5 to double spacing, and the use of numbered paragraphs to help barristers refer to specific sections of the report in court.

The role of the psychiatrist in preparing a report to the court is as an expert witness, and as such he or she is instructed to give an expert opinion, not just provide facts (O'Grady 2004). It therefore follows from this that the opinion is the most important part of the report, and all other information should support that opinion and should be provided in an accurate and brief form. However, this does not mean that information that might contradict the opinion should be excluded. If it is relevant, the report writer should balance the conflicting facts before reaching a final opinion.

Box 16.1 Suggested format for psychiatric report

Introduction: who commissioned the report and for what purpose.

Sources of information:

- interview with patient
- documentation read
- interviews with informants.

Confirm that the limits of confidentiality have been explained and understood.

Defendant's account of the index offence: include any inconsistencies with other evidence or information from the depositions.

Background History:

- family and personal history
- past medical and psychiatric history (including substance abuse)
- past criminal history.

State whether validated from independent sources.

Mental state examination

Opinion and recommendations:

- diagnosis and relevant past psychiatric history
- current mental state
- legal issues (fitness to plead, legal insanity, diminished responsibility, etc. where relevant)
- prognosis of mental disorder
- recommendations for treatment
- medical disposal:
  - how this will be provided and by whom
  - that a bed is available in an appropriate level of security
  - refer to appropriate criteria for detention under the Mental Health Act.

LEGAL ISSUES

Introduction

It is essential to understand the legal issues that arise during the course of preparing a psychiatric report to the courts. However, it is important to remember that psychiatrists prepare reports as doctors and not lawyers. Although the following covers quite complex legal issues, some of which bear little resemblance to psychiatric concepts, all psychiatrists should prepare reports based on their training and experience as clinicians, first and foremost. Although the law has a number of different definitions for mental disorder within statute and case law, psychiatrists should use the diagnostic system with which they are most familiar (in practice this is usually either ICD10 (World Health Organisation 1992) or DSM-IV (American Psychiatric Association 1994)). It is the job of the lawyers and the judge, and not the psychiatrist, to make psychiatric concepts fit legal ones. Legal case law makes it clear that psychiatrists should only give evidence on mental disorder suffered by defendants and should not comment on how a normal person would react to a particular set of circumstances (R v Turner).

Although psychiatrists give evidence as expert witnesses, they still have to keep to the rules of evidence. This principally concerns the inadmissibility of hearsay evidence, which presents psychiatrists with considerable problems, since good psychiatric practice includes interviewing informants. Theoretically, such information, if included in a report, could be inadmissible on the grounds that it is hearsay evidence. However, most, but not all, judges appear to accept that a competent psychiatric assessment should include interviewing informants. Further legal problems arise when an informant may also be a witness in the defendant's case. In such circumstances, it is advisable to discuss this issue with the person who has instructed the report.

The trial process and psychiatric reports to court

A detailed account of the trial process is beyond the scope of this chapter; however, an up-to-date account can be found in the guide to the Criminal Justice System produced by the Home Office (2000a). It may be helpful to consider the various psychiatric issues that might arise in preparing a psychiatric report according to the various stages of the trial process: pre-trial, trial and sentencing. A psychiatric report on the same defendant would have a different emphasis depending on the legal stage at which it is requested. For example, the issue of fitness to plead would not normally be relevant to a report required at the sentencing stage after conviction. For a detailed account of the various psychiatric defences see Mackay (1995).

PRE-TRIAL ISSUES

The principal medico-legal issue at this stage is that of fitness to plead. The criteria for fitness to plead were derived over 150 years ago in the case of a deaf and dumb man who was charged with bestiality (Box 16.2).

Box 16.2 Fitness to plead criteria

Whether the defendant has sufficient intellect to:

- instruct his solicitor and counsel

- plead to the indictment

- challenge jurors

- understand the evidence

- give evidence.

(R v Pritchard)

A number of practice issues arise when considering these criteria. It has been suggested that, rather than considering the concept of fitness to plead, it is better to assess whether the defendant has the ability "to participate to the requisite extent in any necessary trial process" (Archbold 1998, p.341). This will depend on the complexity of the trial and the nature of the alleged offences. Situations have arisen where a defendant is judged to be fit to plead in a trial involving only a guilty plea, yet not fit to plead in a fully contested trial.

One particular problem with the criteria, which probably arises from the fact that they were drawn up in the case of a man who did not have a mental disorder, is the fact that there is no requirement that the defendant suffers from a mental disorder. In practice, particular problems can arise in patients with borderline learning disability, specific reading/language disorders and anxiety disorders. Finally, the legal test is essentially a cognitive test. An example is the criterion of understanding the evidence, but there is no doubt that even the most floridly unwell patient with schizophrenia may, at a cognitive level, understand the evidence against him and will therefore be fit to plead, even though his particular psychopathology may seriously affect his belief in the evidence against him. Using these criteria the severely mentally ill may be judged fit to plead – yet their mental illness would seriously impair their ability to take part in the trial process to the requisite extent. The fact that a defendant may not be able to act in his own best interests does not make him unfit to plead.

The implementation of the Domestic Violence, Crime and Victims Act 2004 has led to significant changes both in the court procedure for determining fitness to plead and the disposal of defendants found unfit to plead. The finding of being unfit to plead according to the above criteria is now made by the judge in the Crown court, not by the jury. If the defendant is found unfit to plead, a special jury is empanelled to decide whether he or she actually committed the acts that led to the offence. This is referred to as a "trial of the facts". It is not a finding of guilt.

The disposal of defendants who have been found to have committed the acts has also been changed by the Domestic Violence, Crime and Victims Act 2004 (Box 16.3).

Box 16.3 Disposal following a finding of insanity or unfitness to plead

- Hospital Order (S 37)+/- Restriction Order (S 41) – if fulfils criteria for detention under MHA

- Supervision Order – allows treatment for physical and/or mental disorder

- Absolute discharge

Domestic Violence, Crime and Victims Act 2004

First, the decision whether to admit the defendant to hospital is now made by the court, rather than the Secretary of State at the Home Office. Second, before making a hospital order under Section 37 of the Mental Health Act 1983 (amended 2007), the court will have to have two medical recommendations supporting that disposal in the usual way. In practice, this means that defendants found unfit to plead can now only be admitted to hospital under the Mental Health Act if they fulfil the criteria for detention under that Act. The court can now order the defendant to be admitted to a specific hospital (unlike in the usual use of a hospital order). The judge can also add a restriction order under Section 41 of the Mental Health Act, and this will continue to be mandatory where the charge was murder.

The remaining two disposal options for defendants found unfit to plead are either a supervision order or an absolute discharge. A supervision order can now be made to provide treatment for physical as well as mental disorders and can no longer include a requirement that the defendant should be admitted to hospital without his or her consent. There continues to be no sanction resulting from breach of the supervision order.

TRIAL ISSUES – LEGAL INSANITY

This is determined by the McNaughten Rules, which state:

> at the time of the committing of the act, the party accused was labouring under such a defect of reason, from disease of the mind, as not to know the nature and quality of the act he was doing; or, if he did know it, that he did not know he was doing what was wrong. (McNaughten Rules)

Most psychiatrists agree that these criteria are so stringent that few mentally disordered offenders will fulfil them. The issue is most often raised during cases of possible "automatism". This is an example in which a legal concept of mental disorder bears little relevance to psychiatry. "Automatism" is legally defined as either insane or non-insane. The difference between the two is determined according to whether the cause of the automatism arose from within the person (for example, post-epileptic automatism) or from outside (for example, post-head injury automatism). The difference is quite significant, since a defendant found to have committed an offence during an insane automatism will fulfil the McNaughten Rules and therefore be found not guilty by reason of insanity, and his disposal will be under the Domestic Violence, Crime and Victims Act 2004 (see Box 16.3). However, if the defendant was found to have a non-insane automatism at the time of committing an offence, he or she would receive an acquittal.

TRIAL ISSUES SPECIFIC TO THE CHARGE OF MURDER – DIMINISHED RESPONSIBILITY

Section 2 of the Homicide Act 1957 reduces murder to manslaughter where there is an:

> abnormality of mind (whether arising from arrested or retarded development of mind, disease or injury or other inherent cause) as substantially impaired [his] mental responsibility.

The defence of diminished responsibility only continues to exist because of the mandatory life sentence for murder. If this were abolished, psychiatrists could provide reports at the sentencing stage, as they do for all other offences. Instead they are asked to fit psychiatric concepts of mental disorder into legal definitions which bear no resemblance to accepted diagnostic criteria (Prison Reform Trust 1994).

TRIAL ISSUES SPECIFIC TO THE CHARGE OF MURDER – PROVOCATION

Section 3 of the Homicide Act 1957 allows the charge of murder to be reduced to manslaughter if the defendant was provoked "whether by things done or by things said or by both together" to lose his self-control. The jury has to determine whether a "reasonable man" would have been provoked to lose his self-control. In order to do so, the jury has to answer two questions:

- Was the defendant provoked to lose his self-control?

- Was the provocation enough to make a reasonable man do as he did?

In answering the second question, the jury is asked to endow the reasonable man with the "relevant characteristics" of the defendant. In practice these include the age, sex and other personal characteristics. The jury uses these characteristics to assess the gravity of the provocation and the degree of self-control that the defendant would have been expected to show. Case law has determined that the relevant characteristics have to be significant enough to be different and permanent. It is not expected they will include exceptional excitability, pugnacity, ill temper or drunkenness. The provocation also has to be connected to these characteristics, but no longer has to immediately precede the loss of self-control. Previously psychiatric evidence was excluded from this partial defence. However, following a number of cases, including a number of "battered women" cases, it is now accepted that psychiatric factors can be taken into account by the jury (Mackay 1995, R v Smith).

TRIAL ISSUES SPECIFIC TO THE CHARGE OF MURDER – INFANTICIDE

This is a partial defence to murder which allows a finding of guilt to infanticide which is defined by the Infanticide Act 1938 as:

> where a woman…causes the death of her child under the age of 12 months, but the balance of her mind was disturbed by reason of not having fully recovered from the effect of giving birth or by reason of the effect of lactation consequent of the birth of the child, then she shall be guilty of infanticide.

A psychiatric report in these circumstances should address the mental state of the woman – for example, whether she suffered postnatal depression or psychosis. If this plea is successful, then the woman is dealt with as if she had been convicted of manslaughter. In practice the courts rarely sentence women convicted of infanticide to prison.

Sentencing

A mentally disordered offender may be sentenced to a hospital order under Section 37 of the Mental Health Act if he has been convicted of an offence punishable with imprisonment and if at the time that he is sentenced, he is suffering from a mental disorder as defined in Section 1. Finally, the judge must be satisfied that, after taking into account the offence, his antecedents and other methods of dealing with him that a hospital order is "the most suitable method of disposing of the case". The mental disorder need not have been present at the time of the offence. A restriction order under Section 41 of the Mental Health Act may be added at the judge's discretion after hearing medical evidence, but he does not have to agree with that evidence. Another option is the hospital direction order under Section 45A of the Mental Health Act that was introduced by the Crime Sentences Act 1997. This is often referred to as the "hybrid order" (Box 16.4).

Box 16.4 Section 45A Mental Health Act 1983 (hospital direction order)

- The court must first consider whether to make a hospital order (S37).

- Admitted to hospital as if detained under a hospital order, but subsequently managed as if on a prison transfer.

- When the patient no longer requires treatment in hospital, he is transferred to prison to complete his sentence.

Mentally disordered offenders who do not fall within the Mental Health Act and are not given a custodial sentence may be treated in the community, either informally or as a requirement of a community order under the Criminal Justice Act 2003. There are 12 different requirements that can be added to a community order, including drug rehabilitation, alcohol treatment and mental health treatment. All of these require the consent of the offender. A community order should only be recommended after discussion with the probation officer preparing the pre-sentence report for the court. This legislation, which was implemented in April 2005, will have far-reaching effects on the sentencing of all offenders. It remains to be seen whether the role of the psychiatrist in assessing and managing non-mentally disordered offenders will increase because of the new public protection sentences for dangerous offenders introduced by this Act.

Summary

Psychiatrists preparing reports to the criminal courts should be aware of the following issues.

- They are acting as clinicians, not lawyers.

- The legal definitions of mental disorder are not the same as clinical definitions.

- The law expects an unequivocal answer.

- It is an adversarial legal system.

- They should keep within their own area of expertise.

THE ROLE OF THE EXPERT WITNESS

The General Medical Council (GMC) (2008) has produced guidance on acting as an expert witness. This defines the role of an expert witness in the following terms: "The role of an expert witness is to assist the court on specialist or technical matters within their expertise. The expert's duty to the court overrides any obligation to the person who is instructing or paying them" (GMC 2008, para. 5). The GMC guidance states that an expert witness should provide a balanced opinion which is within the limits of his or her professional competence and about which the expert has relevant knowledge or direct experience. One area of difficulty is where experts stray away from the area of expertise and express opinions for which they are not qualified. However, psychiatrists can only give expert evidence where the defendant has a mental disorder; this was established by L.J. Lawton:

> Jurors do not need psychiatrists to tell them how ordinary folk who are not suffering from mental illness are likely to react to the stresses and strains of everyday life. (R v Turner)

The GMC (2008) advice to experts is summarised in Box 16.5. It is essential, when a psychiatrist accepts instructions for a report, that he or she has the appropriate training, knowledge and expertise to undertake it. For example, a general adult psychiatrist may not necessarily have had the training or experience to undertake more complex medico-legal cases, such as diminished responsibility or involving defendants who have a learning disability or who are under 18 years of age. The issue of trainees undertaking reports is covered later. Other issues relating to the role of expert witness, including independence, impartiality and the admissibility of evidence, are also discussed later.

Box 16.5 Acting as an expert (General Medical Council 2008)

When giving expert advice and evidence:

- understand exactly what questions are being asked

- in evidence or reports, restrict statements to areas in which you have relevant knowledge or direct experience

- you must give a balanced opinion that falls within the limits of your professional competence

- any report or evidence given must be accurate, must not be misleading, and must include all relevant information

- if you have not examined the subject, justify and explain the limitations of your opinion

- you must be honest, trustworthy, objective and impartial.

PSYCHIATRIC REPORTS REQUIRED WITHIN PRISON

Psychiatric reports required within prison are often provided by psychiatrists working as part of a mental health inreach team in the prison. These psychiatrists have a dual role: they provide psychiatric advice to the primary care service in the prison, and also provide a number of different types of report. Reed (2002) has noted that previously a "significant minority" of these reports were of much lower quality. He went on to say that some were so bad that as a psychiatrist he was embarrassed to read them. One of the causes of the poor quality of these reports is undoubtedly the lack of any clear direction from either the Prison Service or other Home Office departments, e.g. the Parole Board, as to the content and format of these reports. Reports requested from psychiatrists working in prisons may include the following.

Diversion from custody of mentally disordered offenders

This can occur at several levels, from psychiatric assessment following the arrest of a suspect at the police station, to transfer from prison to a psychiatric hospital when on remand or sentenced (Humphreys 2000, Birmingham 2001a). In areas where it is not practical to have a diversion scheme based at the local magistrates courts, a request is often made to the local remand prison for a psychiatric report on defendants who are thought to have a mental disorder. The expectation is that a consultant psychiatrist will prepare the report. However, this can often result in unnecessary delays that prolong the defendant's time in custody. Some courts and services have developed local protocols, which can help to reduce the time on remand (Vaughan 2004). Such protocols could also reduce the need for adjournments for psychiatric reports to be prepared, which, as a Home Office study (1997) has shown, is the second commonest reason for adjournments in the magistrates courts.

A further level of diversion takes place when psychiatric reports are requested under Section 48 and Section 47 of the Mental Health Act 1983 (as amended by the Mental Health Act 2007) for remand and sentenced prisoners respectively. However, situations have occurred when psychiatrists have been under pressure to transfer a sentenced prisoner under Section 47 close to his or her earliest date of release (EDR). Some have described this as a form of "double jeopardy" (Royal College of Psychiatrists 2004c). One possible reason for these cases is the assessment of the risk, which is part of the Multi-Agency Public Protection Arrangements (MAPPA) that is undertaken close to the prisoner's release date. The Mental Health Unit of the Home Office may then choose to direct the prisoner's admission to hospital under the Mental Health Act, including to the new Dangerous and Severe Personality Disorder (DSPD) Treatment Units.

Parole reports

Very little has been written about the psychiatric reports required for Parole Board reviews. Under the Criminal Justice Act 2003, release on licence at the halfway point is

---

Box 16.6 Information requested from Prison Mental Health Inreach teams by Magistrates Courts (Wessex Consortium 2003)

- Mental health history

- Known risks associated with mental health problems

- Details of those currently involved in the care

- Any agreed care package

- Substance misuse issues

- Additional relevant information

---

automatic for prisoners serving standard determinate sentences of 12 months or more. However, the release of mandatory life-sentenced prisoners is still decided by the Parole Board. Discretionary life-sentenced prisoners are dealt with by Discretionary Lifer Panels (DLP) of the Parole Board, which are held at the prison. The DLP are modelled on Mental Health Review Tribunals. The prisoner is legally represented and a psychiatrist may be commissioned by the solicitor to provide an independent psychiatric report and possibly give evidence at the hearing. The psychiatrist working in the prison may also provide a psychiatric report. However, there are no specific rules concerning which prisoners require a psychiatric report be prepared.

Lifers: A Joint Thematic Review (HM Inspectorate of Prisons and Probation 1999) considered psychiatric reports for parole, scrutinising the Life Sentence Plans (LSPs) from 233 prison files. They found that in a fifth of cases the LSP included fully completed psychiatric evaluations. The review noted that general adult psychiatrists completed the majority of psychiatric reports for Parole Board purposes. They went on to state that the reports written by non-forensic psychiatrists added little to the understanding of the case. They were of the opinion that only forensic psychiatrists were likely to have received the necessary training to produce the type of reports required. Following this, one of their recommendations was that "the Prison Service should specify the circumstances in which a psychiatrist's report is necessary and ensure that these are supplied by a suitably qualified forensic psychiatrist to a specified format" (HM Inspectorate of Prisons and Probation 1999, para. 7.34). In 2001 the comprehensive review of parole and lifer processes noted concerns about arrangements for obtaining psychiatric reports for appropriate cases (HM Prison Service 2001). They also echoed the concerns about the quality of these reports noted above. The review stated that the Prison Service was taking forward proposals agreed at the ministerial level for the establishment of a national panel of Risk Assessment Doctors who would prepare these reports in future.

They recommended that monitoring of these new arrangements would be required when they were implemented.

Helpful advice on preparing parole reports was provided in a document giving guidance on the confidential use of health information, produced by the Prison Service in 2002 (HM Prison Service 2002). The document noted that medical reports make a "valuable contribution" to the decision-making of the Parole Board. It was suggested that in order to be "ethically correct" when preparing such reports, the doctor should:

- obtain the prisoner's consent to prepare the report and if this is not given, then the report should state this fact. The report should not contain any information obtained by that doctor during the usual privileged doctor–patient relationship

- only include information which is relevant to the purpose of the report. The document suggests that a comprehensive history would not normally be relevant to a parole report

- not include extracts or copies of documents from the Inmate Medical Record except in the case of disclosed pre-trial reports. But, as a recent legal case has shown (Cornelius v De Taranto), there may still be limits to the disclosure of reports instructed by the defence.

A specific ethical dilemma can arise when the prisoner denies having committed the original offence. This causes particular difficulties, since the information on which the psychiatrist will be relying in his or her risk assessment will derive mainly from the prisoner's account of the index offence and the assessment of his current attitude towards it. Also, the offence-related work is crucial to reducing the risk that a prisoner may pose when released. Although psychiatrists are often advised to tell prisoners that, as far as they are concerned, they have to accept the court's verdict that the person was found guilty of the offence, the number of recent miscarriages of justice which have resulted in the sudden release of prisoners who have served lengthy periods of imprisonment calls into question whether this is an acceptable response to prisoners who state that they have not committed the offence for which they have been convicted.

REVIEW OF CATEGORY A STATUS PRISONERS

Prison Service Order 1010 (HM Prison Service 2004a) recommends that reports which are prepared to inform the review of the security of Category A prisoners may include reports from a psychiatrist. In these circumstances, the report should include the prisoner's psychiatric history and details of the prisoner's contact with psychiatric services during the period of the review. It also requests the following: "please give details and attach reports where possible, subject to medical confidentiality" (HM Prison Service 2004a, Section 4). However, it does not expand further on the issues of confidentiality, and even the guidance on confidentiality issued in 2002 (HM Prison Service 2002) does not specifically refer to this situation. The order states that none of the report writers should make recommendations regarding the change in security category.

Adjudication Reports

The Prison Service considers that it is appropriate for medical information to be required for adjudication hearings. However, some might argue that medical involvement in the discipline and punishment of prisoners has had a long and at times shameful history, which extended up until the twentieth century (Sim 1990). This role is still evident in medical officers' involvement in the examination of prisoners for their "fitness to be punished". The Prison Service advice on confidentiality does not state that the consent of the prisoner is required for the preparation of these reports. However, it does recommend that only information relevant to the adjudication should be included in the report. It is possible that the psychiatrist may be asked to comment, and this raises considerable ethical issues. The reverse argument is that if the psychiatrist does not prepare a report, then this may result in a mentally disordered prisoner being inappropriately punished, if information on his or her mental condition is withheld from the prison governor.

Multi-Agency Public Protection Arrangements (MAPPA)

MAPPA were introduced by the Public Protection Unit of the Home Office to reduce the risk to the public from violent and sexual offenders. The Prison Service, Probation Service and police make up the responsible authority with whom health services have a statutory duty to co-operate. The main group of offenders subject to MAPPA are those about to be released from prison. Psychiatrists may be involved in assessing these prisoners prior to their release and recommending whether psychiatrists in the local catchment area should be involved in their risk management in the community. Useful guidelines on psychiatrists' involvement in MAPPA, including confidentiality issues, are provided by the Royal College of Psychiatrists (2004b).

ETHICS AND REPORT WRITING

Twenty years ago Chiswick (1985) raised a number of important ethical considerations which have to be addressed when preparing psychiatric court reports, and which are still of relevance today. First, he noted that this situation did not constitute the usual patient–doctor consultation, as "doctors' customary concerns for medical welfare of the individual become secondary to the doctor's principal obligation which is to the referring agent who requests and funds the report" (Chiswick 1985, p.975). In order to approach this subject in as ethical a way as possible, he suggested warning the patient of his or her right to silence, and if, after assessing the patient's capacity to consent to the examination, the psychiatrist does not believe that the patient has such a capacity, then the psychiatrist should end the consultation immediately. Chiswick (1985) stated that psychiatrists undertaking this type of medico-legal work were not acting as physicians but as "hired agents", and that the information divulged by the patient was not confidential – a position that has sometimes been called "the forensicist" position.

Second, Chiswick raised concerns that so-called "experts"were not measured against a professional standard, and might be drawn to the legal arena for personal motivation such as money or fame. Joseph (1998) raised similar concerns about the partiality of experts, particularly those who predominantly prepare opinions for one side. From personal experience, it is clear that this is most likely to occur with defence-instructed experts, because the prosecution has to disclose all evidence which may assist the defence. This can include a psychiatric report that the prosecution has instructed, but which they are not intending to rely on because they do not believe that it will support the prosecution case; however, it might support the defence case. In these circumstances the defence are able to call the expert. It is rare that the reverse occurs. The issue of who instructed the report and to whom the report writer owes a duty is most clearly evident in the case of reports to the Parole Board. Reports are prepared by psychiatrists at the request of the Home Office, via the prison. The prisoner can also initiate an independent report via his or her own solicitor.

I would suggest that in all situations, the expert's duty should be to the defendant/ offender. It is instructive to consider a quote from Scott (1953) written over 50 years ago:

> Insofar as this matter can be summarised, the psychiatrist's report to the court should be clearly understandable, accurate, logical, modest, and appearing to be made by a physician and therefore by one who is impartial and genuinely concerned with the welfare of the offender. (Scott 1953, p.97)

The effect of psychiatric reports on sentencing defendants

Bowden (1990) observed that negative comments in psychiatric reports, including comments about treatability, compliance and co-operation, were likely to influence the courts, which would then use them to justify a punitive sentence. He advised against doctors making comments about custodial sentences in reports, unless it was to advise the courts on the inappropriateness of such a disposal. However, ever since the leading case of R v Hodgson the presence of mental abnormality that is considered untreatable has been one of the criteria for imposing a discretionary life sentence. Smith (1998), in a study of 20 such cases, found that where a psychiatrist states that the defendant has a psychopathic disorder that is untreatable, this almost inevitably would lead to a life sentence. The introduction of the Criminal Justice Act in 1991 introduced the concept of the "longer than normal sentence" and Solomka (1996) has shown that the length of sentence is influenced by the psychiatric reports which must be obtained by the court before passing such a sentence. The psychiatric report is expected to focus on the risk assessment of defendants, but since they frequently have no mental disorder, is this an appropriate role for a psychiatrist, and how does it fit with Lord Justice Lawton's judgement from 1975 in R v Turner? Guidance following the introduction of the Powers of Criminal Courts (Sentencing) Act 2000 has taken this further with the suggestion that psychiatric evidence will assist the courts to determine the "correct" sentence. As Padfield (2000) has observed, such psychiatric evidence is often later used by the Parole Board to justify not releasing the defendant.

The Royal College of Psychiatrists (2004c) has suggested that ethical problems arise because of the dual roles of forensic psychiatrists, with their catchment area role (which includes controlling access to secure psychiatric facilities) and their role as expert witnesses in courts. In addition the Multi-Agency Public Protection Arrangements (MAPPA) referred to earlier expect that mental health services will be actively involved in risk decisions about offenders in the community.

Confidentiality Issues

These issues are particularly pertinent to a prison setting, where psychiatric reports often find their way into the main prison file, probation records, psychology files and other non-medical documentation. However, the Data Protection Act has put all of these issues into a sharper focus, not least because of the need to justify keeping of any reports and documentation, which should only be kept for as long as they are needed. On the question of disclosure of reports, once again there is a difference between those psychiatric reports instructed by the defence solicitor at the time of trial and those instructed by the prosecution. The former reports are considered privileged and cannot be disclosed to third parties without the consent of the patient and/or his or her solicitor. However, how often are pre-trial psychiatric reports found in the Inmate Medical Record without clear evidence of consent for disclosure? One practical consequence is the need to make clear to the defendant/prisoner the limits of confidentiality which arise, particularly when the expert is instructed by the prosecution or the Home Office (in the case of parole reports). It is also important to document that this has been explained to the defendant/prisoner and that he or she has agreed with it.

However, a person's right to confidentiality can be overridden in certain clearly defined circumstances (Royal College of Psychiatrists 2000, General Medical Council 2001, HM Prison Service 2002), principally for the reason of preventing serious harm. While the need to obtain consent from the subject of a report (or from his solicitor) is necessary when the defence has commissioned the report, it has not been established that the same duty exists in relation to reports for public bodies such as the Crown Prosecution Service or Home Office (on behalf of the Parole Board).

The Royal College of Psychiatrists' (2000) advice to psychiatrists who prepare psychiatric reports states that the issue of confidentiality differs between those reports requested on patients who are known to the psychiatrist and those on patients not previously known. In the former, while the patient's consent is not required for statutory reports, such as the Mental Health Review Tribunal (MHRT), it is required for other medico-legal reports. In the latter case, the patient may have disclosed information that he or she might have withheld if it was to be used for legal purposes, and in this situation, if the patient does not consent to its disclosure, the psychiatrist should consider whether to proceed with the report. In reports on patients who are previously unknown to him or her, the psychiatrist should not only obtain their consent, but should warn the patient about the limits of confidentiality and who else may see the report. Finally, the Royal College of Psychiatrists advises that any report for the patient's solicitor should not be disclosed to a third party without either the patient's or his or her solicitor's consent, except in the circumstances described above.

Partiality of reports

Joseph (1998) clearly believes that partiality or, to use his word, bias is inevitable in the current Criminal Justice System. Coles (2000) has also acknowledged that bias in reports is a fact and is "widely accepted" by those undertaking such work. As well as being a significant ethical issue that arises when preparing reports for the courts, partiality can also be relevant in the preparation of reports on prisoners for the Parole Board. One suggested way to avoid becoming biased is to make a practice of preparing reports for the court on behalf of both the Crown Prosecution Service and the defence, at different times, and not always for the same side. When preparing reports one should always bear in mind the need to reach the same conclusion regarding the defendant/offender irrespective of who has instructed the report. This can be more difficult to achieve for parole reports. However, reports can have a different emphasis, depending whether they have been instructed by the prisoner's solicitor or by the Home Office. For example, a solicitor who requires a report for a Discretionary Lifer Panel may be more interested in the psychiatric view on suitable after-care arrangements, including accommodation and supervision of the prisoner, than the Home Office would be. When preparing reports for the Parole Board it is essential to avoid recommending continued detention in prison.

TRAINING IN THE PREPARATION OF PSYCHIATRIC REPORTS

It is interesting that none of the "classic" papers or book chapters on preparing court reports makes any reference to the training required in the preparation of reports for courts. This includes the foremost British textbooks of forensic psychiatry.

The Basic Specialist Training Committee of the Royal College of Psychiatrists has recommended that all junior psychiatrists should accompany their consultants when they undertake medico-legal work. Despite the suggestion of the Royal College of Psychiatrists that all psychiatric trainees should acquire competencies in providing reports to courts and giving evidence in court (Royal College of Psychiatrists 2001), only the forensic psychiatry (Box 16.6) and psychiatry of learning disability core competency documents include these competencies. They are noticeably absent from the core

---

Box 16.7 Excerpt from the Royal College of Psychiatrists' forensic psychiatry core competencies for trainees

Be able to act as an expert witness and provide medico-legal opinions.

- Demonstrate detailed knowledge and application of the roles and responsibilities of the expert witness, including relevant ethical issues.

- Demonstrate ability to prepare reports for the criminal and civil courts, Mental Health Review Tribunal and Parole Board.

- Demonstrate ability to give evidence as an expert witness in court and Mental Health Review Tribunals.

---

competencies expected of general adult psychiatry and child and adolescent psychiatry trainees (Royal College of Psychiatrists 2004a).

Reiss and Meux (2000) have emphasised the need for all psychiatric trainees to acquire a range of forensic psychiatry skills, which would clearly include the preparation of psychiatric court reports. They have also emphasised the need for all psychiatric trainees to gain experience in prison psychiatry, and further, the need for all doctors, beginning with medical students, to gain some experience in working in prisons. The Royal College of Psychiatrists has now recommended that all trainees should receive experience in prison work, and it seems logical that this should include report writing in such settings.

Casey (2003) has suggested ways in which psychiatrists could acquire the necessary skills during their training to become expert witnesses. These include:

- observing other experts; consultants should allow trainees to observe the preparation of reports, including giving evidence in court

- presenting medico-legal cases in clinical case conferences for discussion

- attending specific training courses

- preparing medico-legal reports under supervision.

It would be relatively easy to incorporate these recommendations into a psychiatric training scheme. Both basic and higher trainees could observe consultants preparing reports, bearing in mind that a significant number of reports are prepared by general adult psychiatrists, child and adolescent psychiatrists, psychiatrists in learning disability and old age psychiatrists. This would include the assessment of the defendant in prison, the subsequent preparation of the report, and attending court. Higher trainees could present medico-legal cases that they have undertaken, in clinical case conferences including those from general adult psychiatry, child and adolescent psychiatry, learning disability and old age psychiatry. All trainees could also attend a specific training course for the preparation of court reports, though it is fair to say that the majority of these focus on the preparation of civil medico-legal reports in relation to claims for damages. There are very few courses specifically aimed at psychiatrists undertaking medico-legal work in the criminal courts.

Finally, all trainees could prepare psychiatric court reports under supervision from a consultant, with basic trainees undertaking more straightforward work concerned with defendants charged with property offences. Higher trainees, depending on their experience, could take on increasingly complex cases of defendants charged with more serious offences. The opportunity for these types of reports will arise as part of a rotational attachment to a forensic psychiatry training scheme or as a special interest placement.

CONCLUSIONS

It is clear that psychiatrists require a number of skills and competencies in order to prepare all of the various types of medico-legal reports that may be requested of them in a prison context. However, in all situations, it is important to remember that, not-withstanding the considerable ethical problems that can arise, the psychiatrist should still adhere to the principles of good medical practice as defined by the General Medical Council and the Royal College of Psychiatrists. If the psychiatrist is in any doubt about these issues, he or she should always consult a colleague, preferably one with considerable experience in this field. The most important ethical issues arise in the area of confidentiality and partiality. There is now considerable written advice on the former, and the latter can be addressed by asking the question, "How independent have I been in this report, and would it have been different if it had been instructed by someone else?"

Psychiatrists should also consider this aspect of their work when reviewing their own continuing professional development needs. This could involve peer review of their reports by colleagues, who might also observe them as expert witnesses in court. Consultants should also include teaching and training in preparing these reports when supervising both basic and higher trainees in psychiatry.

CHAPTER 17

The Lifer System in England and Wales

Natalie Pyszora

INTRODUCTION

In the UK we sentence more people to life imprisonment than the rest of Western Europe combined (Cullen & Newell 1999). In April 2008, the lifer population in England and Wales was 11,060 (Ministry of Justice 2008c), which represents more than a doubling in the past five years, from 5,419 in June 2003 (Ministry of Justice 2007). The vast majority of lifers are males (10,715), with a small number of females (345). There is an increasing number of young offenders within the life sentence population, and in April 2008, 80 lifers were aged 15–17 and 753 were aged 18–20 (Ministry of Justice 2008c).

There are now three types of life sentences: mandatory, discretionary and imprisonment for public protection (IPP). Automatic life sentences, introduced in 1997, were effectively superseded by IPPs. All lifers have the same basic structure to their sentence. They serve a minimum period of imprisonment (the tariff), to satisfy the demands of punishment and deterrence. Thereafter, release is sanctioned only if prisoners are deemed to present minimal risk to society. The sentence therefore has two clearly defined parts of tariff plus risk. The legal basis for each type of life sentence is outlined below, and an explanation is provided on how the tariff is set in each case.

MANDATORY LIFE SENTENCE

When a judge passes sentence for murder for an adult over the age of 21, a life sentence is mandatory under the Murder (Abolition of Death Penalty) Act 1965. There have been calls to end the mandatory life sentence because of its inflexibility and potential unfairness (Justice 1996, Ashworth 2000), but to date the sentence remains fixed by law.

Significant changes have occurred since 2003 in terms of tariff setting in mandatory life sentences. Prior to 2003, the judge would indicate the term of detention necessary to meet the requirements of retribution and deterrence before the papers would go to the Lord Chief Justice for review. However, the tariff was ultimately set by the Home Secretary, and the views of the trial judge and Lord Chief Justice did not bind him. The Home Office set a higher tariff than that indicated by judges in between 23% and 44% of cases (Justice 1996, Ashworth 2000). Amazingly, until 1993, the prisoner had no right to know the length of his or her tariff. In the case of R v Secretary of State for the Home Department, ex parte Doody (1994), known as the Doody judgement, it was held unanimously that prisoners were entitled to be told the recommendations made by the trial judge, and were entitled to make informed representations on the tariff to be fixed (Justice 1996). They were entitled not only to know their tariff, but also to see the judicial recommendations and the Home Secretary's reasons for departing from those, if he had done so. An effect of this case seemed to be a reduction in ministerial intervention in tariff setting, with tariffs being set higher than the judge's recommendation in only 4% of cases in 1993, and 3% in 1994 (Justice 1996).

Many advocated for a complete separation of powers between judiciary and executive (Justice 1996), and the judgement of the House of Lords on 25th November 2002 in the case of Anderson (R v Secretary of State for the Home Department, ex parte Anderson [2002]) found that the power of the Home Secretary to set tariffs for mandatory lifers, although lawful, was incompatible with the European Convention on Human Rights. As a result of this judgement, the system for tariff setting changed on 18 December 2003, under the Criminal Justice Act 2003. The tariff is now set by the trial judge in open court and, under Schedule 21 of the Act, there are prescribed starting points for consideration of minimum terms, as well as aggravating and mitigating circumstances which the judge may take into account. The four starting points are: whole life (does not apply to those under 21); 30 years; 15 years; and 12 years (for those under 18). Time on remand is taken into account; so if the lifer is given a 15-year tariff but has spent two years on remand, his tariff will be 13 years.

DISCRETIONARY LIFE SENTENCE

The sentence of discretionary life imprisonment may be passed on an offender who has committed a serious offence and whose history suggests that he or she presents a danger of serious offending for an indeterminate time. Thus the basis of the sentence is a prediction of dangerousness (Ashworth 2000).

The criteria for imposing a discretionary life sentence were set out in R v Hodgson (1968). A life sentence may only be imposed (1) where the offence or offences are in themselves grave enough to require a very long sentence, and (2) where it appears from the nature of the offences, or from the defendant's history, that he is a person of unstable character likely to commit such offences in the future, and (3) where, if such offences are committed, the consequences to others may be specially injurious, as in the case of sexual offences or crimes of violence. Although there are no precise thresholds, judicial decisions suggest that the offence in itself must be serious enough to justify a sentence of seven years or more, although it is clear that there is a complex interaction between all elements of the Hodgson criteria (Ashworth 2000). Although there need not be a mental disorder, as defined within the terms of the Mental Health Act 1983 (as amended by the Mental Health Act 2007), to meet the criteria for instability, there must be some evidence of mental disturbance which goes beyond a mere reference to personality disorder. Medical evidence on this matter is not mandatory, but is advisable (Smith 1998).

The tariff for a discretionary life sentence has always been passed immediately in open court as part of the sentencing procedure under Section 34 of the Criminal Justice Act 1991. Section 34 has now been replaced as the governing provision by Section 28 of the Crime (Sentences) Act 1997. In deciding the tariff, the judge considers the determinate sentence that would have been appropriate if a life sentence had not been given. Unless there are exceptional circumstances the tariff should then be set at half of that of the determinate sentence, and then the judge should deduct any period spent in custody on remand.

IMPRISONMENT (OR DETENTION) FOR PUBLIC PROTECTION (IPP)

This new sentence was introduced under the Criminal Justice Act 2003. It came into effect on 4 April 2005 and applies to offences committed on or after that date. It applies to offenders who are convicted of a serious offence (that is, a specified sexual or violent offence carrying a maximum penalty of ten years' imprisonment or more) and who are considered by the court to pose a "significant risk to members of the public, of serious harm". New receptions into prison for those given a life sentence rose from 509 per year in 2003 to 2,158 in 2006 (Ministry of Justice 2007).

For juveniles the public protection sentences are classed as sentences of detention rather than imprisonment. Where a juvenile has committed an offence carrying a maximum penalty of ten years or more, the court must consider whether an extended sentence for public protection (determinate) would be an appropriate punishment before imposing a sentence of detention for public protection (indeterminate).

There is no requirement to prove "mental instability" before imposing an IPP, as in discretionary life sentences, but the judge must have a risk assessment available at sentencing. This may be using the Offender Assessment System (OASys; an assessment tool which gathers information and enables an assessment of risk and need) or a pre-sentence report by probation, but psychiatrists may also be asked to provide reports with risk assessments for the purposes of sentencing. The tariff is set in the same way as in a discretionary life sentence, but short tariffs are typical.

The issue of extremely short tariffs raises significant difficulties in planning the life sentence and ensuring timely moves to prisons which can facilitate the necessary offence-related work. The difficulties surrounding this have been subject to successful judicial review in the High Court on 31 July 2007 and the decision was upheld by the Court of Appeal in February 2008 (Secretary of State for Justice v David Walker and Brett James [2008]). In essence, the Court of Appeal ruled that the Justice Secretary acted unlawfully by not providing some prisoners with access to courses, e.g. anger management and alcohol awareness, needed to prepare for release by the Parole Board. However, the Court of Appeal threw out the earlier High Court finding that the detention of IPP prisoners after the expiry of their tariff was unlawful. It did warn, however, that if prisoners are detained for a long time beyond their tariff without regular review, they may have to be released. This has significant implications for resources within prisons.

AUTOMATIC LIFE SENTENCE

Section 109 of the Powers of Criminal Courts (Sentencing) Act 2000 (formerly Section 2 of the Crime (Sentences) Act 1997) introduced a mandatory and automatic sentence of life imprisonment for a second serious or sexual offence, as long as the offender was aged 18 at the time of the second qualifying offence. The aim of the Government in passing the legislation was public protection (Ashworth 2000), and this function has now been superseded by the IPPs. Thus, automatic life sentences were effectively abolished on 4 April 2005 with the introduction of IPPs. The court was expected to impose a life sentence unless there were "exceptional circumstances relating to either the offence or to the offender which justify its not doing so". Bingham CJ stated in R v Kelly [1999] that "to be exceptional a circumstance need not be unique, or unprecedented, or very rare; but it cannot be one that is regularly, or routinely, or normally encountered". It rapidly became clear that the presence of mental disorder did not qualify as an exceptional circumstance, and mentally disordered offenders who qualified for a life sentence under the 1997 Act would have one imposed and would then require transfer to hospital under Section 47/49 of the Mental Health Act 1983. Tariff setting followed the same guidelines as for a discretionary life sentence.

STRUCTURE OF A LIFE SENTENCE

All life-sentenced prisoners have the same structure to their sentence and are provided with detailed guidance on this following sentencing in the form of the Lifer Manual (HM Prison Service 2006a).

Following conviction, the lifer serves a period of months in a local prison or remand centre where his or her life sentence plan (LSP) will be prepared. The life sentence plan was introduced in 1993, and intended to ensure that all lifers would have (1) a detailed risk assessment, (2) a record of offending behaviour to be addressed, (3) details of the arrangements for addressing offending behaviour, and (4) annual reviews and progress reports. As well as this there was to be a "continuous record of…personal growth and progress, and to what extent behavioural problems, negative attitudes and other areas of concern have been identified and are being addressed" (Cullen & Newell 1999, p.22). At the remand centres confidential summary dossiers (CSDs) are prepared and a Multi-Agency Lifer Risk Assessment Panel (MALRAP) will be held.

Lifers will then move from the remand centres (or local prisons) to the first stage prison, which is Category B, or a dispersal prison if they are Category A. Prison category (from Category A maximum secure through to Category D low secure or "open" prison) is allocated according to the level of risk the lifer is deemed to pose. This first move should take place within a matter of months, but there are considerable delays owing to the lack of capacity within the current prison estate and the rapidly growing number of lifers.

At the first stage prison or dispersal prison, the risk assessment is completed, risk factors are identified and sentence planning takes place, whereby offending behaviour targets are set. When this has been done, prisoners move to a second stage prison, either Category B or Category C, where offence related work will take place. In Category C conditions they will have their first review with reference to suitability for release, experience the introduction of some outside activities at the discretion of the Ministry of Justice, and be tested in less secure conditions. Transfer to a third stage prison (Category D) is in preparation for eventual release on licence. Here resettlement takes place, and there are opportunities for home leave and work in local communities using Release on Temporary Licence (ROTL). Transfer to Category D can only occur on a recommendation from the Parole Board (see later in this chapter).

Throughout the process, progress is assessed through regular reviews, every three years initially. These are called F75 reviews. These examine six key areas: (1) the index offence, (2) the offender's attitude to the index offence, (3) the offender's insight into offence-related behavioural problems, (4) behaviour in prison, (5) external support, and (6) an assessment of suitability for release. These reports are completed by a variety of staff, including probation, personal officer and prison psychologists. Psychiatrists may be asked to prepare a report where there is an issue related to mental disorder.

Release is generally preceded by a period of six to nine months in a Pre-release Employment Scheme (PRES) hostel or in Latchmere House resettlement prison. Here the lifer will undergo final testing in conditions comparable to those of release, be offered work experience in the community, and be subject to final reports prepared by both the hostel staff and the Probation Service. Most lifers end up serving at least one to two years more than their tariff, depending on what "risk" period there is deemed to be. Probation staff are responsible for contacting victims when the lifer is approaching release, to consider any restrictions which might need to be imposed on the lifer as conditions of his or her licence.

All life-sentenced prisoners who are released are subject to a licence, which remains in force for the remainder of their life. In contrast, after release, offenders with an IPP sentence can apply to the Parole Board to have their licence cancelled after ten years, and at yearly intervals thereafter. The licence is subject to seven standard conditions, and sometimes extra licence conditions, for as long as they are deemed necessary, and at least for the first few years. The lifer is monitored by the supervising probation officer, who provides regular reports to the Ministry of Justice. Conditions of the licence and supervision may be cancelled if the Probation Service and Parole Board agree that they are no longer necessary.

The licence can be revoked at any time by the Home Secretary under Section 32(1) of the Crime (Sentences) Act 1997 on the recommendation of the Parole Board, in which case the lifer is returned to prison. A total of 164 life licencees were recalled to prison in 2006 compared with an average of 34 per year between 1999 and 2003 (Ministry of Justice 2007). Most recalls are precipitated by the commission or threat-ened commission of acts of violence, not technical breaches of licence conditions. All lifers now have the right to an oral hearing of the Parole Board following recall. Those released on licence have a low rate of re-offending. For those released between 1972 and 1994, 9% were reconvicted of a standard list offence within two years, including 1% who were convicted for a grave offence; (all indictable-only offences with a maxi-mum sentence of life imprisonment (Home Office 2003a)).

NATIONAL OFFENDER MANAGEMENT SERVICE (NOMS)

The National Offender Management Service (NOMS) was established in 2004 to intro-duce a new case management approach for offenders which would provide greater con-tinuity of involvement through community and custodial settings for offenders. NOMS became part of the Ministry of Justice, when it was created in 2007. Its three key objectives are: (1) to protect the public, (2) to reduce re-offending, and (3) to deliver the sentences of the court. The Public Protection Unit is part of NOMS, and the pre-release section of the Unit is responsible for all issues related to life-sentenced prisoners who are detained in prison. The post-release section is responsible for monitoring progress of those on life licence, and recall to prison when this is required.

PAROLE BOARD

In relation to life-sentenced prisoners, the Parole Board has the powers to (1) direct release, (2) recommend open conditions, and (3) state risk factors.

The Parole Board holds its first review 3–3½ years before tariff expiry. The dos-sier is disclosed at the scheduled review date. The first review will assess suitability for transfer to a third stage, or open prison. Generally these reviews are held as paper panels if the decision is likely to be negative, but if the Parole Board is likely to recommend transfer, an oral hearing is now held, instead of only holding a paper panel. This change in policy followed the enquiry by HM Inspectorate of Probation (2006) into the Anthony Rice case, which identified that one of the key decision-making points was the move from closed to open conditions, and now any preliminary paper decisions that would otherwise recommend release or transfer to open conditions are referred to an oral hearing. This allows the prisoner to be questioned and any residual concerns to be addressed before recommendations are made.

Following the first review, subsequent reviews are held at least yearly. A review occurs just before tariff expiry to consider the question of release. The Parole Board has the power to direct release. The test for release is whether the lifer represents a "more than minimal risk to life and limb", i.e. serious violent offending particularly linked to the index offence.

Intensive case management (ICM) of oral hearings (including oral hearings for life-sentenced prisoners) was introduced by the Parole Board in 2007 to improve the quality of information available to panel members in order that the most informed decisions regarding the suitability of parole can be made. This aims to ensure that panel members are supplied with accurate, pertinent and timely information well in advance of panel hearings in order to be fully equipped to make informed decisions, and avoid cases being deferred both before, and on the day of, hearings.

The process described above represents a significant improvement from the position prior to 2003. Prior to the Criminal Justice Act 2003 any recommendation for release by the Parole Board for mandatory lifers used to be subject to the Home Secretary's approval. If a positive recommendation was received, the Lord Chief Justice and the trial judge (if available) were consulted. The Home Secretary then had the right to reject the recommendation to release if he considered the risk to be unacceptable, or decided that release would undermine public confidence in the criminal justice process. If release was ultimately recommended by the Home Secretary, the date was fixed usually a year ahead. The process created a dependency culture (Cullen & Newell 1999), in which a complex bureaucracy of procedures led to secrecy in contributions towards decision-making (with reports being unavailable to the lifer and therefore unavailable for challenge), and created uncertainty about the timing of procedures and how long decisions would take, uncertainty about the criteria upon which decisions were made (without stated reasons for decisions that were made), lack of clarity about the tariff for many lifers, and lack of clarity about criteria for future behaviour.

In May 2002, in the case of Stafford (Stafford v United Kingdom), the European Court of Human Rights ruled that the Home Secretary's power to authorise the release of mandatory lifers was not compatible with Article 5(4) of the European Convention on Human Rights. Under the Criminal Justice Act 2003 the Home Secretary now has no involvement in the release of lifers, only maintaining his role in recommending transfer to an open prison, as described above.

For discretionary lifers, the Criminal Justice Act 1991 moved the responsibility for decision-making for release from the executive to the judiciary, and Discretionary Lifer Panels (DLPs) were formed. Prior to this, the procedure had been the same as for mandatory lifers. The introduction of DLPs brought about a responsive culture with clear decision-making procedures, openness of reporting, a strict timetable, explicit criteria upon which decisions are made with reasons given for decisions, an explicit tariff, and clearer identification of the areas of risk that the lifer should consider during his sentence. The lifer has access to all reports and can attend the hearing with legal representation.

Prisoners with a "whole life tariff" receive ministerial review after 25 years solely to consider whether the whole life tariff should be converted to a tariff of a determinate period. This review is undertaken entirely by ministers and the Parole Board has no part to play in the process.

LIFE-SENTENCED PRISONERS DETAINED UNDER THE MENTAL HEALTH ACT 1983 (AMENDED 2007)

Lifers may be transferred to a psychiatric hospital for treatment if they are assessed to be suffering with a mental disorder which makes detention for treatment in hospital appropriate and necessary. In these circumstances they will be transferred under Section 47 of the Mental Health Act 1983 (amended 2007), together with a restriction order under Section 49. They are managed by the mental health unit rather than the pre-release section of NOMS, and any applications for leave or transfer must be authorised by the mental health unit.

Lifers detained under the Mental Health Act do not have the same access to the Parole Board as they would if they remained in prison, and are denied access as long as they are deemed to require detention under the Mental Health Act (R v Secretary of State for the Home Department, ex parte Hickey [1995]). Thus, it is only when patients/prisoners receive an absolute or conditional discharge from their detention under the Mental Health Act 1983 that they can have a parole hearing in hospital, although they have access in the usual way if they are returned to prison. This can occur when the responsible clinician advises the Home Secretary that the patient no longer warrants detention in hospital for treatment, or if the Mental Health Review Tribunal recommends that the patient should be discharged, and in both circumstances if the patient would be likely to become unwell if returned to prison. To be eligible for a parole hearing in hospital the lifer must have reached his or her tariff. Time spent in hospital counts towards the sentence for tariff purposes.

SUMMARY

The lifer population in the UK is large and rapidly growing, initially as a result of legislation introducing automatic life sentences for a second serious offence, and more recently with the introduction of imprisonment for public protection. Since 2003 there have been improvements in life sentence planning, greater transparency in tariff setting, and the end of ministerial involvement in release on life licence. However, there are new problems in meeting the treatment needs of the flood of short-tariff lifers entering the prison estate since the introduction of IPPs, in terms of providing them with the opportunity to address their risk factors before the expiry of their tariff. The failure to do so has been the subject of successful Judicial Review but it remains to be seen how the Prison Service will meet the challenge of rehabilitating ever growing numbers of life-sentenced prisoners.

CHAPTER 18

Psychology in Prisons

Graham Towl

CONTEXT

Much of the work currently captured under the rubric of "Psychology in prisons" is actually about some of the roles of psychologists, and often chiefly forensic psychologists (see, for example, Towl 2004). Those roles which appear to have had most emphasis have tended to be activities associated with clinical risk assessment and the related area of clinical interventions designed to reduce the risk of reconvictions. There are some notable exceptions with wider considerations of the role and (potential) impact of an understanding and application of "psychology" in prison settings (Crighton & Towl 2008). The applied psychology sub-specialist Division of Forensic Psychology (DFP) has seen a decade or thereabouts of growth in numbers of members (Towl 2008a). In recent years there has been a broader recognition of the need for a more eclectic mix of practitioner psychologists working in prisons (Towl 2008b).

Between 1995 and 2000 there was a marked growth in the numbers of psychologists directly employed in public sector prisons from approximately 200 to 400, against a backdrop of the increasing influence of New Public Management ideologies and methods in public services (Towl & Crighton 2007). Prisons were no exception to this, with, for example, the new mantra of measurement taking its place within the penal lexicon. In public services measurement often begets manualisation. This may be seen as a prescriptive device for task proceduralisation. There thus becomes a received and routinised way of achieving a numerically expressed organisational goal or target. The growth of such managerialism coincided with an increasing academic enthusiasm for meta-analyses of data thought to be linked to psychological methods associated with achieving reductions in reconviction rates amongst offenders. More specifically, in terms of an application of such research, this period (1995–2000) saw the advent of the expansion of structured, group-based interventions aimed at reducing the risk of reconviction. The dominant theoretical approach that was advanced was cognitive-behavioural. Within the "family" of cognitive-behaviourally based interventions there are some significant variations of emphasis in terms of the therapeutic techniques applied. Indeed this has been the subject of much debate both within the cognitive-behavioural psychological field and from psychiatric commentators too (Gaudiano 2008).

The growth in the numbers of psychological staff accelerated further from 2000 to 2005. One central reason for this five-year period of growth was markedly improved staff retention levels, improved staff supervision arrangements and new pay structures which reflected the capacity for cost-effective delivery, particularly of assessments and interventions. Subsequent to 2005 such directly employed staff numbers appear to have remained much the same. Since 2000 the numbers of psychological staff working with prisoners through health providers and local authorities have been, and appear to continue to be, on the increase.

POLICY DEVELOPMENTS

Currently on the horizon are two key policy developments which will have a direct impact upon psychological services in prisons. The first is the advent of statutory regulation, which, if and when it goes ahead, will be a historical development in UK psychological practice.

The second policy development which will potentially have a significant impact is in relation to the drive to improve access to psychological therapies. Much of what psychology as a body of knowledge has potentially to offer has been unduly limited by the routine policy and practice conflation of "psychology" with "psychologists". In short, if we are to realise the full potential of what "psychology" has to offer the public (including prisoners), then psychological therapies need increasingly to be delivered by staff other than psychologists.

ETHICS OF PSYCHOLOGICAL INTERVENTIONS

There are humanistic underpinnings to much of what is ethical and effective in psychological practice – for example, courtesy, the use of respectful language, demonstrable sensitivity and high professional standards in engaging ethically with prisoners. These are perhaps especially important given the power differentiations which characterise prisons and imprisonment. An understanding and appreciation of the impact of power relationships are important in informing ethical practice in prisons. For example, coercion is the antithesis of consent. Prisons are fundamentally coercive environments.

Therefore there will often be a tension between the environmental context and what we may deem appropriate levels of consent.

There is much real scope to build upon recent developments, particularly in relation to mental health liaison and inreach services, to provide prisoners with the full range of mental health and other services which they may benefit from. The greater range of applied psychology sub-specialisms practising in prisons, whether, for example, clinical or forensic, look set to continue to grow in their diversity. Professional diversity brings with it a substantial benefit in terms of best ethical practice. The British Psychological Society occupational standards project made explicit some of the many commonalities across the sub-specialist areas of applied psychology (Needs 1997). The professional landscape is likely to shift further with the continued growth of staff (and on some occasions perhaps prisoners) who will be in increasingly strong positions to deliver psychologically based interventions.

PSYCHOLOGICAL INTERVENTIONS IN PRISONS

I will focus on clinical aspects of psychological approaches to working with prisoners, an area of work which remains a predominant part of psychological work and characterises much of current psychological practice (for example, Towl & McDougall 1999, Towl 2002, 2004, 2006, 2008c, Crighton & Towl 2008). The work of chiefly (but not exclusively) forensic psychologists in prisons is perhaps more well established than some of the other areas which have seen a recent and very welcome expansion. It will be interesting to read some of the emerging literature from these areas, such as from the work of educational psychologists, which has already began to appear (e.g. Ryrie, Lawrence & Miller 2006) in the forensic field.

Risk assessment

Probably the most prevalent area of individual clinical work undertaken by psychological staff employed by the National Offender Management Service is in the domain of risk assessment. Such risk assessment work has traditionally been undertaken primarily with life-sentenced prisoners in relation to the work involved with estimating their risk of gravely harming others, and thereby informing the management of individual prisoners through "the system" (Towl 1996, Towl & Crighton 1997), and this includes the new Indeterminate Public Protection (IPP) sentences. It is generally acknowledged that one of the main reasons for the significant growth in the prisoner population over the past decade or so has been as the result of more severe sentencing (Prison Reform Trust 2008a, 2008b). It is perhaps less well known that the proportion of the prisoner population represented by indeterminate sentenced prisoners, including IPPs and "lifers", is increasing, underpinning the growth in the overall prisoner population. It is a significant management challenge for prison service staff to ensure that all the relevant risk assessment reports have been completed in a timely, fair and accurate manner for all such prisoners. It is anticipated that there will be a growing onus on practitioner psychologists to undertake such vital risk assessment work.

The Cambridge Framework for Risk Assessment (CAMRA) provides a structure for engagement in the risk assessment process (Brady 2008). The conceptual framework of the CAMRA includes explicit links with risk management. This is imperative if the full benefits of a risk assessment are to be fully realised. The principles of risk assessment are pervasive, not just across the forensic field but well beyond that – we are surrounded by various "risks" in our everyday lives (Breakwell 2007). The current forensic fashion is in increasing the accuracy of structured risk assessment methods or "tools". In such discussions and debates very little is mentioned about the fairness (or otherwise) of the application of particular risk assessment methods (Towl 2005). Ethically, the starting point for an understanding and appreciation of the application of any risk assessment method must surely rest upon issues of fairness. The fundamental point here is that those undertaking "risk assessments" tend to be in much stronger positions of power and influence than those who are the direct recipients of such deliberations. Thus there is a particular duty of care. The duty of care to third parties is implicit in much forensic practice by both the focus and nature of assessments. The term "public protection" is sometimes used in the risk assessment field to refer to those other than the offenders themselves. It is as if the rest of the public are seen to be potential victims, and not the offender him- or herself. This is wrong on two counts. First, offenders are members of the public, and so they are entitled to consideration of their safety and well-being. Second, there is strong empirical evidence to support the notion that lifers and those charged or convicted of violent and sexual offences will have an inflated risk of suicide in prisons (Towl et al. 2000). More broadly, the backgrounds of many prisoners are characterised by social and economic disadvantages which are associated with higher levels of being the victims of crimes (Crighton & Towl 2008).

Much of the individual risk assessment undertaken by psychological staff is in relation to harm to others rather than harm to oneself, yet we know that the rates of suicide in prisons are high. It is widely understood that the period of greatest risk of suicide for prisoners in general is in the first 24 hours of incarceration at a particular prison. This time period numerically accounts for about 10% of all deaths by suicide in prisons (Crighton 2006). Rates of suicide amongst life-sentenced prisoners are appreciably greater than for determinate sentenced or remand prisoners (Towl & Crighton 1998). However, patterns of the timings of suicides amongst indeterminate sentenced prisoners are less well understood. Patterns of suicide which have been observed amongst life-sentenced prisoners have tended to be linked with key decision-making in relation to their futures. From an organisational and practitioner perspective such events are generally reasonably predictable. Thus we have some good information on periods of time for all prisoners associated with an inflated risk of suicide, which can inform our individual work.

I draw this brief section on individual work to a close with two key observations. First, the importance of always preserving a sense of what is the right thing to do.

Psychologists are individually responsible for their professional actions and must fully appreciate their high degree of potential accountability for their actions. Second, it is important that psychologists do not lose sight of the importance of humanity and humility when working with prisoners. The desirable behaviours in question are not dissimilar to what may be required of any health professional working with his or her patients (see, for example, Towl 1991) and indeed the very behaviours that we are often exhorting prisoners to develop and demonstrate too. This means adopting a supportive, considerate and respectful approach to such work. Linked to this is the need for psychologists to actively challenge any inappropriate behaviour from staff (or fellow prisoners) that they witness in relation to the disrespectful, or otherwise unreasonable, treatment of prisoners. Such encounters often require moral conviction and the modelling of effective assertion skills.

Group work

The most common types of group work in prisons reported in the early 1990s were: general offending behaviour (14%), alcohol awareness (14%), drugs (13%), and anger management (10%). Altogether these four types of group work accounted for 51% of the group work being undertaken at the time in prisons. A further 24% were accounted for by anxiety management, social skills, lifer groups and sex offender groups (Towl & Bailey 1995). Much of the diversity in types of group work was undertaken within prisons for women and also, to some degree, within Young Offender Institutions.

In the 1990s much group work in prisons was rebranded as "programmes". This was especially so for the largely imported set of ideas, referred to earlier, which became known as the so-called "What works?" literature, leading to what became known as Offending Behaviour Programmes (OBPs). These "programmes" were not programmes in the sense of an integrated set of interventions, but rather, highly structured and focused, manualised, group-work based interventions. Those marketing such "programmes" were sometimes unequivocal in their bold claims about the effectiveness of their proposed interventions. Such interventions had as their stated purpose to reduce the risk of reoffending amongst course participants. The "programmes" were manualised and training centralised to deliver the courses in a consistent and replicable group work format. An international panel of those involved in such work was set up as an "accreditation body". Some precautions were taken to attempt to ensure that there were reduced conflicts of interest in decision-making around which "programmes" would and would not be "accredited". One example of such a precaution was in relation to individuals with a financial interest in a particular "programme", where they would not be included in panel discussions in relation to their own programme. One parsimonious solution to such potential conflicts of interest would be to bar those with direct financial interests from membership of accreditation bodies.

Also, in prisons, much group work which had previously been undertaken was terminated. In part this was because there was a dearth of evaluation work being undertaken, but also it reflected a renewed tenacity to prioritise group work that was explicitly designed to focus upon the reduction of reoffending rather than other goals. This was an important step because it marked a real shift from what may be broadly termed "prisoner interest" to "public interest". Such an approach marked a sea-change in terms of how (forensic) psychologists would subsequently be regarded by prisoners. The "regard" in this context would be linked to changing roles, in the direction of largely meeting state needs rather than prisoner needs. It has become increasingly important to ensure that psychologists maintain appropriate role boundaries. For example, psychologists involved in delivering specific interventions may, generally, be well advised not to conduct forensic assessments for legal tribunals concerned with the impacts of such interventions.

Some proponents of group work have argued that group-based interventions are a more efficient use of finite public resources in comparison with one-to-one work. However, there have been no clear demonstrations that this is the case. Even if it were true, in some cases, that particular interventions could be run more economically in a group format, economy is not by any means necessarily to be equated with effectiveness. Arguably somewhat crude notions of measurement are used in relation to "accredited offending behaviour programmes" in prisons (Crighton & Towl 2008). The number of "completions" is what is measured in terms of the managerial representation of such potentially therapeutic work. No measures are taken of the proportion of those on the "programme" in terms of their suitability for selection, and the programmes are not necessarily in the places where there would be most therapeutic need for such work.

But what of the evaluation evidence in the UK? There is still a heavy reliance upon international rather than national evidence in support of programmes. There is also a marked dependence upon psychometric testing data in an attempt to demonstrate the effectiveness of the programmes (Towl 2008c). The truth is that the evidence has been rather mixed (and not dissimilar to some of the very group work that the programmes replaced) with some promising early results, but disappointing subsequent large-scale UK studies. The studies have also often tended to lack the degree of methodological rigour warranted for such evidence. In general, the more rigorous the evaluation methods, the less likelihood of being able to demonstrate a positive treatment effect (Crighton & Towl 2008).

Undertaking manualised group-work based interventions aimed at reducing the risk of reconvictions remains one of the most common areas of activity of forensic psychological staff in prisons, and such interventions are much less commonly undertaken by those psychologists not directly employed by the prison service. Within forensic psychology, and perhaps beyond, there have been some concerns that facilitating such highly structured manualised interventions will not serve as sufficient training for those who wish to become fully qualified forensic psychologists. This may very well be true, but it is true for other areas of forensic practice too. Group-work environments can be extremely challenging, in terms both of the organisational skills associated with their planning and implementation and of the high levels of clinical skills required to work effectively in such a therapeutic medium. But the key training problem is that such facilitation roles lack sufficient breadth in their contribution to the training of forensic psychologists.

The big risk in this area of practice, putting aside some of the equivocal research findings, is that we will not build a sufficiently robust research base for such work undertaken in the UK. First, there has been timidity in addressing potential concerns about the implementation of randomised controlled trials. It is unclear whether the barrier to undertaking such work is a misplaced ethical concern about excluding some prisoners from treatment as a function of the research design. Equally the timidity could be linked to a concern that if the research designs are strengthened, then it could be harder to demonstrate positive evaluation results. Second, because of the drive to achieve "completion" targets, perverse incentives have emerged which may directly impact upon the potential evaluation data. For example, if prisoners who do not meet suitability criteria for the particular intervention are included on a particular course, this may distort the data. This is because, if someone not matching the selection criteria is included on the course, the experimental prediction would suggest that we could not anticipate a positive treatment effect. But given that they would count as a "completion", there would need to be proportionately more treatment movement from an appropriately selected course member for there to be a reasonable opportunity to test for the efficacy of the intervention.

CONCLUSION

In this chapter I have outlined some of the key contextual and policy issues in relation to psychological services in prisons. The centrality of ethical concerns to clinical practice within prisons is a pervasive theme, especially given the forensic nature of the work. I have briefly touched upon the clinical mediums of individual and group work in explicating some of the important issues in psychological practice in prisons. Psychological therapies are set to continue to grow in prisons and as such represent a major public health opportunity. The application of "psychology" to prisoners remains a field ripe for further development.

CHAPTER 19

Prison Therapeutic Regimes

Mark Morris

The last two decades have seen a vast expansion of the numbers of people in prison in the UK, in the context of a changing societal culture with a reducing tolerance of recidivism. When an individual creates one victim, there is an expectation that the state prevents it happening again. The expansion itself has been driven partly by changing practice in sentencing, and partly by legislation, particularly "two strikes" legislation with an automatic life sentence for people who reoffend with violent and dangerous crimes, and then indeterminate sentences for public protection.

As a result, prisons are increasingly being filled with people on life sentences who will not be released following a *lex talionis*[1] retributive period in prison as a punishment. They will only be released when, in a Foucaultian sense, they have been internally disciplined, when they can demonstrate that they have been "cured" of their criminal propensity and no longer represent a risk to the public. They will only achieve this with some form of "treatment". This chapter looks at some of the treatment regimes that operate in UK prison settings.

THERAPY IN PRISONS

Broadly, the clinical diagnosis of antisocial personality disorder (ASPD) can be made if an individual has offended against society's mores to the extent that he or she has been imprisoned. So when a patient asks what I, as a clinician, mean by making a diagnosis, what the syndrome comprises, it's broadly that he or she will end up in prison. Prison is

---

1   "law of retaliation", whereby a punishment resembles the offence committed (Concise Oxford Dictionary).

both the symptom and the definition of the behaviour. Diagnostic manuals and schedules provide a little more clarity, which with use identify around 30% of the male prison population as having ASPD (Singleton *et al.* 1998), and 1% of men in the general population (Coid *et al.* 2006), with the psychopathy checklist (PCL-R; Hare 1991) skimming off the most severe 2–5%. Broadly, however, being in prison is tantamount to having an ASPD. The system of crime and punishment is one vast (albeit largely ineffective) behavioural management plan for a society's ASPD population, with, in the UK and a number of other jurisdictions, increasing periods of incarceration being identified as the only and particular effective management strategy, illustrated by the growth of indeterminate sentencing.

These comments are simply to introduce the argument that prison and a criminal justice framework are the natural and correct context for the treatment of people with ASPD. The alternative is to treat ASPD patients under mental health legislation as patients within a medical model of treatment. The disadvantages of treating people with ASPD in hospital under mental health legislation (certainly in England) as opposed to in a custodial environment are as follows:

1. **The invidiousness of the medical model for personality disorder**
    The medical model strips people of their responsibility for their actions: they are not responsible for the "disease" that they have, so that:

    -   the cardinal therapeutic goal of establishing individuals' responsibility and agency over their behaviour is undermined

    -   the adverse behaviour of the patient becomes the responsibility of the clinician rather than the individual

    -   the patient's passivity is amplified

    -   clinicians are reluctant ever to discharge or resettle patients, on account of continuing high risk.

2. **The vulnerability of care ideologies with psychopathic patients**

    -   The perversion/conditioning/duping of care staff who will:

        ○   focus on individuals' history of trauma rather than their criminality

        ○   be more likely to accept at face value when the individuals "fake good"

        ○   have care as a first preoccupation and security second, as security is grafted onto "a core care identity".

    -   Prison staff have a core culture of security and custody:

        ○   safety and security are the more appropriate core task with the maintainence of secure procedures, interactions and interventions

○   care is "grafted onto" this core secure identity and sense of task.

3. **The process of release/resettlement** is guided either by the completion of a *lex talionis* sentence, or, for prisoners about to be released on license, purely on the basis of assessment of public risk *contributed to* but *not determined by* therapeutic and care considerations.

Conceptually, the disease model of ASPD is helpful, as it focuses research on looking at symptoms (for example, leading to the clarification of Cleckley-type psychopathy (Cleckley 1988) in the PCL-R), aetiologies and treatments. Managerially, the disease model of ASPD is a disaster. It fosters the evacuation of responsibility. It distracts from the need to focus on secure containment when incarcerated, and when public risk when released. It consistently dilutes the patient/prisoner's personal responsibility for his or her own criminal and antisocial behaviour. I believe that prison is the place to treat ASPD patients, both in terms of organisational culture, and in terms of legal framework.

PRISON ITSELF AS THERAPY

There is a tendency, within the forensic world, to become overly critical of the practice of others, amplified by the stakes being so high when things go wrong. In this context, in the forensic psychiatry world, one hears dark stories of poor practice in other forensic health settings, but it seems that all forensic health people can agree that the situation in the prisons is worse. For patients with mental illness, there may be some truth in this. There is always a risk that genuine mental illness is interpreted in prisons simply as bad behaviour and managed thus, compounding the psychotic patient's suffering; and second, there is the problem of not being able to medicate people against their will when they clearly need this.

For people with personality disorder, however, the situation is different, and there are various arguments that for this group prison itself is a form of therapy. First, and most obvious, the prison walls prevent (or at least limit) their criminal activity – literal concrete behavioural therapy. Second, this not only benefits society by reducing the number of public victims, but enhances the life of the criminal individual, who is also traumatised by his or her criminal activity. Being in prison minimises the harm in the prisoner's daily routine. People who, "on the street", would be engaged in a cycle of robberies or thefts to buy crack and other street drugs (grafting and scoring), are instead engaged in a cycle of having three nutritious meals a day, with nothing to do but keep up with their dental care and make visits to the GP. Some prisoners will be well known to the staff of a local prison, who will see them arrive in a terrible, battered and malnourished state with a sentence of several months. During this sentence they will be detoxified from a physiological addiction to substances, spend some time in the gym, and eat properly, so they will be released in a much better physical state, only to return several months later, again battered and dishevelled, again to be patched up during a prison stay, and thence to be re-released.

Aside from these general factors, however, there are several more specific ones. Prison disciplinary procedure is a clear and rigorously applied behavioural programme, with a clear set of rules; it enforces these clearly, with clear punishments when rules are transgressed, that act as negative reinforcement to adverse behaviour, thus extinguishing it. Similarly, there is a clear "incentives and earned privileges" scheme, where periods of good behaviour are rewarded with increased freedoms and concessions, reinforcing positive behaviour. For those who break rules, and are recalcitrant, there is the option of physical removal and "time out" confinement in segregation units, and various secure procedures for managing those who rebel against and fight the system itself. Broadly, these systems are effective in containing all but the most disruptive and aggressive of prisoners, so the vast majority can be clear that bullying and aggressive methods that they have used in the past will not be effective, so they desist, and indeed learn other methods.

Prisoners are allocated a "personal officer" in a keyworker system, who will establish a "sentence plan" care pathway, identifying needs and issues. The sequence of security ratings from A category high secure, to D category open prisons constitutes itself a pathway followed by individuals as their sentence progresses, with the final placement in a D category prison involving up to full-time work in the community. Following release, the structure of monitoring through probation work, hostel placement and Multi-Agency Public Protection Arrangements (MAPPA) oversight can be conceived of as a form of personality disorder aftercare programme.

GRENDON UNDERWOOD AND THE DEMOCRATIC THERAPEUTIC COMMUNITIES

Grendon prison is a 240-bed B category prison in Buckinghamshire, opened in 1962. It was built on a wave of optimism following the success of the therapeutic community method with shell-shocked soldiers in the Second World War (Harrison 2000), with a view that a similar recovery might be seen for psychopathic prisoners. From the beginning, Grendon was set up with a quite heavily democratic therapeutic community ethos in the British group psychoanalytic tradition, as distinct from a "concept" or a "hierarchical" therapeutic community culture, more common in the US and in residential drug treatment facilities such as the Phoenix Houses.

The UK democratic therapeutic community model is effectively a prescription for creating a particular culture within a residential environment. Within the managerial literature, the culture has been called a "learning organisation", the cardinal characteristic of which is the facilitation of communication. Within a therapeutic community, daily community meetings have the task of reviewing what has taken place within the unit, and, if appropriate, reviewing its significance. The community meeting has the task of evaluating the requests of individuals (for example, to do particular jobs, attend particular therapies, and so on). The community meeting has the task of sharing all major pieces of information, new clients introduce themselves to the community, and at nodal points in their stay, they give an account of themselves to it; and in particular, the contents of small therapy groups that have taken place on the unit are fed back to the community meeting. In theory, the community meeting is the central hub of information within the unit, a structure enabling everybody to know about everybody.

My belief is that if one creates such a structure within an organisation, within a therapeutic unit, a therapeutic community culture will develop naturally. This culture was described in the 1960s by Rapoport (1960) following an observational study of the Henderson Hospital, where he described four cardinal features:

1. flattening of the authority hierarchy

2. tolerance of behaviour

3. reality confrontation

4. democratisation

– to which Haigh (1999) added a fifth: communalism.

In the late 1990s, in the context of research suggesting a treatment effect of a 20% reduction in reconviction for those staying 18 months or more, against a matched control (Marshall 1997), Grendon, the "experimental prison", was declared to have been a success, and there was a ministerial undertaking to build more such facilities with, early in the new millennium, Dovegate being opened in the Midlands. The Dovegate and Grendon therapeutic communities operate along the same basic lines, comprising therapeutic communities of about 40 residents.

Taking Grendon as an example, there are five relatively autonomous communities, and an additional assessment unit with 25 or so residents. Each of the communities has a multidisciplinary team comprising a community therapist (a group analyst or similar), a forensic psychologist and a probation officer (mirroring the multidisciplinary troika of psychiatrist, social worker and psychologist of mental health teams); and a team of about 14 prison officers who combine the frontline caring role of the psychiatric nurse in an inpatient unit with the secure prison-craft element of their core profession. Two of the prison officers are specialist therapists with group therapeutic training, and facilitate as lead therapists the small groups, along with other multidisciplinary team members and sessional therapists.

The patient group is referred from sending prisons from a variety of sources. Commonly, during the trial process, there has been a recommendation to go to Grendon, either in a psychiatric report, or by the judge, where there is something in the history or facts of the case that indicates a psychopathological contribution to the index offence. Most commonly, there is someone in a prison (e.g. medical, custodial, or chaplain) who has made a connection with the individual, and proposes treatment as part of an ongoing discussion. Others report discussions with a peer who seems to "have their shit together" and discloses that he has spent time there. There are some basics that clearly rule people in or out of treatment, which are as follows.

- **Prisoners have to have at least 18 months to two years to serve**. This is consequent on the empirical evidence that patients who stay in treatment for at least 18 months show a reduction in reconviction following release. Life-sentenced prisoners with long tariffs have to be at least four years into their sentence, so that the therapeutic work is about their lives and offending rather than their trauma at receiving a life sentence.

- **Prisoners cannot be on psychotropic medication**. Appearing simple and arbitrary, this is in fact a very sophisticated filter in a population where there is a high degree of psychiatric morbidity. It means that people who have periods of depression, a history of psychotic breakdowns, or chronic paranoia have to be sufficiently psychiatrically stable to be able to survive without psychiatric medication. Broadly, this barrier means that the prison therapeutic communities have a fairly "pure" personality disorder client group, which in turn is enormously cost-efficient, obviating the need for extensive (and expensive) medical and psychiatric input.

- **Prisoners need to evidence some degree of motivation or reflectivity about their offending**. This is gleaned from the application forms and paper records.

- **For Dovegate, prisoners need to score less than 25 on the PCL-R**. This factor creates a crucial difference between the two therapeutic communities of Grendon and Dovegate, namely that the Dovegate TC does not work with those prisoners with clinical psychopathy, the most dangerous and disruptive. In Grendon, about half the patients score above 25, and are clinical psychopaths.

However, following Freud's reputed method of assessment of a "trial analysis", the main assessment process for new residents takes place in the 25-bed assessment unit, with prisoners taking part in a partial therapeutic community regime, partially modified in that there is not an expectation that they talk about their history or offending, but with the same culture of enquiry about "here and now" events, groups and community meetings. Many prisoners are traumatised by the change of culture from what they have been used to in prisons: simple things, like being expected to address the prison officers by their first names, and the officers being interested and asking them about their reactions to the new culture, and about themselves. For many, the whole process of talking, of using words to express themselves, is novel, and the suggestion that they might use words about personal emotions, or even have emotional reactions, is a shock.

After the first four to six weeks in the assessment unit, prisoners graduate down to their treatment community, where the weekly programme consists of several hours daily in groups, either small groups, or large community meetings. The small groups act like group psychoanalytic groups with an intensity borne out of meeting two or three times weekly. The content of these groups is fed back into the large community meetings, which are the democratised core of the programme. The debate within all of these groups is driven by a strong culture of enquiry, where everything that happens is open to scrutiny and discussion in a "living learning" environment. The residents' behaviour is first tolerated, then deconstructed and discussed as they recount their history (which has often involved considerable deprivation and abuse) in their small group. Eventually, individuals move onto recounting their offending history and cycle, which is explored in the same manner.

In this way, the characteristics of the individual's personality become known and so does the way that, in real time, they are seen dealing with challenges and stresses. Also, in the course of life over 18 months plus, they get into the same situations that have led them in the past to offending. They have an argument that comes to (or nearly comes to) blows on the football field; they are caught or strongly suspected of bringing in drugs, or engaging in some other form of antisocial acquisitive activity. These crises comprise mini offence re-enactments, which can be explored in real time, and can be linked to offending behaviour. There are a number of particular advantages to facilities like Grendon as personality disorder treatment programmes:

- transfer is voluntary: patients lacking motivation or breaking inviolable house rules can be immediately transferred out

- the treatment context is custodial:

  ° the intensive treatment programme is carried out in the legal environment of criminal law rather than the medical model, as discussed above

  ° the intensive treatment programme is carried out in a culture that is primarily security/custody focused, with the frontline care workers being prison officers who are legally equivalent to police constables while in duty (again, as discussed above)

- intensive therapy is carried out on an industrial scale, facilitated in part by the command managerial culture of the disciplined services.

Describing the effect of a Grendon-type treatment is not easy. Between 40% and 50% of those transferred in manage to stay 18 months or more, but anecdotally, the greatest effect is seen with life-sentenced patients who stay two to four years, rather than simply leaving at the end of their sentence – who stay until therapy seems complete, rather than that it's time to "get out of jail free". Like the open-mouthed effort of the patient in psychoanalysis to describe the effect of their treatment, post-treatment Grendon patients have changed, but how is difficult to describe. Family and friends often notice a softening of positions. The individual has the same contours, but somehow less sharp. People may become (paradoxically) more emotional, but less dangerous. Often there is an enhanced ability to describe personal feelings, and there is always a much enhanced ability to give an "I"-centred narrative of their historical (usually traumatic) background, of their antisocial activity, history and attitudes, and of their index offence. Always, there is an enhancement of verbal articulation skills. They will have an enhanced understanding of their vulnerability to substances, although they will probably remain vulnerable to them, and will continue to have the potential for catathymic (Werthem 1927) or instrumental violence in particular constellations of circumstances.

Empirically, while early evidence demonstrated changed social attitudes (for example, a reduction in hostility towards authority) and psychological morbidity, no difference with reconviction rates was found between Grendon graduates and controls (Gunn *et al.* 1978). Later studies introduced the time spent in treatment as a variable, with indications that for patients staying more than 18 months, there is something like a 20% reduction in reconviction at about two years, compared to a matched control (Cullen 1994, Marshall 1997), which treatment effect can still be discerned five years post-discharge, but also with something like a 60% reduction in the rate of recall of lifers discharged on license for graduates, compared to controls (Taylor 2000).

COGNITIVE-DIDACTIC "PRISON PROGRAMMES"

In the UK the Prison Service has two core tasks, the first being safe custody, and the second being the rehabilitation of offenders. Apparently, in the 1960s and 1970s, a "rehabilitative ideal" held sway – that offenders needed to be understood, and that they would stop offending if offered treatment – at the time in a variety of liberal-minded guises. Martinson's (1974) influential paper that concluded that "nothing works" in the actual reduction of recidivist offending seems to have been an articulation of the "collapse of the rehabilitative ideal" rather than its precipitating catalyst, as the rehabilitative meta-narrative in criminal justice had been being undermined for some time by the ever-rising crime statistics. The idea that "nothing works", in the hands of public administrators, led to a cost-saving decimation of custodial therapeutic programmes across the jurisdictions of the developed world.

Forensic psychology fought back in the 1990s with the "What works" movement (e.g. McGuire & Priestley 1995). These new "What works" programmes had several characteristics that made them highly successful:

- a focus on their evidence of effectiveness in terms of reduction in reconviction, this having been demonstrated

- a clear criminological meta-theory, where programmes had to specifically address cluster analytically derived "criminogenic factors", themselves associated empirically with offending

- centrally developed and written programmes based upon the best evidence, and devised by leaders in the field, rather than the more usual local and home-grown style of psychology group treatments

- a rigorous audit system to ensure local adherence to the programme manual and delivery "by the book", supported by a rhetoric that "programme drift" led to poor treatment results

- a clear strategy for obtaining investment, based upon the evidence of effectiveness.

This fight-back was so successful that in the late 1990s, first, "What works" became a byword for legitimate public investment; and second, in the prisons, it seemed that all rehabilitative investment was being ploughed into these programmes, with a massive expansion. There is no empirical evidence that teaching someone a trade such as plastering or bricklaying while in prison reduces that person's involvement in crime at the end of his or her sentence. Clearly, it makes intuitive sense that if you've a legitimate means of income, you're less likely to resort to illegitimate ones such as crime. Also, it makes intuitive sense to suppose that a trade and a job role reduce the sense of anomie, detachment from, and resentment of a society that one then feels justified in stealing from or offending against. These conjectures are obvious, but based upon lofty ideals and the life work experience of generations of custodians rather than tick-box, controlled outcome studies. Without the empirical evidence, many "governor's workshops" were closed down, the money instead being used to pursue national targets for the number of offending behaviour psychology programme "completions".

Albeit a rather gross simplification, within the psychological therapies, cognitive therapy occupies the middle ground between psychodynamic work (looking at emotional and deeply hidden motivations and fears) on the one hand, and pure behaviourism (changing or preventing behaviour – for example, stopping bank robberies by putting people in a locked prison cell) on the other. Cognitive theory consists of theories about thinking, and the therapy derived from it is in large part about explaining to people how they think. As a therapy, therefore, it lends itself well to structured programmes, delivered in two-hour seminar settings which combine some experiential learning and self-reflection, with delivery with a more straightforward "chalk-and-talk" type teaching of basic concepts. Many of the theories that are taught are highly instructive to individuals in understanding themselves (for example, the stages of change model (Prochaska & DiClemente 1982), or the cycle of offending (Finklehor 1984)). The length of the programmes varies from as few as 20 sessions for some of the basic "thinking skills" type programmes, to 90 sessions for the more elaborate Sex Offender Treatment Programme (SOTP).

These cognitive programmes have their critics, but from the perspective of a consultant psychiatrist in psychotherapy, they can only be a good thing. Violence can be understood as born out of a lack of mentalisation, a lack of being able to have ideas and thoughts, so that one acts instead. Instead of thinking about what's been said, and why it makes you feel angry, you hit out without thought or feeling. The simplest of these cognitive programmes opens up prisoners to the idea of their having choices, to the idea of making decisions about how they react to things, about understanding that they have a mind, and that this mind affects and governs their actions, so that if they understand and manage their minds, they might be able to manage their violence. The more complicated and in depth ones (such as the SOTP) look in detail at the witness statements of prisoners' offences, taking prisoners through these line by line, in the hope of bringing into cold, hard reality the crimes and excesses of the index offence, so often fogged by minimisation, rationalisation, denial or drunkenness at the time.

These cognitive-didactic programmes do have several drawbacks. They rely on, and assume, genuine motivation in the subject. The courses, like studying for public exams and qualifications, require hard work and dedication, concretely in terms of the programmes; patients are given homework to complete. From a psychodynamic perspective, the motivations for doing something are always multiple. Prisoners will be more motivated to complete these programmes "to get out", than in order to understand themselves better, or to understand, or reduce their offending. If told that they need to do such-and-such a course if they want parole, they'll do it. Furthermore, in terms of completing the course, they will submerge any motivation they might have to understand themselves, or even to reduce their offending, beneath an overriding wish to be seen to be doing well on the course, faking good in front of the course facilitator, singularly motivated to get a good report that will be passed to the parole or release board. Appropriate, honest and straightforward motivation is assumed, by definition, from a population of criminals. This is to be contrasted with a psychodynamic approach, where the issue of truth in motivation is the central problem, where even non-criminals and psychoanalytic trainees are assumed to be trying to dupe the therapist with the same tenacity that they are assumed to be duping themselves.

Aware of this, in the UK there was a practice of excluding people scoring above 25 on the PCL-R from these programmes, on the grounds (with some justification) that high PCL-R scorers, namely psychopathic people, were more likely to act as described above, manipulating the course, its content and context, rather than engaging with it genuinely to understand themselves better and reduce their criminality. This situation led to an invidious position for policy makers. Given that about 5% of a prison population scores above 25 on a PCL-R, and that this group is *de facto* excluded from the only rehabilitative activity available in prisons (following the collapse of other programmes in favour of the "effective" psychology programmes), these people effectively had no chance of ever being released on license, being specifically excluded from the sorts of programmes that might enable them to be rehabilitated. It may be that this situation contributed to the need to develop specific programmes for these patients, namely the DSPD pilots briefly described below.

THE DSPD (DANGEROUS AND SEVERE PERSONALITY DISORDER) PROGRAMMES

Over the last decade in the UK there has been a development of services for people in prison and secure settings whose criminality seems more centrally linked to their personality than to more malleable sets of pro-criminal cognitive sets, or accidents of socialisation that might be modifiable though the sorts of offending behaviour programmes and security step-down and resettlement noted above. In the UK in the 1990s, the few remaining inpatient personality disorder treatment units (the Henderson and Cassel hospitals) needed to distinguish between the groups of severe self-harmers that they treated, and the groups of chronically dissatisfied people to be found on any general practitioner's list, who would probably receive a personality disorder diagnosis. The former group was described as "*severely* personality disordered". Similarly, in distinguishing between the many dangerous people in prison, the many personality disordered people in prison, and the identified group targeted for special treatment, the term "dangerous and severe personality disorder" (DSPD) was coined. Further on in the project, the term was more closely defined, such that, to have DSPD, there was a need for individuals to have either:

- severe psychopathy, with a score above 30 on the PCL-R, or

- a score above 25 on the PCL-R and another personality disorder diagnosis.

In addition to fulfilling one of these criteria, there must be a clear functional link in the offending pattern between the personality disorder and the offending. The functional link might, for example, be that an element of the borderline personality problem is impulsivity, and that the offending pattern has a clear impulsive element.

The dilemma for policy makers was that the majority of the DSPD patients were in prison, and the culture of maintenance of responsibility by the individual was to be found in the prison sector, while the treatment expertise was to be found in the health sector, to access which prisoners need to become patients, and to be detained under the Mental Health Act, with all the baggage of the medical model, and the "responsible medical officer" culture of divesting the individual of responsibility for his or her own actions. The compromise was to fund different pilots, two high secure pilot sites in prisons and two in health, then to fund four medium secure personality disorder units in health, as well as identifying facilities such as Grendon as a prison therapeutic step-down pathway. Seeing that the majority of the DSPD programme, therefore, is within the health sector, it is beyond the scope of this book.

Policy makers, as well as piloting DSPD treatment in different settings, prison and health, gave the programme leaders on the sites a relatively free hand to develop their therapeutic programmes. From a psychotherapeutic perspective, there are two particular "technological" developments that have contributed to the effectiveness of these treatments, and which have indeed moved the whole of the personality disorder treatment world forward.

The first is the extension of the "motivational interviewing" (Miller & Rollnick 2002) literature and techniques to people with psychopathy. The application of motivational interviewing ideas to psychopathic people is not about instilling enthusiasm into participants like a warm-up act gees up a TV audience, which can be a caricature in its normal form. Motivational interviewing confronts the psychopathy problem noted above with the cognitive programmes head-on. It posits that the reason why more psychopathic people are not "responsive" to cognitive programmes is because they are contemptuous of them, and because more deeply, they have no wish to change their habits and values. Indeed, they are contemptuous of the sad, middle-class "nine to fivers" advocating these changes. Motivational interviewing acknowledges these attitudes and confronts them head-on, for example, that the individuals are unlikely ever to be free again if they continue with their current attitudes. Furthermore, it is not assumed that these attitudes will change following a set of 10 or 20 didactic sessions, or a certain number of interviews. It is assumed that the individual is cemented into his or her pre-contemplative denial of the need to change, and patiently, the motivational message is repeated until the penny drops. Once more genuine motivation has been, or can be, established, the reason why the individuals cannot benefit from the more standard cognitive therapy programmes has been removed, and these programmes become potent. Consequently, the DSPD therapy programmes seem from the outside a mixture of cognitive/didactic programmes, Grendon therapeutic community elements (to both facilitate the environment and treat a social dimension of need), and motivational/ introductory sessions.

The other highly significant idea is, within the psychopathy concept, separating the psychological aspects of the syndrome (lack of empathy, etc.) from the criminal ones (enacting violence). Psychopathic people are problematic and dangerous almost exclusively because they are violent. If a programme can stop psychopathic people being violent, effectively it has done its work. There are lots of unempathic people in the community living quite safely, because violence is not a part of their repertoire. Clearly, this is an oversimplification of the situation, but it seems to be a central idea behind the two leading programmes described for this group, Wong & Hare's (2005) psychopathy programme, and Wong's (2000) Violence Reduction Programme.

OTHER THERAPEUTIC ACTIVITIES

There are two final therapeutic activities that deserve mention within the rubric of prison therapeutic activities: first, the Close Supervision Centres (CSC), and second, the Drug Strategy. The CSC comprises about 40 beds, with a central hub in HMP Woodhill and a second unit in HMP Whitemoor, then with several beds in each of the high secure prison segregation units. The purpose of the system was to find a better way of dealing with the most difficult and dangerous prisoners – most difficult, that is, in terms of their institutional behaviour, the sort of person who would formerly be moved every six to eight weeks from one segregation unit to another to allow the officers in that unit respite. People are considered for management in the CSC system if, for example, they have killed in custody, if they are frequently and severely violent towards officers or peers, if they engage in severe self-harm repetitively, or if they are extremely difficult to manage for other reasons, for example being highly manipulative, litigious, and so on. Clearly, within the UK prison population of about 80,000, there will be many people who are difficult to manage, and both the culture and structures of management are highly resilient, tolerating and processing large volumes of difficult behaviour. The CSC works with activities that, one way or another, have broken through these containing systems.

Broadly, the philosophy within these units has three pillars. First, prisoners are held in highly staffed, small, physically maximally secure units, enabling both rigourously secure procedural management of individuals (for example, a proportion requiring six officers to unlock), and a high level of individual work with prisoners and officers. The units are small enough and well enough staffed for officers to really get to know their wards, both developing dynamic security, and allowing the prisoner to see staff as human as well as the uniform, much like the introductory period at Grendon. Second, the group has specialised forensic psychiatric input, as there is evidence of considerable psychiatric morbidity in this group, albeit somewhat refractory to treatment. Third, embedded across the units is a violence reduction strategy, based upon the Violence Reduction Programme (Wong 2000), and with this programme running for some prisoners. The aim of the CSC system is to work intensively with very difficult and dangerous people to enable them, after a year or two, to return to normal location, or move on to developing their therapeutic activity in a facility such as Grendon. Obviously, for some, their historical risk, refractory difficulties or political notoriety necessitate a longer stay.

CONCLUSIONS

HMP Grendon hosts a series of open days, where a frequent discussion point raised by prisoners is about how they will survive back "in the system" when they leave. The complaint is that in Grendon they have learned less psychopathic ways of functioning, and they feel that in returning to more default prison environments they will have to become psychopathic again. Anecdotally, post-Grendon prisoners are more work for staff, being more garrulous with custodial and probation staff, and more hungry for therapeutic or psychologically supportive input than their peers. They do survive and maintain what they have learned in treatment, but they require support and seek this out (using appropriate channels of enquiry, lobbying and complaint) in the settings in which they find themselves. In common parlance, "prison" is not synonymous with "therapy", but there is therapy going on and available if one seeks it out, as the post-Grendon group do.

CHAPTER 20

Death in Custody

Andrew Forrester

The term "death in custody" is used to refer to deaths in prison or police custody or in immigration detention centres, or relates to deaths of those detained under the terms of the Mental Health Act. This chapter will, however, largely focus on deaths in prison custody unless otherwise specified. The prison term "self-inflicted death" refers to those who have taken their lives in custody, while the coroner's term "suicide" represents the outcome of an inquest, recognising that not all self-inflicted deaths result in a suicide verdict.

When an individual dies in custody, the event automatically raises questions of the state and the extent to which it cares for those whom it chooses to incarcerate. Such questions form an important part of our democratic structures, allowing us to examine the way we collectively deal with those whose freedom we curtail in the interests either of society, or of themselves. The ways in which we ask, or try to answer, such questions hint strongly at the very nature and purpose of our world. In England and Wales there is a history of relatively strong and robust inquiry, traditionally focused through the coroners' courts (with the involvement of other bodies such as the independent prisons and probation ombudsman). The Human Rights Act 1998, which enshrines the rights contained in the European Convention on Human Rights, guides this inquiry process through a number of articles (Table 20.1). By prohibiting torture, setting out the right to a fair trial and preventing arbitrary punishment, the Act affirms the tone and content of our criminal justice system. It also adjusts the parameters for detention and provides a measure by which we can review deaths in custody when they take place.

Table 20.1 Relevant articles of the Human Rights Act 1998

Article 3 – Prohibition of torture	No one shall be subject to torture or to inhuman or degrading treatment or punishment.
Article 6 – Right to a fair trial	Everyone is entitled to a fair and public hearing within a reasonable time by an independent and impartial tribunal established by law. Everyone charged with a criminal offence shall be presumed innocent until proven guilty. Everyone charged with a criminal offence has a prescribed set of minimum rights.
Article 7 – No punishment without law	No one shall be held guilty of any criminal offence on account of any act or omission which did not constitute a criminal offence under national or international law at the time when it was committed.

THE SIZE OF THE PROBLEM

In the five-year period to 2008, there were 381 self-inflicted deaths and 444 non self-inflicted deaths in prisons in England and Wales (Inquest 2008). This figure represents a drop in numbers from the preceding five-year period, when there were 434 self-inflicted deaths. It has taken place within the context of a dramatic increase in the size of the prison population since the early 1990s, from just over 40,000 to over 80,000 (National Offender Management Service 2008b), meaning that the relative numbers of self-inflicted deaths have fallen considerably in recent years.

In order to work towards preventing deaths in custody in the future, it is important to understand who is likely to be at risk, and why. In an attempt to answer those questions, the *National Confidential Inquiry into Suicides and Homicides by People with Mental Illness* looked at 172 suicides between 1999 and 2000, and found clear links with substance dependence and mental illness (Shaw, Appleby & Baker 2003b). Later, the Joint Committee on Human Rights (2004) reviewed self-inflicted deaths that took place in 2003, and found that younger age groups (mainly those aged 25–39), women and white prisoners were over-represented. They were more likely to be imprisoned for violent offences, and much more likely to be unsentenced. Most were not considered at risk of self-harm or suicide in the period before their death, but the majority had been in prison for only a short period. Most such self-inflicted deaths took place in Category B local prisons. Elsewhere (Royal College of Psychiatrists 2002), asphyxiation has been described as the most commonly used method, generally at night.

In considering prevention, HM Inspectorate of Prisons (1999, p.57) has clearly stated the view that "the total experience of imprisonment affects suicidal behaviour" and called for an "appropriate balance between security, control and justice" within the wider criminal justice system. Setting out the key components of a "healthy prison" (defined as a prison in which "prisoners and staff can remain healthy"), and then outlining a commitment to measure these components through the inspection process, has put preventing suicide at the front of the agenda. The key components now being measured, recorded and made publicly available for each prison are as follows:

- safety of the environment

- treating people with respect

- a full, constructive and purposeful regime

- resettlement training to prevent re-offending.

INVOLVED AGENCIES

A number of agencies have a direct interest in the conduct and outcome of deaths in custody. Key involved agencies include the National Health Service (NHS), with the main point of contact at primary care trust (PCT) level; HM Prison Service; the Prisons and Probation Ombudsman (PPO); HM Chief Inspector of Prisons (HMCIoP) and the coroners' courts. Other less directly involved agencies include charities such as the Howard League for Penal Reform, the Prison Reform Trust and Inquest, and a cross-government expert task force, the Forum for Preventing Deaths in Custody.

Each of the above agencies has an interest in the outcome of death in custody inquests. How they fit together to provide a way forward, however, remains a work in progress. The roles and requirements of involved agencies are discussed below.

The National Health Service (and primary care trusts)

The NHS is divided into two main sections – primary and secondary care. Primary care is responsible for delivering what are often called frontline services, while secondary care is usually accessed following referral from a primary care professional such as a general practitioner (GP). PCTs are presently at the core of the NHS, controlling almost 80% of the overall budget. As local, devolved bodies, they are charged with understanding and delivering the health care needs of a community. Since 2006 they have also been responsible for understanding and commissioning health care services inside prisons. When an individual dies in custody, the local PCT becomes responsible for liaising with the Prisons and Probation Ombudsman and undertaking a Serious Untoward Incident investigation, in the form of a clinical review (HM Prison Service 2004b). Guidelines regarding the level of expertise required for this review, and its content, are not presently available. Once complete, the report is made available to the PPO, and then to HM Coroner.

The Prisons and Probation Ombudsman (PPO)

The PPO has responsibility for dealing with complaints from prisoners, immigration detainees and those on probation. He also investigates deaths in prisons, immigration removal centres and Probation Service approved premises. After a death in custody occurs, a lead investigator and family liaison officer are appointed. The remit of the lead investigator includes questions such as the safety, standards and governance arrangements of the institution, accessibility of services, suitability of the environment and the promotion of health and social well-being in a people-centred way. Following investigation, a draft report is produced, followed by a final report which is sent to HM Coroner.

HM Prison Service

Following a death in prison custody, the prison governor is responsible for taking immediate action, including reporting the death, providing support for staff and prisoners, notifying next-of-kin, providing support for the family and dealing with funeral arrangements. An immediate assessment of what went wrong takes place, with remedial action to be invoked without waiting for the report of the PPO. Each prison must appoint an investigation liaison officer, who is then responsible for enabling the investigation of the PPO.

In terms of prevention, Prison Service Order 2700 (HM Prison Service 2007b) provides instructions for identifying and supporting prisoners considered at risk of suicide or self-harm, and for training and supporting the staff who work with them. All staff in contact with prisoners must receive training and support, and safer custody team leaders hold key responsibility for local suicide and self-harm management and prevention. Suicide prevention co-ordinators ensure that responses on the ground match up with the agreed strategy.

Coroners' courts

The office of coroner was first established in 1194 to investigate many and varied aspects of medieval life (mainly those that could benefit the Crown through revenues). By the nineteenth century, however, many of the fiscal responsibilities of the coroner were removed by the Coroners' Act of 1887. Since then the role of coroner has focused on sudden, violent and unnatural deaths.

A key attribute of the coroner is judicial independence: coroners can only be removed from office by the Lord Chancellor or the courts. Appointment requires qualification as a solicitor, barrister or medical practitioner for a minimum of five years, but most have legal qualifications. There are presently around 120 coroners in England and Wales, but few of them are full-time, the rest being mainly solicitors in private practice working part-time.

The Coroners Act 1988 creates, under Section 8(1), a duty to hold an inquest in cases of violent, unnatural and sudden deaths of unknown cause. This duty includes death in prison custody, when the inquest must take place before a jury regardless of the cause of death. These requirements also hold if the death takes place in hospital, the deceased having been transferred there from prison custody (R v HM Coroner for Inner North London, ex parte Linnane).

THE INQUEST

The process of the inquest, the public face of HM Coroner, is intended to be inquisitorial rather than adversarial in nature. The intention is to establish the facts, rather than to undertake a trial of involved parties with different interests. Therefore, no formal allegations are made, and no pleas are expected or delivered. The events are managed within the terms of the Coroners Act 1988 and the Coroners Rules 1984 (the latter functioning as a statutory instrument). The coroner is able to run events as seen fit, being "the master of his own procedure" (R v HM Coroner for East Kent, ex parte Spooner). The remit is therefore to conduct an inquiry to find the facts, with the aim of answering four specific questions (R v HM Coroner for North Humberside, ex parte Jamieson):

- Who was the deceased?

- Where did the death occur?

- What was the time of death?

- How did the deceased come by his death?

The last question is usually, but not always, the most significant. Intended to cover all "acts and omissions which are directly responsible for the death" (R v HM Coroner for Western District of East Sussex, ex parte Homberg), it can therefore have a wide application, at the discretion of the coroner.

The hearing

The Coroners Act 1988 requires that all inquests are held in public, except in cases where evidence might jeopardise national security. Members of the public and journalists have the right to attend, but there is no obligation to provide additional access if the courtroom becomes full. Rule 20 of the Coroners Rules (1984: SI No. 552) sets out the entitlement to examine witnesses, as follows:

> Without prejudice to any enactment with regard to the examination of witnesses at an inquest, any person who satisfies the coroner that he is [an interested person] shall be entitled to examine any witness at an inquest either in person or by [an authorised advocate].

The following individuals have the above rights, opening up the potential for many witnesses and points of representation:

- a parent, child, spouse and any personal representative of the deceased

- any beneficiary under a policy of insurance issued on the life of the deceased

- the insurer who issued such a policy of insurance

- any person whose act or omission or that of his agent or servant may in the opinion of the coroner have caused, or contributed to, the death of the deceased

- any person appointed by a trade union to which the deceased at the time of his death belonged, if the death of the deceased may have been caused by an injury received in the course of his employment or by an industrial disease

- an inspector appointed by, or a representative of, an enforcing authority, or any person appointed by a government department to attend the inquest

- the chief officer of police

- any other person who, in the opinion of the coroner, is a properly interested person.

Giving evidence

The coroner is responsible for opening and closing inquests formally. Once open, she must ascertain who the interested parties are before outlining the purpose of the inquest. She then outlines the format of evidence to be given, including witnesses to be called and documents to be taken.

Evidence is given on oath and must be recorded by the coroner, either by tape or in writing. Given the inquisitorial nature of proceedings, the coroner is usually the first to question a witness. Although statements may already be available, and therefore the answers to many questions may already be known, it is considered important that the facts are aired in public. Indeed, such an airing forms part of the coroner's responsibility. It should be done with a view to resolving as many unanswered questions as possible (R v HM Coroner for Coventry, ex parte O'Reilly), while being mindful of witness credibility and reliability (R v Avon Coroner, ex parte Bentley). After the coroner has questioned a witness, interested parties are invited to ask questions. Sometimes questioning will proceed with future criminal or civil proceedings in mind, even though this is clearly contrary to the spirit of the coroner's inquest (R v Poplar Coroner, ex parte Thomas). Further questioning may also be undertaken by interested persons who are not legally represented, and this will often require the close assistance of the coroner, who should be careful to remain neutral.

In order to be a competent witness, a person must be able to understand the nature of what is required. Such an individual can be compelled to attend and give evidence, and all summoned witnesses must answer the coroner's questions, unless one of the following four exceptions apply:

- answering the question will incriminate the individual (this has a bearing on possible future criminal, but not civil, proceedings)

- the information is protected by legal privilege

- a journalist is protected from revealing an information source unless certain overriding concerns (e.g. national security) apply

- public interest immunity can be demonstrated (i.e. a balance between public interest and the administration of justice must be considered (Conway v Rimmer)).

Evidence should be given in a clear and precise fashion, without speaking too quickly (given the necessity to record). It is best to exude a calm, professional appearance, sticking to facts without being emotive. Arrogance is unhelpful. Witnesses should, where possible, use simple language, while remaining within the field of their own knowledge.

The verdict

The use of the word "verdict" often leads to a misunderstanding of the nature of the coroner's inquiry, suggesting, as it does, an adversarial process. As a consequence, coroners have increasingly moved towards narrative verdicts for appropriate cases, instead of the more traditional verdicts (e.g. misadventure, open verdict, etc.). In some cases criminal or civil liability will become clear as the inquest unfolds. The narrative verdict might then offer a springboard for future litigation, but should, nevertheless, retain the use of neutral language to prevent future prejudice.

Commonly used non-narrative verdicts include "natural causes" (usually referring to the normal progression of a natural illness), "accidental death" (death arising from an unnatural event), "misadventure" (after starting a task that then goes wrong) and "suicide" (a voluntary act requiring intent). An "open verdict" is also available if other conclusions cannot be satisfied.

CHAPTER 21

Prisons Inspection

Tish Laing-Morton and Colin Allen

INTRODUCTION

The *modus operandi* and effectiveness of the work of the independent Chief Inspector of Prisons in England and Wales has been observed with envy by those interested in the proper treatment of prisoners in other countries in the developed world.

The qualities of the last three post-holders have earned the post a reputation for integrity, common sense and persuasiveness that has helped the Prison Service improve its treatment of prisoners, even against the background of unremitting overcrowding. Perhaps above all, the inspectorate has earned the respect of prisoners and of prison staff for being apart from politics and therefore able to focus on the internationally agreed standards for the treatment of prisoners.

HISTORICAL CONTEXT

The first independent inspectors of prisons were appointed in 1835. Then, as now, they reported directly to the Home Secretary and these reports were in the public domain. They played an important role in standardising the prison system and introducing rules about the way that prisoners should be treated.

Their independence was removed in 1877 by Sir Edmund Du Cane, who was responsible for the new national prison system. He perceived that the inspectors would undermine his authority. Consequently the work of the inspectors was subsumed into the Prison Commission, later to become the Prison Department. The situation remained unchanged for over a hundred years until the late 1970s, when a crisis of gigantic proportions over disputes between managers and the Prison Officers Association brought the prison system to its knees and prompted Lord Justice May's inquiry (Home Office 1979). One of his major recommendations was to appoint a Chief Inspector with the authority to report independently about the treatment of prisoners. This was set in statute by Parliament in 1982. This also gave the Chief Inspector the right of access to any part of a prison, day or night. Despite having no executive authority over the Prison Service, the power of the post has been to have direct access to ministers over prison issues and the freedom to publish what has been found during inspections. Within public services, independence rests primarily with the post-holder rather than with the post. Over the past two decades, whether by intention or default, successive Home Secretaries have chosen for the role of Chief Inspector of Prisons people with both the ability and the willingness to act independently.

After early years of comparative calm, the profile of the post was raised and became very influential during the tenure of Judge Sir Stephen Tumim. He co-operated with Lord Woolf in the report of the major riots at Strangeways (Home Office 1991a) and went on to challenge the negativity of prison life and many of the underlying and residual practices of a Prison Service that was perceived by many to have lost its way in a modern world. He strongly believed that the way to encourage prisoners to move away from criminal behaviour and to claim a respectable stake in society was through enabling them to gain a sense of achievement by way of educational qualifications and artistic expression. By constantly bringing this to the attention of politicians and the public through his inspection reports and appearances on the media, he played a big part in making education and art in prison both respectable and desirable. By challenging the *status quo* Sir Stephen was frequently in conflict not only with Prison Service officials but also with ministers, much of it in public view over the airwaves and in print. His eccentric but respected judicial image became very effective in influencing the press and broadcasting media. As a result the public began to understand more about what prisons and imprisonment were about. Despite this, prisons in England and Wales, as in other parts of the world, were overcrowded and starved of resources because they were not seen as areas of public administration where improvements lead to governments gaining popularity. Consequently, after eight years in the post, Sir Stephen's contract was not renewed.

Stephen Tumim was succeeded by Sir David Ramsbotham, recently retired from a very distinguished career in the British Army. One of his first actions was to publish a paper that made the case for the National Health Service to take over responsibility for the health care of prisoners (HM Inspectorate of Prisons 1996). This was largely accepted by the Government, but has taken many years to be implemented (HM Prison Service & NHS Executive 1999). This is discussed more fully later.

Following the inspection of Holloway prison in 1995, which profoundly disturbed him, Sir David produced a thematic review on the treatment of women prisoners. This and other published reviews on young prisoners, life-sentenced prisoners, elderly prisoners and pre-trial prisoners produced the criteria which were to guide his prison inspections. Like his predecessor, Sir David never flinched from challenging senior officials and ministers about what he found during his inspections, and throughout his tenure in office the public were kept well informed about what was taking place in prisons and his recommendations about how they should be improved. In turn, Sir David's contract was not renewed.

Close observers of the Home Office predicted that ministers would next choose someone as Chief Inspector of Prisons who would be less energetic and publicly challenging of the system. These predictions proved to be wrong. In selecting Anne Owers, the first woman to hold the post, ministers appointed someone who had already had a distinguished career as director of the all-party campaigning organisation Justice and had previously been director of the Joint Council for the Welfare of Immigrants. Anne Owers' style has perhaps been more cerebral than that of her two predecessors, but no less challenging, and her pace of work has been no less energetic. This has been demonstrated by the robust way in which she defends the independence of the role and the informed insight that she has brought to improving inspection.

CURRENT INSPECTION

Since 2000, the Inspectorate has extended its role well beyond the boundaries of prisons and young offender institutions in England and Wales. Under the Asylum and Immigration Act 1999 it was given a statutory duty to inspect immigration removal centres (IRCs). In 2003 ministers further extended this remit to include immigration short-term holding facilities (STHFs) at air- and seaports. In 2004 the Inspectorate was commissioned to inspect the Military Corrective Training Centre, Colchester, and the Sovereign Base Areas prison, Cyprus. Since 2005 there have been further commissions to inspect prisons in Northern Ireland, the Channel Islands, the Isle of Man and Canada. Closer to home, a range of joint work is being undertaken with other criminal justice inspectorates, including looking at police and court cells in the context of criminal justice area inspections, and inter-prison escorts with the Magistrate Courts Service Inspectorate (now the Inspectorate of Court Administration).

Broadening the scope of inspection has demanded the recruitment of increasingly diverse and specialist staff. The Chief Inspector is a Crown appointment and was, like her predecessors, drawn from outside the Home Office. Below her, the majority of inspectors are still drawn from the Prison Service but, increasingly, they come from medical, nursing, probation, social work, drug treatment and legal backgrounds. In addition, to minimise the burdens on establishments and to maximise available expertise, full inspections are conducted jointly with Ofsted, the Royal Pharmaceutical Society of Great Britain and the Dental Practice Division of the Business Services Agency of the NHS, the latter two as part of the health care inspection team. This diversity enhances the validity and quality of inspection and reflects the "normalisation" of service provision in prisons, where education and health services are increasingly funded, managed and delivered in much the same way as they would be in the community.

Just as individual specialists have been recruited, so the five inspection teams have been required to specialise to increase consistency and professionalism. Thus, while prisoner numbers dictate that all teams inspect some adult male establishments, specialist women's, young adult, juvenile and immigration detainee teams have been established. Individual inspectors are also expected to develop a policy interest and take part in thematic inspections on particular topics, as well as cross-cutting reviews with other inspectorates.

Historically, ministers have required that the Inspectorate conduct a full inspection of each adult prison and young offender institution every five years, and of each juvenile facility and immigration removal centre every three years. In order to assess progress, follow-up inspections are conducted in the interim. Full inspections are usually announced and follow-ups unannounced. Unannounced inspections are an important tool in the effective scrutiny of closed institutions. They allow the Inspectorate to pursue public, parliamentary and ministerial concerns without advanced warning or preparation time and, by the same token, can provide powerful evidence that vindicates prisons if assertions about their performance are ill-founded.

In line with the Government's principles for the inspection of public services (Office of Public Services Reform 2003), the Inspectorate has developed an impartial, transparent and evidence-based methodology. The aim is to support the improvement of services by revealing actual, as opposed to intended, outcomes for service recipients. This means going well beyond the mere auditing of processes to test what is really happening by using confidential detainee survey and prisoner groups, interviews with prisoners or detainees, staff and visitors, and painstaking observation. Published assessment criteria guide inspectors and allow judgements to be made against the Inspectorate's four tests of a "healthy prison": safety, respect, purposeful activity and resettlement (HM Inspectorate of Prisons 1999). A new volume of generic inspection criteria, or *Expectations*, was published in 2003 to provide a transparent basis for making judgments. A volume of *Expectations* for IRCs and STHCs was published in 2005, as were *Expectations* specifically for juveniles. In general, *Expectations* mirror the outcomes sought by Prison Service and Immigration and Nationality Directorate standards, but they are also explicitly grounded in and referenced to international human rights instruments. As an independent inspectorate concerned with the qualitative and holistic inspection of outcomes for detainees, there are occasions when *Expectations* must expand on the nature, detail and adequacy of internal standards. This creates an inherent tension, although recent analysis by the Prison Service suggests that less than 5% of our criteria diverge from internal standards, but also provides a constructive stimulus for policy and performance improvement.

A key element of the Inspectorate's methodology is the deployment of confidential surveys to a random and representative proportion of detainees. These generate data from service recipients which can be triangulated against other types of evidence to test whether "healthy prison" tests are met. Establishment survey results are compared to the comparator figure for other establishments of that type, and significant differences between the figures highlighted to inspectors to indicate apparent areas of concern and of good practice. Inspectors are also able to use the survey to look at the different perceptions of particular groups – for example, black and minority ethnic or foreign national prisoners. The surveys also allow variations in the views of residents in different wings of large establishments to become apparent. Since their introduction in 1997 these surveys have provided a unique, comparative database of detainees' perspectives. Commendably, in 2003 the Prison Service introduced a similar tool designed by Cambridge University, the Measurement of the Quality of Prison Life Survey, to enable prisoner perceptions of life inside to inform prison management.

Good inspection distils huge quantities of evidence into clear, consistent judgements that stakeholders can understand and which can help managers as they pursue performance improvement. Inspection reports contain a healthy prison summary divided into safety, respect, purposeful activity and resettlement. In 2004 this was further refined by the introduction of a formal, four-point assessment of outcomes for detainees under each healthy prison heading and, therefore, of the establishment's performance against each test. (See Table 21.1. For IRCs amended healthy establishment assessments are made.)

Table 21.1 Healthy prison assessments

Numeric	Definition
4	The prison is performing well against this healthy prison test. There is no evidence that outcomes for prisoners are being adversely affected in any significant areas.
3	The prison is performing reasonably well against this healthy prison test. There is evidence of adverse outcomes for prisoners in only a small number of areas. For the majority there are no significant concerns.
2	The prison is not performing sufficiently well against this healthy prison test. There is evidence that outcomes for prisoners are being adversely affected in many areas or particularly in those areas of greatest importance to the well-being of prisoners. Problems/concerns, if left unattended, are likely to become areas of serious concern.
1	The prison is performing poorly against this healthy prison test. There is evidence that the outcomes for prisoners are seriously affected by current practice. There is a failure to ensure even adequate treatment of and/or conditions for prisoners. Immediate remedial action is required.

With resources ever tighter and demand growing, and the need for smarter, less burdensome inspection, simply maintaining a chronological cycle is neither affordable nor effective. As a result, the Inspectorate has sought to balance chronology with risk assessment: in other words, targeting resources where they are most needed. This has inherent difficulties: multiple audit and inspection bodies tend to descend on higher-risk establishments, while the lower-risk receive, in effect, "inspection holidays". Such holidays are inappropriate in the context of protecting human rights in changeable, closed institutions. So a balance is required. The Inspectorate has sought to achieve this by retaining the current chronology of full inspections, but applying risk assessment to determine the type of follow-up inspections required. Risk is judged using a new intelligence system underpinned by healthy prison assessments.

Since April 2005 the Inspectorate's programme of inspections has been based on a mixture of chronology and risk assessment. Full inspections continue unchanged on their five- or three-year cycles, but this can only be afforded by rationalising the resources devoted to unannounced follow-up inspections on a risk-assessed basis. A full inspection requires maximum resources, it is preceded by a full prisoner survey, involves a team leader and four core inspectors, plus specialists and partner inspectorates, and lasts a week. By contrast, follow-up inspections are resourced on the basis of risk assessment. Those deemed higher-risk are revisited within 12–36 months of a full inspection to assess progress against previous recommendations, and place particular emphasis on areas of concern. They usually include a full team of inspectors and researchers. Fresh healthy prison assessments are made and an inspection report published with a full healthy prison summary. Lower-risk establishments are revisited 24–36 months after their last full inspection. A smaller team of inspectors focuses purely on progress against previous recommendations. Short reports are placed on the Inspectorate website with a brief healthy prison summary which confirms or amends the previous assessments.

HEALTH CARE INSPECTION

As with the rest of the Inspectorate, the inspection of health care in prisons has evolved and developed in recent years. The core health team has grown from two part-time inspectors (a Medical Inspector and Nurse Inspector) to a full-time Head of Health Inspection with a full-time deputy, with added support from contracted part-time health inspectors. As well as this increase in size, the change of titles was deliberate to signal a broader focus of inspection on the health of prisoners generally in a custodial environment, not just on the services provided in the health care centre. Consequently, health care expectations are cross-referenced with many others, such as suicide and self-harm, substance use, physical activity and resettlement.

Members of the health team may work with any of the specialist inspection teams and also fully contribute to health care aspects of thematic reviews and joint working. For full inspections, a core member of the health team and one of the two substance use inspectors will be joined, usually for half a day, by a pharmaceutical and dental inspector. The latter visits are timed for when the relevant practitioners are present in the establishment. The subsequent dental and pharmaceutical reports are then integrated into the health care chapter of the inspection report.

Another aspect by which health team inspectors differ from other inspectorate teams is that, apart from substance use inspectors, all members of the health team have specific professional responsibilities to report clinical concerns to their registration bodies. Fortunately this has rarely occurred. Occasionally, the health team has invited guest inspectors to add expertise in highly specialised areas, such as forensic child and adolescent psychiatry.

The transfer of responsibility for commissioning health care from the prison service to the NHS has brought further complexity to health inspection, not least because it is only publicly run prisons that are now the responsibility of the primary care trust (PCT) in which they are located. Organisationally, financially and culturally the Prison Service and NHS are unequal partners, facing different pressures. There is evidence that partnership working is beginning to improve the health care available to prisoners, but it is probably too soon to judge whether these improvements will result in better health and social outcomes for prisoners (Boyington 2005).

As the Healthcare Commission (HCC – to be replaced by the Care Quality Commission in April 2009) is responsible for assuring the quality of NHS health care, there was the potential for confusion of responsibility for inspection where custodial care is commissioned and provided by the NHS. To avoid this, a Memorandum of Understanding (MoU) was drawn up between the Inspectorate and the Healthcare Commission. This makes it clear that the Inspectorate health team will continue to inspect the delivery of health care within custodial settings, whilst the HCC inspect the commissioning arrangements at the relevant PCT (see Figure 21.1). The combined findings are submitted as part of the inspection report that is published after every inspection.

INSPECTION OUTCOMES

In 2003, the Inspectorate introduced post-inspection exit surveys and an annual stakeholder survey to try to find out stakeholders' views of inspections. The exit survey gives those inspected a chance to voice concerns (or indeed praise) about the inspection process, which can be fed into our internal performance management. When aggregated, this feedback has also helped drive specific change. For example, the Inspectorate has responded to concerns from governors and directors about clashes with internal audit bodies by working closely on programming with other scrutiny bodies. The annual stakeholder survey has a wider internal and external audience and focuses on the quality of inspection reports. Again, findings have been used to drive change – for example, influencing the new report formats introduced in 2004.

In an effort to assess whether inspections make a difference, all our follow-up reports are closely monitored to see, first, the take-up of our recommendations by inspected bodies, and, second, implementation of recommendations since the last full inspection. Analysis for 2006–2007 revealed that 94% of our recommendations were accepted and that 67% of recommendations had been implemented wholly or in part by

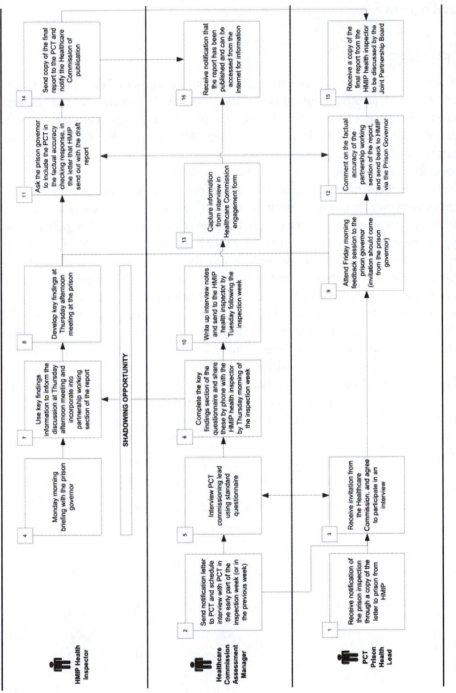

Figure 21.1 Process for the joint project between HM Inspectorate of Prisons and Healthcare Commission on commissioning prison health services (Healthcare Commission 2006)

the time of our follow-up inspection visit (HM Inspectorate of Prisons 2007a). These are impressive indicators of our effectiveness and suggest that the Inspectorate is making a real difference.

THE FUTURE

In 2005 the Government put forward a proposal to amalgamate HM Inspectorate of Prisons with the four other criminal justice inspectorates. The creation of the National Offenders Management Service (NOMS) inevitably raised questions about the existence of separate inspectorates for prison and probation. Although the five CJS Inspectorate amalgamation did not materialise, there has been an increase in the levels of joint inspections, formalised in the Police and Justice Act 2006.

The Government has made clear that it accepts the unique importance of independent inspection of custody: a function required by international law as a safeguard against human rights abuse and an essential source of reassurance to the public about the appropriateness of what goes on in their name in the hidden world of detention. Recent events across the globe illustrate how rapidly behaviour towards those in custody can spiral away from decency and respect. It is therefore of no surprise to see such an eminent commentator as Lord Hurd argue that "nothing must be done to impair the professionalism, independence and the integrity of the Inspectorate of Prisons. The Inspectorate is a fortress of independent analysis and good sense on which all of us rely. That fortress must not be weakened by mining and sapping from Whitehall" (Hurd 2004, p.3). It remains to be seen whether the fortress will be weakened. Certainly the Chief Inspector of Prisons, Anne Owers DBE, has been vociferous in demanding that the Government honour its public commitment to maintain "the nature, efficacy and extent" (Scotland 2004) of independent prison inspection.

CHAPTER 22

International Perspectives (I) – An Overview of US Correctional Mental Health

Charles Scott and Barbara McDermott

INTRODUCTION

The overall mission of the US correctional system is multifaceted and includes retribution for law-violating behaviors, removal of the offender from society, deterrence of future criminal acts, and rehabilitation. As the US correctional facilities increase in number and size, rehabilitation has become an increasingly important component of correctional systems. At midyear 2006, more than 2.2 million individuals were incarcerated in the United States and one in every 133 US residents lived in a jail or prison (Sabol & Harrison 2007).

This chapter reviews types of US correctional facilities and provides a brief overview of treatment interventions for inmates with mental illness, substance use disorders, and developmental disabilities.

TYPES OF US CORRECTIONAL FACTILITIES

The United States correctional system is complex and includes a federal system, 50 separate state systems, and thousands of local systems (Silverman 2001). Correctional housing facilities vary and are broadly classified into three types of facilities: lockups, jails, and prisons. Lockups are local, temporary holding facilities that constitute the initial phase of the criminal justice system in a significant number of jurisdictions. The lockup is the most common type of correctional facility, with an average stay usually lasting less than 48 hours. Lockups are often located in the local police station, where only temporary detainment (such as with arrestees charged with drunk driving) is required.

Jails are locally operated correctional facilities that confine persons before or after adjudication. Individuals who are convicted of a misdemeanor (minor crime) may receive a sentence of a year or less and complete their sentence in a jail, not a prison. Prisons are confinement facilities that maintain custodial authority over individuals who receive a sentence greater than one year. Prisons are operated by both state and federal governments and are typically large facilities, often with over 500 beds (Beck & Harrison 2006).

At some point after an individual is placed into a US correctional facility, a process known as "classification" occurs. Classification attempts to match inmates with the appropriate level of security, custody supervision, and services necessary to meet their needs For individuals who are serving time in jail, the classification procedure typically occurs in the jail in which they are housed. As a result of this process, the inmate may be placed in a particular housing unit within the jail, based on either security, medical, and/or mental health needs For those individuals sentenced to prison, the location of the classification process depends largely on the inmate's jurisdiction. In some areas, inmates are sent to a central reception and diagnostic centre after they are sentenced. After an evaluation of the level of security and special services required, the inmate is transferred to the most appropriate matched facility. In other jurisdictions, inmates undergo the classification process in a prison reception unit where they are kept until this process is completed. They are then placed in general population or transferred to another facility if needed.

Facility security level refers to the type of physical barriers designed to manage inmates and prevent escape. Whereas the security level refers to the number of environmental barriers to prevent escape or manage behavior, an inmate's custody level is determined by the degree of staff supervision necessary to provide adequate control of the inmate (National Institute of Corrections 1987).

During the last few decades, several US jurisdictions have built or modified existing prison facilities that create highly isolated environments for those inmates considered too dangerous to be maintained in a general prison population. These facilities are known by various names, to include "extended control facility," "supermax," "maxi-max," or a "security housing unit" (SHU). Often labeled a prison within a prison, these tightly managed facilities provide control of inmates who have exhibited violent or seriously disruptive behavior while incarcerated and as a result cannot be maintained in a less restrictive environment. In 1963, the United States Penitentiary at Marion, located in southern Illinois, was opened to replace Alcatraz and was the highest maximum security prison in the United States. Inmates in these types of facilities are often kept in their cell for up to 23 hours a day with minimal, if any, interaction with other inmates.

MENTAL DISORDERS

Correctional facilities are quickly becoming the new mental health treatment centers for individuals with mental disorders. According to E. Fuller Torrey (1999), the Los Angeles County Jail houses 3,400 inmates with mental illness, making it the largest psychiatric inpatient facility in the United States. The prevalence of mental illness among US inmates is substantial. According to a 2005 nationwide survey of jails and prisons conducted by the US Department of Justice, more than half of all prison and jail inmates had a mental health problem. Female inmates had higher rates of mental health problems than male inmates. Mental health problems were defined by a recent history or symptoms of a mental illness during the 12 months prior to the interview. Inmates qualified as having a recent history of a mental health problem if they had a clinical diagnosis or had received treatment by a mental health provider. Symptoms of a mental disorder were based on criteria specified in DSM-IV. Despite the significant prevalence of mental illness in this surveyed population, only one in three state prisoners and one in six jail inmates with a mental health problem were noted to have received treatment since admission. In reviewing types of treatment received, 15% of state prisoners were prescribed medication for a mental health problem, and nearly 15% also reported some type of mental health therapy (James & Glaze 2006).

The types of psychotherapy available to US inmates vary widely and may include individual psychotherapy, group and recreational therapy, cognitive-behavioural therapy, and dialectical behaviour therapy. Behavioral incentive programs (BIPs) and token economies are utilised by some US correctional facilities to alter inmates' maladaptive behaviors. The Tamms Correctional Center in Illinois and two prisons in the California Department of Corrections utilise such programs by allowing inmates to earn various privileges through demonstration of appropriate behaviors and adherence to recommended treatment plans. Examples of privileges contingent on specified behaviors include use of radios and television, out-of-cell time to clean the unit, use of small group yards, and access to canteen and packages (Chaiken, Thompson & Shoemaker 2005).

Several states, such as Colorado, have also established residential community corrections centres (RCCCs) for inmates approaching parole. RCCCs function as decentralized residential programs that assist in the reintegration of inmates into the community. RCCCs utilize the "self-help" approach characterized by therapeutic communities and provide intense supervision prior to the inmate's release into the community. Although RCCCs are not restricted to inmates with mental illness, they often provide many services important in assisting offenders with mental disorders, such as monitored medication administration, case management, individual counseling, psychotherapy, and substance abuse treatment (Chaiken et al. 2005).

To prevent individuals with mental illness from entering the criminal justice system, numerous states and local jurisdictions have developed mental health courts. These courts are a division of the criminal court system established to identify nonviolent offenders with mental illness who are appropriate for diversion into mandated treatment programs as an alternative to incarceration. Over the last ten years, approximately 120 mental health courts have been created in the United States. The efficacy of such courts shows promise in increasing access for offenders with mental illness to appropriate services and in decreasing costs associated with incarceration (Kuehn 2007).

SUBSTANCE USE DISORDERS

Substance use and substance use disorders (SUDs) are extremely common among US inmates. In a 2004 national survey of state and federal prisons, the United States Bureau of Justice Statistics for the first time included specific measures of substance use and dependence based on the DSM-IV criteria. The survey results indicated that 53% of state and 45% of federal prisoners met the DSM-IV criteria for drug dependence or abuse. Nearly a third of state and a quarter of federal prisoners committed their offence under the influence of drugs (Mumola & Karberg 2006).

Because of the nearly epidemic presence of substance use disorders in this population, treatment interventions are essential in diverting individuals with substance use disorders away from the criminal justice system. To address this need, an increasing number of jurisdictions in the US have developed special drug courts within the criminal justice system. These courts seek to provide mandatory alcohol and drug treatment programs as an alternative to incarceration. Defendants who commit nonviolent crimes related to their drug use are candidates most commonly considered for drug diversion programs. Participants who complete mandatory treatment programmes ordered through drug courts have a substantially reduced risk of future criminal recidivism (Cooper 2003).

For those individuals with a substance use disorder who do not qualify for a diversion programme and are subsequently incarcerated, substance use treatment within a correctional facility is vital. However, surveys examining the actual availability of substance use treatment for US inmates range from 28% (Peters & May 1992) to 70% (Wilson 2000). Do jail-based drug treatment programmes decrease recidivism rates? Some early outcome studies suggest cautious optimism. For example, Turley *et al.* (2004) found that three different cohorts of nonviolent jail inmates who participated in a drug treatment programme were substantially less likely to be criminal recidivists during a one-year follow-up period, when compared to an inmate control group.

Substance use treatment needs of prison inmates are also substantial. In their analysis of data from over 14,000 inmates in 275 US prisons, Belenko & Peugh (2005) estimate that one-third of male and half of female prison inmates need residential treatment for a substance use disorder. These authors recognize that the actual treatment capacity is inadequate and suggest four levels of treatment that correspond to intervention programmes potentially available in prisons:

1. no treatment – appropriate for inmates with no or little history of actual substance use and no consequences of involvement in drug-related behaviors

2. short-term intervention – programmes such as self-help, drug education, treatment readiness, or short-term motivational interventions

3. "outpatient treatment" – moderate duration of either individual treatment and/or group counselling, though not necessarily in a separate housing unit in the correctional facility

4. residential treatment – long-term, intensive clinical intervention where inmates reside in a separate treatment housing unit. This more intensive treatment is recommended for those inmates with recent histories of frequent hard drug use, three or more drug-related consequences, or a relatively high number of other drug-related problems.

The few studies that have examined the efficacy of a prison-based therapeutic community in treating substance use disorders also show promising results. For example, in their analysis of data from the California Substance Abuse Treatment Facility therapeutic community programme for California prisoners, Prendergast, Farabee & Cartier (1999) found that enrolled inmates had lower institutional infraction rates compared with inmates in the general population, had no positive drug tests on random drug testing, and that correctional officers had a more positive view of their unit compared with officers working in non-treatment settings. Similar findings were noted in an analysis of Delware's in-prison therapeutic community, known as KEY, which houses approximately 120 inmates, with a length of stay ranging from 6 to 18 months (Dietz, O'Connell & Scarpitti 2003).

The majority of studies following inmates after their release from prison indicate that rehabilitation-oriented treatment for substance use can lead to favorable outcomes following incarceration (Gendreau 1996, Knight, Simpson & Hiller 1999), especially if aftercare is provided (Griffith *et al.* 1999). In their study of over 4,000 male and female parolees (who received a California prison-based therapeutic community substance abuse treatment program), Burdon *et al.* (2007) found that released individuals benefited equally from outpatient and residential aftercare, regardless of the severity of their drug/alcohol problem. These authors emphasize the importance of an uninterrupted continuum of community care following inmates' participation in prison-based treatments.

DEVELOPMENTAL DISABLITIES

In the correctional system, the developmental disability most often encountered is mental retardation, and the majority of inmates with mental retardation are in the mild range

(Noble & Conley 1992). Some research has indicated that mental retardation is over-represented within the criminal justice system (e.g. Santamour & West 1982a, Petersilia 1997, Cockram, Jackson & Underwood 1998) although others have found no differences from the general population (MacEachron 1979, New York State Commission on Quality of Care for the Mentally Disabled 1991, Conley, Luckasson & Bouthilet 1992). The considerable variability in estimates may be secondary to differences in assessment, definition, and methodology as well as regional differences. Santamour & West (1982a) reported that the rate of adults with mental retardation in prison ranged from 8% to almost 30%. Specifically, the South Carolina Department of Corrections indicated a rate of 8%, Texas reported a 10% rate of offenders with mental retardation, and Georgia reported 27%. Petersilia (1997) estimated that 6,400 adult and juvenile inmates have mental retardation in the California corrections system. An estimated 4–10% of individuals in prison or jail in California are developmentally disabled (Petersilia 2000). However, some reports suggest that the prevalence of individuals with mental retardation in corrections is comparable to the prevalence in the general population. For example, the New York State Commission on Quality of Care for the Mentally Disabled (1991) reported that 2% of approximately 53,400 inmates are developmentally disabled. Noble & Conley (1992) reported that approximately 14,000–20,000 inmates have developmental disabilities, constituting roughly 2% of all inmates in state and federal prisons. They also noted that rates of mental retardation ranged from 0.5% to almost 20% within state and federal prisons, asserting that the differences are secondary to methods of assessment.

The management of inmates with developmental disabilities has presented correctional systems with significant problems. One controversy has been whether inmates with developmental disabilities should be housed in the general prison population. Those in favor of housing with the general prison population adhere to the principle of normalization, suggesting that individuals with mental retardation should be treated like others as much as possible (Santamour & West 1982a). As such, it is most often the case that prisoners with developmental disabilities are housed with the general population (Smith et al. 1990, New York State Commission on Quality of Care for the Mentally Disabled 1991, Giamp & West 2003). This housing situation places the inmate with developmental disabilities at risk for victimization by other inmates. Prisoners with mental retardation are more likely to be exploited, victimized, abused, and injured secondary to the previously noted cognitive deficits (Santamour & West 1982a, Ellis & Luckasson 1985, Smith, C. et al. 1990, Stavis 1991, Petersilia 1997, Müller-Isberner & Hodgins 2000, Giamp & West 2003). Petersilia (1997) reported that offenders with mental retardation who are housed with the general population are victimized in such ways as having their property stolen, being raped, or being manipulated by other inmates to violate the rules. They have difficulty understanding the rules, which also increases the likelihood of disciplinary action.

Hall (1992) estimated that fewer than 10% of inmates with such deficits receive specialized services. Unlike programmes for offenders with mental illness, the goals of specialized programs for offenders with developmental disabilities are not remediation of their disability. The goal of most programs is education, training, and skills enhancement tailored to the specific needs of the inmate. As with any other disorder, the diagnosis of mental retardation provides no information about the needs of the specific individual. For these reasons, assessment is a critical component in any specialized program. For example, as a result of Clark v State of California (1998), prison officials in California developed a "remedial plan" (known as the Clark plan) for identifying prisoners with developmental disabilities and providing them with access to a variety of programs that would make early release more likely. This plan includes:

1. screening for developmental disabilities

2. housing developmentally disabled inmates together based on level of functioning

3. providing additional staff to these housing units

4. training staff on interacting with developmentally disabled inmates

5. providing instructors with special education credentials for each Developmental Disability Program responsible for developing individually tailored programmes as necessary

6. providing parole agents to ensure that developmentally disabled inmates understand the terms of parole and are aware of services available in the community.

Programs for offenders with mental retardation generally focus on improving the functioning and adaptation of the inmate while incarcerated and upon release (Santamour & West 1982b, Santamour 1987). The vulnerabilities outlined in the previous sections lead to logical interventions that include skills training, educational/vocational rehabilitation, and counselling/treatment specific to the needs of each offender. Model programs in several states have been developed that incorporate many of the mentioned treatment approaches. In each of these programs, several basic functions are performed, including assessment, intervention and discharge planning.

CONCLUSION

In the United States, an increasing number of individuals with mental disorders and mental defects are living behind bars. As a result of these various societal forces, many mental health professionals are discovering that their new workplace is located inside a jail or prison. Mental health practitioners play a variety of vitally important roles in the assessment, treatment, and management of offenders at virtually every point along their journey through this unique and complex world.

CHAPTER 23

International Perspectives (II) – Delivery of Mental Health Services in New Zealand Prisons: Context and Approaches

Ceri Evans and Phil Brinded

THE NEW ZEALAND CONTEXT: FORENSIC PSYCHIATRIC SERVICES

The impetus for the development of forensic psychiatric services in New Zealand was provided by the 1988 Mason Report (Mason, Bennett & Ryan 1988), a wide-ranging inquiry into psychiatric procedures which followed an incident in which a patient with a diagnosis of schizophrenia and a known history of serious violence was refused hospital admission and on the same night killed two fellow patients at his supported accommodation and seriously injured two members of the public. This report was comparable in influence in the New Zealand context to the impact of the Butler report in the United Kingdom at an earlier stage (Home Office & Department of Health and Social Security 1975). The recommendations of the report focused on establishing mental-health based facilities to care for mentally disordered offenders and potential offenders, which has ultimately led to the building of five regional secure units to serve a national population which passed the four million mark during 2004. The secure units act as the focal points for forensic psychiatric services, which include secure inpatient beds, outpatient services, court liaison services and psychiatric clinics within the regional prisons.

THE NEW ZEALAND CONTEXT: CORRECTIONAL SERVICES

The Department of Corrections currently oversees the running of 19 public prisons in New Zealand. Six specialist units operating within the prison system include three drug and alcohol treatment units, two sex offender treatment units, and one violent offender treatment unit. There are also 15 prison units with a special focus, including five Maori focus units and four Young Offenders Units.

The most pressing issue facing the Department of Corrections at the current time is that of coping with a rising national prison muster, which in April 2005 reached approximately 6,800 inmates. This represents a high rate of imprisonment of 155 inmates per 100,000 population for 2003–2004, higher than comparable countries other than the United States (Department of Corrections 2005). The Department of Corrections is currently forced into using both court and police cells to cater for the demand for prison beds Several factors have contributed to the current pressure, including population growth; more stringent bail conditions; more prosecutions and cases being finalised as more judges are appointed; inmates serving greater proportions of imposed sentences following the Parole Act 2002; increased numbers of inmates serving preventive detention or longer non-parole periods; a gradual increase in imprisonment rates and average length of sentence, at least in part due to the prevailing social and political climate; increased number of remanded inmates; and extended supervision order legislation, for example, up to ten years for sex offenders.

The Department of Corrections is also challenged by significant demographic trends apparent in the prison population. There is over-representation of Maori and Pacific Island peoples, with about 50% of the prison population being accounted for by these ethnic groups, which comprise just 20% of the overall population (Department of Corrections 2005). There is increased pressure on female facilities because of an increase in serious female offending and increased incarceration. There has been an increase in males in the 16–40 age range, especially related to serious offending in the younger 16–20 age range. An ageing population and longer sentences have combined to create a challenge in caring for inmates with dementia (several inmates have been released to hospice care). There are relatively high re-offending rates, with 42.3% of all inmates released from prison in 2002–2003 being reconvicted, and 28% being re-imprisoned (Department of Corrections 2005).

The high rate of imprisonment in New Zealand has fuelled debate over the purpose of incarceration. This is, in part, answered by the new Corrections Act 2004, which outlines the purpose and guiding principles of the New Zealand corrections system, principles which focus on public safety, victims' interests and the prevention of re-offending through rehabilitative programmes, sentence planning to facilitate successful reintegration into the community, and the use of restorative justice processes where appropriate.

New Zealand has recently compared relatively well internationally in terms of unnatural prison deaths, with a rate of 0.10 per 100 inmates being reported in 2000–2001 (Department of Corrections 2002).

THE INTERFACE BETWEEN CORRECTION AND PSYCHIATRIC FACILITIES

Psychiatric care for prisoners, both within prison and in hospital secure beds, is the responsibility of the regional forensic psychiatry services. The standard approach used by all five regional forensic services within New Zealand is based on the "inreach" model, with a multidisciplinary team based with community forensic services also providing mental health care in prisons. For the four regional services outside Auckland, this involves mentally disordered inmates being seen in nurse- and psychiatrist-led prison clinics. In the event that admission to hospital is deemed necessary, transfer can usually be effected within a matter of days. The Auckland forensic service, which has the greatest national demand for inpatient beds, uses a slightly different approach, with some consultant psychiatrists working solely within the prison team, as opposed to having primary or additional outpatient or inpatient responsibilities. The Auckland Regional Forensic Psychiatry Service carries out over 330 new inmate assessments each year, and typically has a waiting list for psychiatric admission of about 13 or 14 inmates, some of whom have to wait for several weeks or even months before gaining admission to psychiatric hospital for assessment and treatment of major mental illness, including psychotic conditions. In comparison, other regional secure units have small or non-existent waiting lists.

Therefore, there are large regional variations in terms of the demand and access to such services. There is a limited degree of co-operation across the country, with one unit assisting the Auckland service by taking non-local admissions, although this results in geographic isolation from families and *whanau* (extended family) for those transferred, an important consideration in the New Zealand cultural setting.

In New Zealand, psychiatric treatment pursuant to the Mental Health (Compulsory Assessment and Treatment) Act 1992 cannot be enforced in prison, although the Act does have provision for compulsory and voluntary transfer of mentally ill inmates to psychiatric hospital for such care. Under civil conditions, the Act enables a patient to be under compulsory assessment and/or treatment either in hospital or in the community.

New Zealand has been the site of some of the most methodologically sound prison epidemiological research in terms of mental disorder. Arising from an earlier local Christchurch study (Brinded *et al.*1999), a national prison study identified high unmet need among mentally disordered prisoners (Brinded *et al.* 2001). In accordance with findings in other countries, rates of schizophrenia, bipolar disorder, obsessive-compulsive disorder and alcohol and drug abuse and dependence were grossly elevated compared to community prevalence rates. Using conservative calculations based on Gunn *et al.* (1991) group, it was estimated that 135 inmates were detained in prison who would require hospital care for acute psychotic illness. This would require an approximate doubling of the secure hospital bed capacity nationally. It was further estimated (through self-report) that only about one third of inmates with schizophrenia and related disorders and one half of those with major depression are receiving any treatment for the condition, irrespective of whether this is caused by a lack of recognition of major mental illness or by other patient-related factors, for example, non-compliance with medication, or treatment refusal.

One interesting feature of the New Zealand legislative context is that judges have the power to order immediate admission of a defendant to a secure mental health facility for psychiatric assessment and provision of a court-ordered report. Aside from the Auckland forensic service, which has to deal with a larger population base and New Zealand's only maximum security-level prison within its catchment area, the impression is that admission to psychiatric hospital can be facilitated without undue delays in most cases, a situation characterised by the relative absence of waiting lists for admission to psychiatric hospital from prison in most areas of the country.

The aspect that would most likely strike visitors to the New Zealand context as a point of differentiation from other countries in terms of provision of mental health care in prisons is the unique cultural mix of its population, although over-representation of ethnic groups within the prison setting is a pattern that has been well recognised elsewhere. This has implications for the design of New Zealand mental health services, most notably with each forensic service having access to input from "cultural workers" employed by the district health boards rather than correctional services (which also provide a cultural service). Epidemiological studies show that Maori and Pacific Islanders in prison manifest rates of psychiatric disorder similar to the rest of the prison population. What differentiates them, however, is that they have fewer prior psychiatric admissions, fewer community outpatient appointments and less treatment in prison for the same degree of psychiatric morbidity, compared to non-Maori inmates (Simpson *et al.* 2003). Some high-level initiatives have focused on the mental health needs of Maori in general terms (Ministry of Health 2002).

RESPONSES AND STRATEGIC INITIATIVES

Correctional services are attempting to respond to the challenges set out above with several strategic initiatives. First, new prisons are being built and opened and existing facilities are being extended to provide significantly increased regional capacity. Three new corrections facilities in Auckland, Otago and Waikato will be under construction during 2005–2006 and the Auckland Regional Women's Correctional Facility is due to open during this period. Further construction at existing facilities will provide additional accommodation.

Second, a major strategic focus for the Department of Corrections in terms of interventions in the management of offenders is "reintegration", a generic term used to refer to "removing blockages to remaining offence-free". This includes increased focus on development of basic living skills, parenting, budgeting skills, links to community support services, day and work release, relapse prevention programmes, and involvement of family/*whanau*, *hapu* and *iwi* (tribal connections) in reintegration plans. There are also programmes which address victim empathy and offenders as victims. Reintegration is conceptualised as occurring parallel to rehabilitation. Two programmes, *Straight Thinking* and *Tikanga Maori*, are designed to address motivation and responsivity. In addition, there are some local opportunities for alcohol and substance use, and violence prevention programmes. There are two special treatment units, one in each island, which specifically deal with sex offender rehabilitation. Both rehabilitation and reintegration initiatives are being developed, while increased attention is also being placed on development of safe, secure and humane containment, and education and employment skill development, including basic numeracy and literacy skills.

Despite these strategic initiatives, deficits within the current service provision for mentally disordered offenders persist. There is limited ability of correctional staff to work effectively with people with long sentences. As for most correctional services, the management of inmates with severe personality disorder is a problematic issue, but this is compounded in the New Zealand context by the current emphasis on risk assessment over therapeutic interventions by psychologists employed by the Department of Corrections. This situation has also highlighted ethical concerns over the "double agency" issue, for instance, with information gained in a therapeutic context later being disclosed in risk assessment evaluations by the same or other psychologists. There are also significant difficulties in providing effective interventions for those with dual diagnosis.

For their part, forensic psychiatric services continue to seek to develop regional services, although the low population and local employment challenges (e.g. nurses providing care in the community and prisons are currently paid considerably less than their hospital colleagues because of the absence of shift-work allowances) provide significant hurdles. Despite this, three initiatives warrant mention.

First, the Auckland Regional Forensic Psychiatric Service has been awarded additional funding by the Ministry of Health to develop an enhanced prison psychiatric service. Although this is still in the early stages of development, the intention is both to reduce caseloads of multidisciplinary staff by simply employing more mental health professionals, and to provide additional training so that, in particular, nursing staff develop the capability to deliver increased therapeutic input more in line with inpatient provisions. Special focus will be placed on psycho-education, alcohol and drug interventions, risk assessments, and linkage with community services by way of release planning. Of note, two prisons in Auckland, including the only privately run prison in New Zealand (although the Government has indicated that management will shortly be returned to the public sector), have employed psychiatric nurses, who, although liaising closely with the local prison psychiatric team, provide commendable input that originates within the prison structures, as opposed to being inreach in nature. Other prisons rely on general trained nurses and prison GPs to carry out referrals and initial assessments.

Second, current prison screening procedures simply are not commensurate with the rates of significant mental disorder in New Zealand prisons as identified by the national prison study involving a large cohort of both remand and sentenced prisoners (Brinded *et al.* 2001). A working party involving representatives from all regions with forensic mental health services and from the Departments of Health and Corrections is developing a protocol that is likely to lead to a national prison screening study, in an attempt to improve the identification of inmates in need of immediate mental health interventions.

Finally, perhaps the most unique feature of the New Zealand context is the nature and importance of cultural issues, not just in terms of the delivery of mental health services but more pervasively in terms of the national psyche. Indeed, the requirement for mental health services to address the needs of Maori people in particular is enshrined in the contents and interpretations of the Treaty of Waitangi, which addresses historical grievances and also requires specific current attention to be placed on Maori needs There are various ways in which this requirement is addressed. Each forensic mental health service employs cultural advisors and workers, some of whom provide input into prison team functioning. In most regions, each new inpatient will receive both a clinical and a cultural assessment, which is generally conducted within a framework of four related aspects: *Te Taha Tinana* (physical well-being and attributes), *Te Taha Hinengaro* (mental well-being), *Te Taha Whanau* (family/extended family) and *Te Taha Wairua* (spiritual well-being). One new prison based at Nga Wha in Northland has been built within an area of relatively high Maori population density and will place additional focus on incorporating Maori protocols and procedures into care plans.

OVERVIEW

In general terms, New Zealand's greatest advantage in delivering effective mental health care in prisons, the relatively low population base, is also its greatest weakness. On the one hand, the size issue means that New Zealand has relatively less well developed general infrastructure, and practical issues such as obtaining suitable staff become relevant. On the other hand, the small absolute size of the issue in international terms means that there are relatively fewer layers of bureaucracy, and good opportunities for regional co-operation, collaboration and even cohesion, and local services can be well organised and efficiently run. National studies and approaches to problems are possible and have been achieved, for example, in prison epidemiological work. Most services are able to assess new referrals within two or three days, arrange admission to hospital relatively quickly if needed, and address release planning issues to some extent – a practice facilitated by the nature of the population distribution.

Overall, New Zealand's provision of mental health services into the prison setting, while not offering much that would mark it out from similar services internationally, other than the strength of the cultural approach, would be characterised as relatively orthodox but relatively effective in delivering adequate prison assessments, timely interventions, and release planning. The areas that require the greatest focus include reception screening to identify those in need of mental health assessment, and potentially treatment and treatment interventions for those detained in prison either prior to transfer or in the longer term.

CHAPTER 24

Inside–Outside: Ethical Dilemmas in Prison Psychiatry

Gwen Adshead

THE PRISON AS A TYPE OF COMMUNITY

Prisoners are a particular group of people, those excluded from society and deprived of liberty as a punishment for offences against the wider social group. Doctors are expected to provide health care services to the community as a whole, including the prison community, since the National Health Service (NHS) reforms of prison care in 2006 (Department of Health 2005b). Psychiatric services are especially necessary because of the high prevalence of mental disorders in prisons (Fazel & Danesh 2002), considerably higher than the general community at large (Singleton *et al.* 2003a).

From a sociological perspective, prisons function as containers for social disturbance that place an emphasis on individual deviance, rather than social and political disorganisation. It is comforting to many people to think that the "badness" of society is (a) being punished justly (Janoff Bulman 1985) and (b) safely tucked away behind a big wall. Medical ethics, however, has always been ambivalent about prisons because of the harm and distress that detention often causes. Detention is frightening and stressful, especially for vulnerable prisoners, such as the young or those with histories of mental illness. Physicians may be ambivalent about the whole process of punishment at all, and reluctant to see medical practice as colluding with the state in exerting control over individuals. Traditional medical ethics has placed so much emphasis on individual autonomy and experience that state intervention in the life of the individual can seem like a dangerous challenge to professional identity and practice. Medical ethics has also been profoundly affected by the Nuremberg trials of the doctors involved in the abuse and murder of those the state deemed to be "unworthy of life" or "enemies of the Reich", and anxiety about collusion with state cruelty is real among doctors (Caplan 2005). In simple consequentialist terms, doctors may also simply want to argue that prison does no good, and a great deal of harm, so it is their duty not to be involved in prison work.

Of course, there are important counter-arguments to these, not least from a utilitarian perspective. Those detained in prisons are ill and in need of help; if psychiatrists were to refuse to do prison work, there would be untreated sick people effectively ignored by health care services, just because physicians don't agree with the social system that put them there. Doctors have always had a public health role, as well as a duty to sick individuals. Improving the health of prisoners generally may have positive long-term consequences for society – for example, assisting prisoners with substance misuse problems not only benefits the prisoner healthwise, but also has a potentially positive effect on risk reduction by reducing substance misuse. It is not unreasonable for the state to seek to use health care services to improve the care of those detained in prison. The punishment, after all, is the loss of liberty, not the experience of detention. This point is especially germane for the mentally ill, since acutely disturbed and distressed prisoners are not likely to get the moral message, and it is not just to punish those who cannot appreciate justice. Finally, it has often been argued that doctors who come into prisons to assess and treat prisoners are in a good position to comment on what they see there, and thus to improve poor care and conditions. Doctors are therefore usefully involved in visiting prisons, not only to provide care but to report on conditions and check the welfare of prisoners.

Bowden (1976) makes the point that the personal attitudes of doctors are likely to have more of an impact on how ethical dilemmas are resolved than professional codes of ethics, which may in any case conflict with each other. He also makes the point that prison psychiatry involves activities that work to the benefit of the individual prisoner, the prison as a whole, and for the state; they are not necessarily alternatives.

ROLES AND RELATIONSHIPS

It has been suggested that psychiatry needs a particular framework of ethical reasoning and theory to assist with the types of dilemmas and conflicts met in daily practice (Robertson & Waller 2007). The most useful ethical theory for psychiatric practice is relational and care-based, partly because therapeutic relationships are central to successful treatment, and also because dysfunctional interpersonal relationships are a key feature of many psychiatric disorders. This is particularly so in prisons, where so many of the prisoners are profoundly antisocial in their outlook on life, and in their relationships with others.

It is worth taking a moment to consider what being "antisocial" really means. For many people, it literally means being "anti-the-social", against anything that connects people in relationships. Laws and rules are ways in which individuals are connected into groups that function across time and space. Laws regulate the relationship between the individual and the group. Laws can obviously be tools for diminishing individual freedom or dissent, but most antisocial people who break the laws are not seeking political change or social improvement. Their rule-breaking arises from the attitude that only their happiness and welfare matters, and all other consequences and issues are not particularly real to them. Other people's welfare, in particular, is not real to them, and this lack of empathy for others makes rule-breaking more likely.

Two key questions therefore are (a) what is the role of the prison psychiatrist? and (b) what is his or her relationship with the prisoner? Traditionally, prison psychiatrists have principally concentrated on treating people who are mentally ill in prison, and restoring them to the best mental health possible. However, prisoners frequently have to wait long periods for treatment because their care is not allocated much financial resource. Resource allocation dilemmas are among the commonest ethical dilemmas in psychiatry, yet they are rarely discussed. When it comes to getting access to treatment resources, it is not unusual to find that prisons come off badly, presumably because the health needs of others are seen as more deserving of scarce resources. But it might be argued, in terms of the role of the prison psychiatrist, that they have an interest in making prisoners not only feel better but behave better. A utilitarian argument might be that proper investment in the "treatment" of antisocial and unempathic attitudes (let alone mental disorders) would be much more cost-effective and beneficial socially than the treatment of, say, childhood cancers or Alzheimer's disease. In terms of quality of life years saved, the psychological and psychiatric treatment of prisoners makes much better economic sense than treating diseases that are currently irreversible, such as the dementias. The cost-benefits include reduced needs for prison places and reduced future legal costs; the social benefits include not only less crime, but fewer frightened and victimised people. It is even possible that the individual prisoners might feel better in themselves, and live longer, happier lives. There is some limited evidence that pro-social behaviour makes people happier, and being antisocial is a potent risk factor for early death.

It is surely not cynicism, but rueful acceptance of the fact of human vengefulness that makes one certain that no such investment will be forthcoming for the prisons. Health care resources are finite, and primary care trusts, which are meant to commission services, are not familiar with the multiple needs of prisoners (Birmingham, Wilson & Adshead 2006), and probably do not wish to be. At present, nearly all therapeutic work on helping prisoners change their antisocial views and values is mainly done by psychologists in prisons. Psychiatrists usually take the view that they only treat illness, not deviant behaviour, so their role in the prison is to identify and assist prisoners who are mentally ill. However, with the current emphasis on psychiatrists as risk managers for psychiatric patients, there may be a role for psychiatrists to get more active in treating antisociality more generally (Royal College of Psychiatrists 2008b).

The psychiatrist also has a role in liaising with the other staff in the prison who are overseeing health care, including prison officers who have a role in security and discipline in the prison. They may even have a role in assisting in the organisational running of the prison, especially in remand prisons or prisons with therapeutic communities. I will discuss the issue of prison discipline below, but there are general complexities in the relationships with prison staff. Prison officers may be more similar in attitudes and values to the prisoners they contain than to the health care professionals who come to "help" the prisoner, and this can lead to ethical conflict over how a prisoner should be treated. Within prison inreach teams also, composed of nursing and other non-medical staff, there may be real clashes of values and attitudes between different professionals. Clashes in ethical viewpoints within a team are often covers for different emotional reactions to a difficult situation. In these situations, it is often useful to set aside reflective practice time so that all the different value perspectives can be heard and considered, and the different emotions explored.

At a more individual level, the relationship with the prisoner is in itself complex, partly because of the uncertainty of the doctor's role, and partly because of the psychology of distressed and angry men. Many prisoners are highly suspicious of those who claim to be offering them help, especially if they appear to have the support of the prison staff. It will take all the best professional skills available to make good quality relationships with them, and it may be emotionally difficult to do so (Birmingham et al. 2006). Relationships cut both ways, and the antisocial attitude of many of the men means that they find being a "patient" very disturbing, because it means having to depend on others. In the literature on prison medicine, there is sometimes a rather idealised view of vulnerable prisoners who are longing for some kind doctor to listen and understand them. No doubt this is true for some prisoners, but often the ethical challenge is to maintain a therapeutic and compassionate relationship with someone who needs your help, but attacks you for it.

The complex nature of the prison psychiatrist's role is often exposed in relation to issues of confidentiality. Prisoners are often either wary of disclosing information, because they perceive the prison doctor to be part of the prison, or they may be very trusting of the visiting psychiatrist, unaware that there are real limits to confidentiality in medicine generally, and custodial settings in particular (Royal College of Psychiatrists 2000, Department of Health 2003). Visiting psychiatrists have to decide for themselves how much they want to ally themselves with the institution, and this decision will affect how they respond to dilemmas about information given to them by prisoners about illicit activities, past or present. In the current climate, it seems that the perception that risk might be ameliorated by disclosure of information seems to be justification for doing so. However, it seems unjust not to inform the prisoner of the disclosure. It is the experience of this author that it is the deception of prisoners by professionals about disclosure decisions that causes most unease.

Participation in justice: punishment, protection and investigation of crime

Psychiatrists in prisons may already feel uneasy about the extent to which they are colluding with punishment of individuals by the deprivation of liberty. Their anxiety may or may not be eased by the thought that this punishment is a just one, agreed and carried out in the context of due democratic and legal process. However, their anxieties are likely to be raised still further if they are asked to be involved in disciplinary procedures within the prison, for example, judging someone fit for solitary confinement or reviewing someone in seclusion. The European Commission requires that prisoners are not treated in an "inhuman or degrading" way, but it may be left to the individual doctor to decide whether a prison discipline is inhuman or degrading.

In some countries, prison psychiatrists may have to declare whether prisoners are mentally fit for punishments that include flogging or death. To simply state that carrying out such assessments is "unethical" is rather to miss the complexity and tragedy of such dilemmas. As Bowden (1976) suggests, for every person who is declared fit for such punishments, there may be at least one who is saved from such punishments by medical intervention. The most explicit and stark example of medical involvement in punishment is in relation to the death penalty. The American Medical and Psychiatric Associations have declared that participation in the death penalty, including declaring someone mentally fit for execution, is ethically unjustifiable for doctors. However, there are other countries apart from the USA which have the death penalty, and it is not clear that their medical associations have taken the same view.

The key ethical tension seems to be around the question of whether all doctors ought to be opposed to legitimate punishment of an individual on health grounds. The problem with this argument is that it sets up the medical profession against the rest of the body politic, who have voted in a democratic process for these punishments. It commits the medical profession to a political/criminological opinion that not all its members may share. The point also remains that if the medical profession is not involved in these social controls, much worse harms may follow. Another version of this ethical argument has been raised recently in relation to the treatment of political detainees in prisons. For example, there has been considerable concern about the involvement of psychiatrists and psychologists in the interrogations of political prisoners at Guantanamo Bay prison (Lewis 2005). There are really two concerns: first, that mental health professionals are declaring people fit for "interrogation", which may actually involve torture, and second, that mental health professionals are actually using their skills to assist in the torture process. Full exploration and discussion of these issues could be a book in itself, but it is of interest to consider the professional responses to these allegations. Internationally recognised professional bodies, such as the American Academy of Psychiatry and Law and the Royal College of Psychiatrists were invited to criticise the individuals involved and state their opposition to such practices. At the same time, a group of psychiatrists in the UK criticised the British Government for the unlawful detention of men suspected of terrorist offences, many of whom were detained without charge for months on end through the implementation of new anti-terrorist legislation (Robbins *et al.* 2005). Interestingly, the psychiatrists based their criticism on the grounds that they could provide evidence that indefinite detention without charge was causing psychological distress and psychiatric disorders in the detainees. It is not clear whether they would have been opposed to indefinite detention without charge if it had not caused mental harm to prisoners.

Further, these psychiatrists did not oppose lawful detention in prison, which, as we have seen, also causes harm in the form of distress and increased risk of mental disorder more generally. There is a type of inconsistency of moral argument here which is related to the uncertainty of whether medicine can be a critic of state policy, purely on health grounds, without becoming an alternative political system in its own right, but without a public mandate (Wilson 2005). The Royal College of Psychiatrists (2005) supported this criticism of the Government, despite the fact that a number of these "prisoners" are also held in psychiatric secure units, which are therefore party to the detention.

At present, prisons and prison policies are part of a social structure which has been democratically created. Staff who work in prisons operate one part of the social structure that investigates and punishes crime, especially crime that carries a risk of serious harm to others. If what is being argued is that no doctor should ever be involved in social punishment of any kind, then some doctors will refuse to work in prisons at all. Others might argue that they are there purely to attend to the health needs of prisoners, and have no role to play in upholding prison discipline. This position is harder to maintain for those psychiatrists who are employed by the prisons. Even if they have no role in maintaining discipline, they equally have no role in undermining it. There is a danger that doctors, in their fear of colluding with what they see as oppressive prison practices, will demonise prison staff who are lawfully charged with making sure that prisons are reasonably safe places to live for everyone. Doctors should undoubtedly speak out against brutality or cruelty, but need to beware of being critical of prison staff just because they have a punitive role that doctors do not.

However, psychiatrists also have a professional commitment to crime prevention and punishment – Section 30 Annex B of the *NHS Confidentiality Code of Practice* (Department of Health 2003) states that staff are permitted to breach confidentiality in the "*detection, investigation and punishment* of violent crime" (p.34, my italics). The Royal College of Psychiatrists' (2008b) recent guidance on risk management clearly takes the view that it is part of a psychiatrist's professional duty to prevent violence by patients through risk assessment processes, and government mandated inquiry reports have been highly critical of individual professionals who failed to prevent patients from acting violently. There is real public ambivalence in doctors about this role. When it comes to child protection work, doctors, including child psychiatrists, have been exposed to criticism and public condemnation for raising the possibility (which is clearly evidence-based) that some parents can and do pose a real risk of serious harm to their children (Dyer 2004).

Risk management and prison psychiatry

Psychiatrists will also visit prisons for the purpose of preparing reports for third parties, usually relating to the risk the prisoner may pose to others on release. Although these assessments may not be done by psychiatrists employed by the prison, they may be involved in the process nonetheless. The obvious ethical issue here is transparency of intention of assessment, and the extent to which the prisoner knows why this assessment is taking place. Although in theory consent to the assessment, and consent to disclosure of the assessment, need to obtained, it is often suggested that prisoners will not appreciate that the doctor is not operating as "their" doctor, a custodial version of what Appelbaum & Lidz (1982) called in another context "the therapeutic misconception".

The general ethical question, however, is the extent to which psychiatrists give opinions for non-therapeutic purposes. This is another variation on the theme outlined above; namely, should doctors use their professional skills and expertise to assist in the state's function of public protection? The current professional position appears to be that doctors do have a duty to contribute to public protection, which they fulfil by providing risk assessments. Since risk assessments may cause injury to the prisoner's liberty, it is ethically unjustifiable not to warn the prisoner of the nature and purpose of the assessment, and not to allow the prisoner to refuse to participate. It is also unjustifiable to deceive the patient into thinking that the assessment is a purely therapeutic one. Given the involvement of health care professionals in risk assessment, it must be a moot point as to whether risk assessment is in fact a medical intervention, which in theory competent individuals could refuse.

It is often suggested that it does people good to be prevented from harming others. Quite apart from the fact that this "good" is not universally applied to all citizens, most prisoners who are detained on the grounds of preventive detention do not experience it as a "good". In relation to longer than normal sentences, these appear to be more likely in cases of personality disorder and perceived "untreatability" (Solomka 1996). The difficulty here is that lack of treatability may be a function of services and resources, not the condition itself (Adshead 2001a). Conversely, although the "ghost train" prisoners may be transferred under the Mental Health Act for unspecified "treatment", the treatment may not actually exist.[1] In theory, the 2007 revisions of the Mental Health Act require that there be appropriate treatment for the prisoner; but in practice, these types of transfer make preventive detention possible for particularly troublesome or worrying prisoners.

The overwhelming ethical concern is that other people's anxiety drives detention decisions which result in loss of liberty. Psychiatric risk assessment procedures contain none of the due process elements that are usually required in a democratic society before a man's liberty is removed. Anxiety at the thought that a man who has committed a particularly bizarre offence will be released may lead to his detention, despite the

---

1   The "ghost train" is the term used for prisoners who are transferred ("ghosted") to hospital at the end of their sentence, ostensibly for treatment of a mental disorder, but really for public protection by continuing to incarcerate them.

fact that he has served a sentence. For very bizarre and rare offences, there can be no sensible "evidence" that could justify further detention, yet it is precisely these offenders who will be detained using psychiatric evidence. It will be interesting to see whether psychiatrists who are opposed to being involved with state punishment procedures will also to the same degree oppose being involved in public protection.

CONCLUSION

Professional identity is made up of training, experience and attitudes. Doctors are not separate from the general body politic by virtue of their professional identity, and are part of the social system that puts men, women and children in prison. If we do not like it, there are political ways to change this, but holding oneself aloof is not an option. Both professionally and personally, we benefit from the detention of many of these prisoners, and we subscribe to the system of moral beliefs that expresses condemnation of wrong-doing. It may well be that punishment does not help in changing those who break the rules, and that changes in social policies and structures would help many not to do so. But while there are prisoners in custody, we are part of the system that put them there, and we therefore cannot walk away.

CHAPTER 25

Prison Language as an Organisational Defence Against Anxiety

Gabrielle Brown and Julian Walker

In the early 1990s the psychoanalyst Hinshelwood wrote two papers on the limitations of working as a therapist within prisons resulting from the structuring of defenses against anxiety within such institutions (Hinshelwood 1993, 1994). Unable to balance the custodial role with the remedial potential of imprisonment, he suggests that the institution developed a defensive structure which marginalised the therapeutic endeavour and the therapist (Hinshelwood 1994, p.289).

The psychoanalytic study of anxiety's impact on task performance in organisations stretches back to Menzies Lyth's (1959) much cited work on underperformance and burnout in nursing. She found the seemingly rational organisation of tasks and hierarchy in nursing to be generated by unconscious defences against anxiety. The anxiety was provoked by the core task in nursing, care of those in physical distress. Centrally she found that defensive systems are self-perpetuating: "The social defence system itself arouses a good deal of *secondary anxiety* as well as failing to alleviate *primary anxiety*" (Menzies Lyth 1959, p.65; our emphasis).

All organisations have cultural defences which may skew their ability to perform the full range of their "core business" (Armstrong 2005). Understanding the culture enables purposeful change, porousness to new ideas and adaptation to new clinical and custodial challenges. In large institutions like prisons, "secondary anxiety" is consciously experienced and relates to concerns with the smooth running of the institution as a whole, captured in the prison phrase "good order and discipline" (GOAD: a monitoring and punishment/reward system for inmates). "Primary anxiety", running beneath the surface, often unconscious, responds to the reality that "good order" may rarely equate to good outcomes, especially for a client group with longstanding and complex problems, needs and disadvantages (Nurse, Woodcock & Ormsby 2003). A prison's failure impacts, in different ways, on both the morale of its staff and the prospects of its inmates. The language in prisons forms part of a "manic defence" which protects the institution and its inhabitants against the sense of helplessness and persecutory blame in the face of failure – "anxiety, guilt, depression" (Rycroft 1968, p.86).

A LOCAL PRISON

Our experience is largely from a local male prison in an inner city area. Our roles were as communicable disease social worker and clinical psychologist respectively, both with a brief to provide therapy to individuals or small groups to alleviate distress and promote change. In the prison we were categorised as "civilians", as distinct from "officers". In what follows we use the term "visiting professionals" loosely to denote "civilians" whose core training was not in the prison service, but in the NHS or elsewhere.

The prison holds a half-and-half mix of prisoners awaiting trial or sentencing and those who have been sentenced. The dominant debate about prisons at the time of writing is of "overcrowding" (de Silva 2005). An exponential rise in the numbers imprisoned has an impact upon the individualised projects of rehabilitation, such as education, therapy and therapeutic activity.

Problems of overcrowding were evident in this local prison. There were frequent "lock-outs", when the prison reached capacity during the day and was unable to take back those who had left for court in the morning, disrupting their care. Paradoxically, high rates of recidivism and relapse created a flow of familiar faces over time, especially in drug users and the mentally ill. This gave the impression that both staff and prisoners existed in a closed community, with fleeting contact with the locality beyond its walls. We suggest that the prison language supported this impression of a "closed system".

THE LANGUAGE – VOLUME AND TYPE

Like many visiting professionals working in prisons, we found that we had passively acquired over 1,500 prison linguistic terms within our first year. This was considerably more than the NHS, social care, therapeutic and managerial jargon which we brought from previous settings. The pervasiveness and exclusive use of prison terms struck us forcefully, initially as confusing and mystifying, and subsequently as burdensome, restrictive to communication, case discussion and project development, even in our "non-custodial" roles. We came to think of the language in three categories. First, it is well known that groups of inmates bring their own slang or *patois* into the institution, such as "bird" or "doing bird", meaning "prison sentence". Second are terms used by staff, which effectively replace common language used in the community with a prison-specific term, such as "canteen" meaning prisoners' rations and shop (not staff diningroom, which is termed "the mess"). The third and largest category consists of terms that denote the abstruse functions and activities of prison life, for which no equivalent exists outside. "Bedwatch", the procedure for guarding and chaining prisoners admitted to an NHS hospital, is an example in this category. The second and third of these linguistic categories are the subject of our discussion here.

We focus little on prisoner language, because prisoners were sparing in the slang to which they gave us access, and presented as more "bilingual" than staff. It is known that prisoners' language often imports terms used in the drug world, terms used by criminal culture, and language specific to ethnic groups.[2] However, in conversation with us, prisoners tended to translate prison terms as they went along, if they used them at all, e.g. "I'm getting my *bracelet*, you know, [electronic] *tag*, next week." Evidence of prisoners' tendency to translate or suppress slang and prison terms and to maintain politeness in conversation with us was provided by prisoners who spoke little English and therefore lacked this flexibility of register. For instance, those who had learnt their English exclusively inside the institution, from cellmates, would refer to one of us as a "bird" (slang for woman). Often formality was improvised by these inmates, indicative of the pervasive attention to appropriate terms in conversation within the hierarchy. Thus "bird" became "Professional Bird" or "Lady Bird". Within the culture it is the role of staff/officers to maintain the language barrier, as it is to maintain the physical barriers. Prisoners, then, addressed us as designated "outsiders" to the language, long after we had acquired fluency. In reflecting on our acquisition of fluency we noted that it brought few rewards in terms of communication, because we remained outsiders in terms of how both the prisoners and the staff related to us – we clearly lacked the uniform, even if we could speak the language. While an early fluency with prison language decreased our initial confusion, it was not helpful in furthering discourse on primary anxiety within or around the therapeutic work.

PRISON TERMS REPLACING TERMS USED "OUTSIDE"

The language used by staff to denote the functions and activities of the institution was hegemonic and monolithic from the first. The formidable barrier is particularly noticeable where a different term is used in prison language from that which exists in common language. These sites of non-equivalence create the "insider–outsider" divide. Examples of different terms are "treatments/treats" (nurses' clinic), "swinger" (suicidal prisoner), "slasher" (prisoner who cuts himself), "IMR" (inmate medical record, patient's notes), "body" (prisoner), "body count" (roll-call), "break off" (shift change). Additionally, as we discuss later, the floors of the buildings have a non-standard numbering system. These aspects of the discourse mystify prison life even at points of apparent equivalence with tasks of other institutions. Intentionally or unintentionally, the effect of this

---

1   Important considerations of prisoners' linguistic presentation of self across divides of social class, gender and professional status have been studied by Mayr (2004), and a full list of prisoner terms can be found in Devlin (1996).

mystification is to put anxiety into the confused outsider, whilst allowing those "inside" to feel part of something exclusive, communal and "safe".

PRISON-SPECIFIC TERMS

A third type of staff language consists of coined terms, neologisms and euphemisms to denote the abstruse and sometimes controversial activities of prison life. Such terms formed the bulk of our learning, indicative of a general preoccupation in the institution with its daily functioning and struggles, above all else (secondary anxiety). An example is "lock-out" (no vacancies), explained above. "Discipline" (the discipline office) denotes the administrative area. "Discipline officers" describes all uniformed officers. "The team" is the prison's riot squad, who may "play" (fight) with prisoners. "The draft" refers to the list of prisoners who will be transferred, "shipped out", to other establishments (prisons) across the "estate" (English prisons). Many activities are referred to by the paperwork or form that records an activity, for instance "E man" (on the Escape list) and "on an ACCT", meaning suicidal, to which we return below (see page 268–269). Radio designations are also used to describe staff roles, "Hotel 6" being the on-call nurse, "Oscar 1" their custodial equivalent. These terms domesticate even the most abstruse and complex aspects of custody, ensuring that nothing is "unspeakable". It is the plethora of such terms we wish to emphasise here.

LANGUAGE AS SYMPTOM

In focusing on language, we are aware that we are choosing a shifting symptom in defensive structures. Efforts to introduce "decency" into prisons have led to a "clean-up" in terms considered appropriate (Home Office 2007). For example, in multidisciplinary case conferences, the term "fraggle" was on the wane as a term for a mentally ill patient, although still in use in less formal settings. In the context of directives for change, terms and discursive interactions which resist change could be seen to be held in place by their defensive function in the culture, and symptomatic of its underlying tensions. As David Jones, writing on "humane prisons", comments, "exhortations to 'decency' do not necessarily resolve the staff fears and anxieties which gave rise to previous behaviours" (Jones 2006, p.34), although they may shift their manifestations. If the plethora of prison terms is seen as indicative of underlying, primary anxiety, removing the symptom (cleaning up the language) does not allay underlying tensions.

DEFENSIVE STRUCTURES RESISTANT TO CHANGE: DEPERSONALISATION

It is not surprising to find overcrowded jails using linguistic defences which relate to dealing with human beings *en masse*, to the warehousing functions of prison institutions. Menzies Lyth noticed that terms which depersonalised or "dehumanised" nursing patients seemed particularly intransigent to change, because of their role in underpinning defences against anxiety: "nurses often talk about patients not by name, but by bed number or by their diseases or a diseased organ: 'the liver in bed 10...'. Nurses themselves deprecate this practice, but it persists" (Menzies Lyth 1959, p.52). From another perspective, we often wondered how it would be possible do anything other than dehumanise and warehouse inmates, as the only officer on duty for a busy wing with a long list of tasks, innumerable relationships to consider and unthinkable criminality and pathology to contain. What impressed us was that many officers of different grades did manage humanity and thoughtfulness. It is important for the "outsider" to recognise (as we detail in our discussion of care for the suicidal below) that a dehumanising language does not equate to off-hand attitudes to prisoners on the part of individual staff. However, it does equate to an institutional culture whose focus does not always value, develop and support these aspects of its staff's contribution.

In the prison, staff deprecate use of the term "feeding/feeding time" (meal times/ serving meals) with its connotations of prisoners as zoo animals. However, both staff with highly developed therapeutic skills, and those with routine duties, used the term "feeding" daily. Likewise, prisoners dealt with *en masse* are termed "bodies". Such terms may protect staff from the anxieties aroused by the conflict between helping prisoners and rendering them humiliatingly powerless, "just a number", to which Hinshelwood (1993, p.433) refers. "Bodies" also proved an intransigent term: for instance, in a coroner's court, despite legal briefing to avoid prison terms, an officer recounted "finding the [dead] body" whilst "counting the bodies [undertaking a roll-check]". No awareness was shown of the confusion caused by the language in this testimony. Such lapse of self-consciousness is consistent with the unconscious nature of the defences in which the language system serves.

As in many institutions, therapeutic work itself takes place with individual prisoners in the interstices of a daily regime in which they are dealt with, counted, fed, etc., *en masse*. Even rehabilitative therapy (Anger Management or Enhanced Thinking Skills) is delivered *en masse* for good economic reasons, despite the economic outcomes being equivocal or unknown. The underlying dilemma becomes whether the institutional defences prevent inmates from having and meeting simultaneous needs, both as individuals and as "numbers" within it. Examples of the difficulty for the institution in allowing the masses individuality are given by Hinshelwood (1993, 1994), in the form of the prisoner who cannot be found by officers and therefore misses his therapy session. Although recounted in both his papers, the anecdote is not specifically discussed. Over a decade later, the failure to locate a prisoner will be frustratingly familiar to visiting professionals. It represents an enactment of the persistent depersonalisation of prisoners in the face of attempts to provide individualised care or assessment. Part of the mechanism of depersonalisation lies in the fact that officers eschew prisoners' first (more personal) names and shout only surnames when calling prisoners out from the noisy, crowded wings. This renders inmates with common or mispronounced surnames particularly hard to find, and therefore work with. This is an enduring example of defence against contact with the experience of the "warehoused" – therapeutic services representing a point of such contact. The defence seems to have impacted on service provision over considerable time.

CREATING "OUTSIDERS"

Much prison language disrupts the translation of prison life into common human experience through a refusal of common language. A sense of impermeable "inside" is created by the language, with renunciation of old (linguistic) ways demanded on entry into prison. An example of such discontinuity is the alternative numbering of the floors of the buildings, where the ground floor is termed "the ones", the first "the twos", and so on. The origins of this system remained unknown. No alternative directions are offered by staff, so that transactions in the language actively create disorientation.

We will examine floor numbering in some detail as an example of a lack of common language, and as emblematic of the functions of prison language. On the one hand, by using such language with visitors, prison staff can be seen to create a distinction between "insiders" and "outsiders" (who do not understand the language). On the other hand, the experience of getting lost on a prison wing is sufficiently troubling to force the visitor to notice the nature of the miscommunication that has occurred, and provoke thought. There is therefore considerable *unspoken* communication in prison language; in this instance, in the simple act of giving bad directions. Whatever its origins, the numbering of prison floors gives the impression of an extra floor, and therefore of greater capacity than is really available. Revising this impression brings contact with the crowded "warehouse" nature of the wings, as do frequently documented difficulties in finding suitable and safe interview space for individual work (Nurse *et al.* 2003, Broderick 2007). Again, the misunderstanding created by the insistent use of prison-specific language enacts the "culture-clash" between warehousing the many, as a purpose of imprisonment, and the project of working with the few, the therapist's potential contribution to the prison sentence.

An additional communication provided by staff's unintelligibility is that "in the wider prison, most of the time spoken language is of little use", as writer-in-residence Kathy Page comments (2006, p.13). This is a particularly salient message for "talking therapists" to receive: "People blot out the words and read the body. They gesture: draw a line across the throat...push their chair back so it screams on the floor, then add a few expletives for emphasis" (Page 2006, p.13). The "message" in the use of prison terms is unspoken, but often has an impact. In work with forensic patients the lack of use of words and discursive exploration is of central concern: most patients can be seen to have impacted on others too much and spoken too little (Welldon & Van Velsen 1988). Therapeutic work seeks to redress this. Putting feelings into words is designed to prevent their being "acted out" reactively, enabling communication at the level of thought rather than impact (Hyatt Williams 1998). The impulsive discharge of emotion in violence, flight into drugs and alcohol, obliteration of neediness in theft or sexual encounters, can all be seen as symptoms in need of further elaboration.

Moreover, apparent failure by staff to notice or anticipate confusion created by prison terms enacts a cut in empathy with their interlocutor. Hinshelwood posited that therapists/"outsiders" come to represent unbearable contact with the internal, psychological world of prisoners. These moments of failure of empathy with the "outsider", enacted through obscure prison terms, are axiomatic of the functioning of a "manic defence": "purchas[ing] freedom from guilt and anxiety at the expense of depth of character and *appreciation of the motives and feelings of others*" (Rycroft 1968, p.86; our emphasis). We return to the theme of defences against empathy in the following section.

Finally, the impact of the sudden loss of common language is to situate staff as "good" at something which outsiders become "bad" at, in this example, orientation on the wings. Much as in Hinshelwood's experience of the stereotyping of the therapist as "gullible" (Hinshelwood 1993), the language enacts a projection of stupidity and vulnerability onto the "outsider" (Britton 1998). Menzies Lyth (1959) noted the projection of incompetence and "irresponsibility" downwards in defensive professional hierarchies. These projections can be seen as a defence against feeling overwhelmed and vulnerable (lost/at a loss) on the wings (Rycroft 1968, p.28). An emphasis in the culture, which we discuss below, on the non-communicative aspects of guarding prisoners, such as surveillance, makes the potential of disorientation particularly unthinkable.

UNMENTIONABLE DISTRESS

One of the effects of prison language is to prevent discussion and discursiveness between multidisciplinary staff, reducing most transactions to a brevity more appropriate for radio communication. This makes clinical work difficult, given the complexity of individual pathology and of the psychosocial consequences of imprisonment itself, both of which need to be addressed and drawn out. A troubling example is the tendency for the institution to avoid both the word "suicide" and discussion of suicidal states, despite very high rates of completed and attempted suicide (Owers 2006, p.181). Rather, a prisoner experiencing suicidal feelings is described by the reporting form used to monitor his behaviour: he is "on an ACCT" (spoken "act"). This form accompanies the prisoner everywhere, to enhance vigilant surveillance. It therefore receives constant reference in transactions but little comment, except in specialist forums. Furthermore, actual suicide is termed "death in custody" or colloquially "a death", not "suicide", pending the coroner's decision.

ACCT stands for Assessment, Care in Custody and Teamwork, and about 5% of the prisoners were "on ACCT" at any one time. The document is equally used for those who self-harm without suicidal intent, such as those who habitually cut or burn themselves under stress. Thus being "on an ACCT" designates a large range of emotional states and possible outcomes. Like many prison terms, "on an ACCT" precludes discussion, but aids categorisation and subsequent surveillance: an "ACCT" is either "open" or "closed", a prisoner is either "on an ACCT" or "off" it. In terms of defences, the discursive use of categorisation ("on an ACCT") rather than description (e.g. suicidal ideation/plan/ states) can be seen as part of a fantasy of omnipotent (bureaucratic) control, which defends against the helpless and persecutory feelings aroused in others by suicidal states (Campbell & Hale 1991). Persecutory feelings are exacerbated by the prospect of an appearance in (coroner's) court, where courts are generally seen as the preserve of wrongdoers. The language of categorisation thus privileges surveillance of the suicidal over psychological understanding or formulation.

If the use of prison terms acts as a defence against exposure to achingly difficult emotions, as in the above example, it does so at the expense of the experience and psychological expertise of staff who use it, which the terse language prevents from being aired or shared. Avoiding the term "suicide" denies staff's skill and insight in managing a vulnerable population. The defensive language sets up a split in risk management between "outsiders" who are seen to understand the inner world of prisoners and "officers" who come to provide only surveillance. In reality, untoward events are usually prevented by the mix between set procedures, intuition, and psychological understanding (Shaw et al. 2003b). However, staff anxiety remains consistently high when the possibility of human error in surveillance is unmitigated by confidence in humane efficacy and learning from experience over time (Menzies Lyth 1959, p.75). Researchers such as Liebling (2004) have convincingly shown that it is the humane and personal qualities of prison officers, rather than simply their bureaucratic functions, which enable them to meet both prison service targets and prisoners' needs Similarly, Birmingham et al. (2006) have noted the designation of prison staff as "naïve" in case discussion, and as unhelpfully replicating and perpetuating defensive pathologies: "Good communication is essential between those managing complex patients. Consistency, honesty and attempts to reduce 'splitting' that can emerge in the team are vital. Dividing staff into the 'good guys' from health who are allowed to know about the patients and the 'bad guys' in uniform who must be kept in the dark is a good example of acting-out the patients' unconscious view of the world" (Birmingham et al. 2006, p.4).

"MOTHERESE"

Prison language often gives the sense that there is a word for everything, but little to be said about anything. When prison staff and inmates converse, they use the formulaic and terse language that we have described. The language provides banter between staff and prisoners, diffusing anxiety directly through humour, in transactions from which "outsiders" are excluded. In banter, officers who "spin" (search) cells for contraband are called "the burglars"; the most exposed and risky staff office on the wing is designated the "wendy house" (doll's house). Many professional slang systems, such as "doctor slang", serve to obscure the mechanisms of a professional system from its recipients/ service users (Fox et al. 2003). By contrast, prison language highlights and flaunts the procedural, with prisoners equally conversant with terms for security and control as staff. It shifts the institution's focus solely onto its procedures for the processing of prisoners. The language reduces the "balanced system" (Jones 2006), reducing the space in which to consider or voice a fuller range of methods for addressing criminality, disease and distress.

Rycroft describes defences which operate through "identification with objects from whom a sense of power can be borrowed" (Rycroft 1968, p.86). The defensive fantasy that routine, order and control in prison are in themselves rehabilitative, prevent recidivism and promote health in a highly morbid population, is evident in both the institution's language and procedures. Many prison terms are drawn from military might and procedures, and these terms permeate aspects of prison life beyond control and "regime", such as health care activities. Terms such as "sick parade" (doctor's clinic), "MO" (GP, medical officer) and "fitting" (certified in good health, as in "fighting fit") provide a linguistic continuum with "officers/men" (guards/prisoners) "night orderly" (officer in charge at night), "canteen" (prisoners' rations/shop), "officers' mess" (staff diningroom/canteen), "kit" (clothing). Procedurally, there is a gravitational pull on "outsiders", and particularly medical staff, away from health concerns and towards operational roles and preoccupations (Birmingham *et al.* 2006). Cases which necessarily disrupt the order of the "regime" , such as an infectious prisoner's need for a single (not the ubiquitous shared) cell, meet with seemingly irrational resistance throughout the staff hierarchy. We return here to the defensive fantasy that "good order and discipline" can prevent all untoward events, including disease running riot. In this model, prison language becomes a protective and defensive barrier against the complexity of both the "outside" world ("the community") and internal mental states. With its seamless continuity of terms across a wide range of professional disciplines, it acts as a sort of "motherese" – the comforting sounds and words in the exclusive communication between a baby and its primary caregivers, before the child is subject to the rules of grammatical common language (Reber 1985). Psychoanalytically, we might think in terms of dyadic (motherese) as opposed to three-person relationships (common language in which "outsiders" are included), where the former allow little space for thought, perspective and choice (Britton 1998).

CONCLUSION

There are several ways to account for the defensive structures in an institution. Menzies Lyth (1959) posits defences as responding to the impact of a patient's physical and existential condition. We have traced such defences in the "warehousing" language of the institution. We commented on how a language system which privileges operational procedures perpetuates high anxiety by silencing and dismissing staff abilities in understanding and intuitive foresight. The institution is then rendered dependent upon visiting professionals as "experts" who protect it from calumny, particularly in managing patients presenting mental distress. This dependence is perpetuated by a resistance in the institution to engage with the "outsider" in mutual collaboration and learning from experience.

Many forensic commentators, however, see the patients' psychopathology as unconsciously contributing to defences, "infecting" staff and institutional defences. For instance, Welldon & Van Velsen link staff machismo with the reactive impulsiveness of patients/criminals: "Many prisoners feel at home in a prison with its walls, guards and macho culture as it actually matches their internal world so well; thinking is still unavailable and impulses are acted out rather than addressed" (Welldon & Van Velsen 1988, p.4). In this model the "treatability" of prisoners (often termed simply "men" in prison langauge) is diminished by the defensive environment in which they find themselves. The "motherese" described above allows "being inside" (being in prison) to replace any notion of individual psychic "interiority", so that change is conceived as resulting magically from "time served". Hinshelwood, however, suggests more active collusion between parties within the institution (staff and prisoners) than mutual "infection". In the trajectory that he describes, this collusion serves to drive the therapist/therapeutic out: "sets of attitudes have become locked together into a joint system *co-operatively worked* by the prisoners and the officers" (Hinshelwood 1994, p.286; our emphasis). Such *co-operation* is in evidence in the rapidly acquired, shared language system between officers and prisoners. In such a defence, the enormous complexity of the prison's task is oversimplified or split. The risk is that links with the "outside" world and with internal psychic reality of inmates then come to be conceived as tangential to the institution's purposes – in language terms, not part of its mother tongue.

However, we found the language, as a defensive system, to be far more meaningful and rich in (unspoken) communication than it is obscure as a set of unfamiliar terms. We are therefore not providing a glossary of terms here, for several reasons. First, as we commented, absorption of the discourse is rapid for the "outsider", as is acquisition of skills for managing the procedural complexity of the prison (responding to secondary anxiety). Second, local prisons particularly have unusually high tolerance of misunderstanding, chaos and individuals "at a loss", and therefore of confounded "outsiders". In this tolerance also lies the institution's ability to contain and, broadly speaking, manage prisoners with high levels of illiteracy, lack of fluency in English and chaotic internal worlds and external circumstances. Practically, it is probably safer in a prison to be confused and ask for help or guidance, than to appear fluent before procedural security has been proficiently learned. It can be more useful for the "outsider" to experience the impact of chaos than to arrive "word perfect" at the prison gates. In particular, tolerating the mixed emotions of frustration and empathetic understanding that contact with the language provokes can translate into skills in clinical work with individuals. The most important objection to a glossary lies in the need to preserve a sense that there are differences between prisons and other institutions which require detailed efforts of translation. In the period since Hinshelwood's papers, prisons and NHS institutions have been put under obligation to meet a standard of "equivalence" in care provision (HM Prison Service & NHS Executive 1999). "Equivalence" means that "prisoners should receive the same level of health care as they would were they not in prison – equivalent in terms of policy, standards and delivery" (Wilson 2004, p.5). Achieving this requires dialogue, mutual understanding, and mutual empathy or "mentalisation" (Bateman & Fonagy 2004).

The language barrier we have described actively resists the dialogue required for "equivalence" in care and replaces it with a kind of "psychic equivalence", an unconscious assumption that other minds hold identical thoughts to one's own or, in our examples, speak the same language (Nathan & McClean 2007). Such mental functioning typifies the defences of traumatised individuals, for whom difference (as opposed to sameness) is equated with threat and with misunderstanding and the possibility of abandonment (Bateman & Fonagy 2004). Prison language can be seen, in the context of "equivalence", to enact an urgent and voluble defence against imminent misunderstanding, including "one size fits all" assumptions by "outside" agencies and guidance. Services in prisons are often subject to dismissive and hostile projections by "expert" community provision, despite the fact that high rates of recidivism and relapse in the community raise important questions of services there. Moreover, recent commentators such as Wilson (2004) have traced the failure of the NHS framework to understand or "mentalise" the specificity of the prison environment in detail. For instance, the Mental Health Act 1983 has limited application to those in custody and therefore does not provide a "common language" for psychiatric work (Wilson 2004). In daily service provision, core health care values such as confidentiality and protection from stigma need to be reconfigured where patients share their living space (cell) with a stranger, have letters censored, or are monitored "on an ACCT" (Edwards *et al.* 2001). The prison language signals the difficulty of engaging with the institution and with those housed within it.

The Contributors

Gwen Adshead is a forensic psychiatrist and psychotherapist. She has worked in a maximum security hospital for ten years. She has a longstanding interest in ethics in psychiatry and was chair of the Royal College of Psychiatrists' ethics committee.

Colin Allen worked for many years as a prison governor before becoming Deputy Chief Inspector of Prisons for England and Wales in 1989. He retired from full-time work in 2002. Colin has wide experience of all prisons in England and Wales and takes a particular interest in women prisoners and juvenile prisoners.

Phil Brinded is Associate Professor of Forensic Psychiatry at the Christchurch School of Medicine and Health Sciences, University of Otago, and also Chief of Psychiatry for the Canterbury District Health Board in New Zealand.

Gabrielle Brown is a psychodynamic therapist trained at Westminster Pastoral Foundation, where she now teaches on the Advanced Diploma in Psychodynamic Counselling. Originally trained as a social worker, she worked in prisons and the community, including as Communicable Disease lead for Brixton prison until 2006.

Preeti Chhabra is a specialist registrar in forensic psychiatry on the Maudsley Hospital training scheme in London.

David Crighton is currently Acting Chief Psychologist at the Ministry of Justice and visiting Professor of Forensic Psychology at Roehampton University, London. He was previously a consultant forensic psychologist in the NHS and visiting Lecturer in the School of Medicine at the University of Newcastle upon Tyne.

Ian Cumming is Consultant Forensic Psychiatrist at HM Prison Belmarsh and Oxleas NHS Foundation Trust.

Raj Dhar is a consultant forensic psychiatrist in medium security at Oxleas NHS Foundation Trust and a qualified barrister with a broad interest in clinicolegal study.

Ceri Evans is Clinical Director for the Canterbury Regional Forensic Service and Clinical Senior Lecturer with the Christchurch School of Medicine and Health Sciences, University of Otago.

Seena Fazel is Clinical Senior Lecturer in Forensic Psychiatry at the University of Oxford and an Honorary Consultant Forensic Psychiatrist.

Andrew Forrester is a consultant in forensic psychiatry, employed by South London and Maudsley NHS Foundation Trust at HM Prison Brixton since 2005.

Maria Fotiadou is Consultant Psychiatrist with the South London and Maudsley NHS Foundation Trust, working at the Lambeth Community Forensic Team and at the Women's Medium Secure Unit.

Don Grubin is Professor of Forensic Psychiatry at Newcastle University, and Honorary Consultant Forensic Psychiatrist in Newcastle Tyne and Wear NHS Trust. He trained at the Maudsley Hospital, the Institute of Psychiatry and Broadmoor Hospital.

Dominic Johnson is a specialist registrar in forensic psychiatry on the Maudsley Hospital training scheme in London.

Tish Laing-Morton was the head of Healthcare Inspection at HM Inspectorate of Prisons from 2002 to 2006. During that time she helped to shape the changes in health care inspection, including the work with the Healthcare Commission on joint inspections. She is also a non-executive director on the Board of Secure Health Care, a social enterprise organisation providing primary health care in HMP Wandsworth.

Barbara McDermott is Professor of Clinical Psychiatry in the Division of Psychiatry and the Law at the University of California, Davis School of Medicine. She is also Research Director at Napa State Hospital.

Rebecca Milner is a chartered forensic psychologist and has worked for HM Prison Service since 1996. Her current role is national clinical lead for the Extended Sex Offender Treatment Programme (a programme for high-risk sexual offenders) and the Booster Sex Offender Treatment Programme (to prepare sexual offenders for release).

Mark Morris is a psychiatrist and psychoanalyst. He now leads the Partnerships in Care Kneesworth House Personality Disorder Service, a 15-bed medium secure unit with rehabilitation step-down beds attached. His research area is looking at how psychopathic traits are employed in leadership and management.

Glynis Murphy is joint Chair of Clinical Psychology and Learning Disability at the Tizard Centre, University of Kent, and at Oxleas NHS Foundation Trust. Previously she was Academic Director of the Clinical Psychology Training Course at the Institute for Health Research at Lancaster University. She is co-editor of the *Journal of Applied Research in Intellectual Disability*, a fellow of the British Psychological Society, and President of the International Association for the Scientific Study of Intellectual Disability (IASSID).

David Ndegwa is Clinical Director and Consultant Forensic Psychiatrist at River House, South London and Maudsley NHS Foundation Trust.

Janet Parrott has led the development of forensic psychiatry services at the Bracton Centre, Oxleas NHS Foundation Trust. At a national level Dr Parrott is Chair of the Forensic Psychiatry Faculty at the Royal College of Psychiatrists.

John Podmore has worked in the Prison Service for over 20 years and governed three prisons – Belmarsh, Swaleside and most recently, Brixton. John left Brixton in May 2006 and after a secondment as Senior Operational Advisor in the Department for Offender Health he was appointed as Head of the Corruption Prevention Unit in the National Offender Management Service in September 2008.

Natalie Pyszora is a consultant forensic psychiatrist working at Broadmoor Hospital, a high-security psychiatric hospital in England. Prior to this she worked in a high security prison and her research interest involved assessing life-sentenced prisoners in 20 prisons across the country.

Crystal Romilly is a consultant forensic psychiatrist at South West London and St George's NHS Trust, based first at HMP Wandsworth, and then at the Shaftesbury Clinic Medium Secure Unit. Before medicine, she graduated in economics from the London School of Economics. She has written on male genital self-mutilation, restriction orders, sexual behaviour in high security, and prison mental health.

Charles Scott is Chief, Division of Psychiatry and the Law, Forensic Psychiatry Training Director, and Professor of Clinical Psychiatry at the University of California, Davis. He is board certified in general psychiatry, child and adolescent psychiatry, addiction psychiatry and forensic psychiatry.

Huw Stone is a consultant forensic psychiatrist at Ravenswood House Medium Secure Unit. He has been visiting consultant psychiatrist to a lifers prison; clinical director of a forensic psychiatry service for ten years, and the clinical lead for the development of a 20-bed adolescent secure unit. He is currently Deputy Medical Director for the Adult Mental Health directorate of Hampshire Partnership Trust.

Danny Sullivan is a psychiatrist in Melbourne, Australia, where he is Assistant Clinical Director of the Victorian Institute of Forensic Mental Health (Forensicare), and Adjunct Senior Lecturer, School of Psychology, Psychiatry and Psychological Medicine, Monash University. He trained in psychiatry in the UK and Australia and also holds masters degrees in bioethics and in medical law.

Richard Taylor is a consultant forensic psychiatrist at the North London Forensic Service, Camlet Lodge Regional Secure Unit.

James Tighe is Senior Nurse for the substance misuse programme at the Forensic/Prison Mental Health and Challenging Behaviours Directorate at Oxleas NHS Foundation Trust.

Graham Towl is Principal of St Cuthbert's Society at Durham University and Chair of Psychology. Previously, he was Chief Psychologist at the Home Office and most recently with the Ministry of Justice.

Julian Walker is a consultant forensic clinical psychologist at Fromeside Medium Secure Unit and Honorary Research Fellow at the Department of Psychiatry, University of Bristol.

Simon Wilson is Consultant Forensic Psychiatrist at Oxleas NHS Foundation Trust, and Honorary Senior Lecturer in Forensic Psychiatry at the Institute of Psychiatry in London. He was formerly a consultant forensic psychiatrist at the South London and Maudsley NHS Foundation

Trust, and at HM Prison Brixton. He is also Associate Editor of the Journal of Forensic Psychiatry and Psychology

Julie Withecomb has worked as a consultant in adolescent forensic psychiatry for 14 years. During that time she has been involved in the development of teams and services across a range of settings where young people present with mental health difficulties, including young offender institutions, secure training centres, local authority secure children's homes and the National Adolescent Medium Secure Network.

Kiriakos Xenitidis is a consultant psychiatrist with the South London and Maudsley NHS Foundation Trust. He works at the Mental Impairment Evaluation and Treatment Service (MIETS), and is lead clinician at the Adult Attention Deficit Hyperactivity Disorder Service.

Jessica Yakeley is a consultant psychiatrist in forensic psychotherapy at the Portman Clinic, Tavistock and Portman NHS Foundation Trust, and a consultant psychiatrist in psychotherapy in the Camden Psychotherapy Service, Camden and Islington NHS Foundation Trust. She is also an Honorary Senior Lecturer in the Department of Mental Health and Behavioural Sciences, University College London, and a member of the Institute of Psychoanalysis.

References

Aday R (1994) Golden years behind bars: special programs and facilities for elderly inmates. *Federal Probation* 58, 47–54.

Aday R, Rosefield HA (1992) Providing for the geriatric inmate: implications for training. *Journal of Correctional Training* 14–16.

Adesanya A, Ohaeri JU, Ogunlesi AO, Adamson TA, Odejide OA (1997) Psychoactive substance abuse among inmates of a Nigerian prison population. *Drug and Alcohol Dependence* 47, 39–44.

Adshead G (2001a) Murmurs of discontent: treatment and treatability of personality disorder. *Advances in Psychiatric Treatment* 7, 407–415.

Adshead G (2001b) Ethical and public policy issues in the management of Muchausen's syndrome by proxy (MSBP), in Adshead G, Brooke D (eds) *Munchausen's Syndrome by Proxy: Current Issues in Assessment, Treatment and Research*. London: Imperial College Press.

Advisory Council on the Misuse of Drugs (1979) *Report on Drug Dependants within the Prison System of England and Wales*. London: HMSO.

Advisory Council on the Misuse of Drugs (1996) *Drug Misusers and the Criminal Justice System Part III: Drug Misusers and the Prison System: An Integrated Approach*. London: HMSO.

Advisory Council on the Penal System (1968) *The Regime for Long-term Prisoners in Conditions of Maximum Security*. London: HMSO. [The Radzinowicz Report.]

Agbahowe SA, Ohaeri JU, Ogunlesi AO, Osahon R (1998) Prevalence of psychiatric morbidity among convicted inmates in a Nigerian prison community. *East African Medical Journal* 75, 19–26.

Ahmad M, Mwenda L (2004) *Drug Seizure and Offender Statistics. United Kingdom, 2001 & 2002*. Home Office Statistical Bulletin. London: Home Office.

Aiyegbusi A (1996) Thinking under fire, in Jeffcote N, Watson T (eds) *Working Therapeutically with Women in Secure Mental Health Settings*. London: Jessica Kingsley Publishers.

Altun G, Akansu B, Altun BU, Azmak D, Yilmaz A (2004) Deaths due to hunger strike: post-mortem findings. *Forensic Science International* 146, 35–38.

American Psychiatric Association (1994) *Diagnostic and Statistical Manual of Mental Disorders*. Fourth Edition. (DSM-IV). Washington, DC: APA.

American Psychiatric Association (2000) *Diagnostic and Statistical Manual of Mental Disorders*. Fourth Edition. Text Revision (DSM-IV-TR). Washington, DC: APA.

Anderson JC, Morton JB (1989) Graying of the nation's prisons presents new challenges. *The Aging Connection* 10, 6.

Andrews DA, Bonta J (1998) *The Psychology of Criminal Conduct*. Second edition. Cincinnati, OH: Anderson.

Annas GJ (2006) Hunger strikes at Guantanamo – medical ethics and human rights in a "legal black hole". *New England Journal of Medicine* 355, 1377–1382.

Anonymous (1974a) Ethical statement: artificial feeding of prisoners. *British Medical Journal* iii, 52–53.

Anonymous (1974b) The Hunger Striker. *Medico-legal Journal* 42, 59–60.

Anonymous (2000) Marion Price: voice of extremism. *The Daily Telegraph* 12 Dec 2000.

Appelbaum P, Lidz C (1982) The therapeutic misconception: informed consent in psychiatric research. *International Journal of Law and Psychiatry* 5, 319–329.

Archbold (1998) *Criminal Pleading, Evidence and Practice.* London: Sweet and Maxwell.

Arendt M, Rosenberg R, Foldager L, Perto G (2005) Cannabis-induced psychosis and subsequent schizophrenia-spectrum disorders: follow-up study of 535 incident cases. *British Journal of Psychiatry* 187, 510–515.

Armstrong D (2005) *Organization in the Mind.* London: Karnac.

Arndt S, Turvey CL, Flaum M (2002) Older offenders, substance abuse, and treatment. *American Journal of Geriatric Psychiatry* 10(6), 733–739.

Arrigo BA, Bullock JL (2008) The psychological effects of solitary confinement on prisoners in supermax units. Reviewing what we know and recommending what should change. *International Journal of Offender Therapy and Comparative Criminology* 52, 622–640.

Arscott K, Dagnan D, Kroese B (1999) Assessing the ability of people with a learning disability to give informed consent to treatment. *Psychological Medicine* 29, 1367–1375.

Arseneault L (2004) Causal association between cannabis and psychosis: Examination of the evidence. *British Journal of Psychiatry* 184, 110–117.

Arsenault L, Cannon W, Poulter R, Murray R, Caspi A, Moffitt T (2002) Cannabis use in adolescence and risk for adult psychosis: longitudinal prospective study. *British Medical Journal* 325, 1212–1213.

Ashworth A (2000) *Sentencing and Criminal Justice.* Third edition. London: Butterworths.

Australian Institute of Health and Welfare (2006) *Towards a National Prisoner Health Information System.* Cat. no. PHE 79. Canberra: AIHW. Available at www.aihw.gov.au/publications/phe/tnphis/tnphis.pdf, accessed 1 August 2009.

Babor TF, de la Fuente JR, Saunders J, Grant M (1992) *The Alcohol Use Disorders Identification Test: Guidelines for use in primary health care.* WHO Publication No. 92.4. Geneva, Switzerland: World Health Organisation.

Bailey S, Marshall R (2004) Perspectives on substance misuse in young offenders, in Crome I, Ghodse H, Gilvarry E, McArdle P (eds) *Young People and Substance Misuse.* London: Gaskell.

Banerjee S, O'Neill-Byrne K, Exworthy T, Parrott J (1995) The Belmarsh Scheme. A prospective study of the transfer of mentally disordered remand prisoners from prison to psychiatric units. *British Journal of Psychiatry* 166, 802–805.

Baroff G, Gunn M, Hayes S (2004) Legal issues, in Lindsay WR, Taylor JL, Sturmey P (eds) *Offenders With Developmental Disabilities.* Chichester: John Wiley & Sons.

Barratt A, Trevena L, Davey HM, McCaffery K (2004) Use of decision aids to support informed choices about screening. *British Medical Journal* 329, 507–510.

Barron P, Hassiotis A, Banes J (2002) Offenders with intellectual disability: the size of the problem and therapeutic outcomes. *Journal of Intellectual Disability Research* 46, 454–463.

Barron P, Hassiotis A, Banes J (2004) Offenders with intellectual disability: a prospective comparative study. *Journal of Intellectual Disability Research* 48, 69–76.

Basoglu M, Yetimalar Y, Gurgor N, Buyukcatalbas S, Kurt T, Secil Y, *et al.* (2006) Neurological complications of prolonged hunger strike. *European Journal of Neurology* 13, 1089–1097.

Bateman A, Fonagy P (2004) *Psychotherapy for Borderline Personality Disorder: Mentalisation-based Treatment.* Oxford: Oxford University Press.

Bean P, Nemitz T (1994) *Out of Depth and Out of Sight.* London: Mencap.

Beck A (2000) Prison and jail inmates at midyear 1999. *Bureau of Justice Statistics Bulletin,* U.S. Department of Justice, NJC181643.

Beck AJ, Harrison PM (2006) Sexual violence reported by correctional authorities, 2005. *Bureau of Justice Statistics Special Report,* U.S. Department of Justice, NCJ 214646.

Beck AJ, Shipley B (1997) *Recidivism of Prisoners Released in 1983. Bureau of Justice Statistics Special Report.* Washington, DC: Department of Justice.

Beech AM, Erikson C, Friendship C, Ditchfield J (2001) A six-year follow-up of men going through probation-based sex offender treatment programmes. *Home Office Findings* 144, 1–4.

Beech AR, Fisher D, Beckett RC (1999) *Step 3. An Evaluation of the Prison Sex Offender Treatment Programme.* London: HMSO.

Beech AR, Ward T (2004) The integration of etiology and risk in sex offenders: a theoretical model. *Aggression and Violent Behavior* 10, 31–63.

Belenko S, Peugh J (2005) Estimating drug treatment needs among state prison inmates. *Drug and Alcohol Dependence* 77, 269–281.

Benson BA, Ivins J (1992) Anger, depression and self-concept in adults with mental retardation. *Journal of Intellectual Disability Research* 36, 169–175.

Benson BA, Johnson Rice C, Miranti SV (1986) Effects of anger management training with mentally retarded adults in group treatment. *Journal of Consulting and Clinical Psychology* 54, 728–729.

Berridge V, Edwards G (1987) *Opium and the People: Opiate Use and Policy in 19th and Early 20th Century Britain.* London: Free Association Books.

Birmingham L (2001a) Diversion from custody. *Advances in Psychiatric Treatment* 7, 198–207.

Birmingham L (2001b) Screening prisoners for psychiatric illness: who benefits? *Psychiatric Bulletin* 25, 462–464.

Birmingham L (2003) The mental health of prisoners. *Advances in Psychiatric Treatment* 9, 191–201.

Birmingham L. Gray J, Mason D, Grubin D (2000) Mental illness at reception into prison. *Criminal Behaviour and Mental Health* 10, 77–87.

Birmingham L, Mason D, Grubin D (1996) Prevalence of mental disorder in remand prisoners: consecutive case study. *British Medical Journal* 313 (7071), 1521–1524.

Birmingham L, Mason D, Grubin D (1998) A follow-up study of mentally disordered men remanded to prison. *Criminal Behaviour and Mental Health* 8, 202–213.

Birmingham L, Wilson S, Adshead G (2006) Prison medicine: ethics and equivalence. *British Journal of Psychiatry* 188, 4–6.

Black L, Novaco RW (1993) Treatment of anger with a developmentally disabled man, in Wells RA, Giannetti VJ (eds) *Casebook of the Brief Psychotherapies.* New York: Plenum.

Bland J, Mezey G, Dolan B (1999) Special women, special needs: A descriptive study of female special hospital patients. *Journal of Forensic Psychiatry* 10, 34–45.

Bluglass R (1990) Recruitment and training of prison doctors. *British Medical Journal* 301, 249–250.

Bluglass R (1995) Preparing a medico-legal report. *Advances in Psychiatric Treatment* 1, 131–137.

Boer DP, Tough S, Haaven J (2004) Assessment of risk manageability of intellectually disabled sex offenders. *Journal of Applied Research in Intellectual Disabilities* 17, 275–284.

Bogue J, Power K (1995) Suicide in Scottish prisons: 1976–1993. *Journal of Forensic Psychiatry,* 6(3), 527–540.

Borrill J, Maden A, Martin A, Weaver T, Stimson G, Farrell M, Barnes T, Burnett R, Miller S, Briggs D (2003) Substance misuse among white and black/mixed race female prisoners, in Ramsay M (ed.) *Prisoners' Drug Use and Treatment: Seven Research Studies.* Home Office Research, Development and Statistics Directorate. London: HMSO.

Borthwick-Duffy SA (1994) Epidemiology and prevalence of psychopathology in people with mental retardation. *Journal of Consulting and Psychology* 62, 17–27.

Boudreaux MC (2000) Child abduction: an overview of current and historical perspectives. *Child Maltreatment* 5, 63–71.

Bowden P (1976) Medical practice: defendants and prisoners. *Journal of Medical Ethics* 2, 163–172.

Bowden P (1990) The written report and sentences, in Bluglass R, Bowden P (eds) *Principles and Practice of Forensic Psychiatry.* London: Churchill Livingstone.

Bowden P (2002) Personal communication.

Bowers PE (1913) Prison psychosis. A pseudonym? *American Journal of Insanity* 70, 161–173.

Boyington J (2005) Health & offender partnerships. *British Journal of Forensic Practice* 7, 56–58.

Bradley EA, Summers JA, Wood HL, et al. (2004) Comparing rates of psychiatric and behaviour disorders in adolescents and young adults with severe intellectual disability with and without autism. *Journal of Autism and Developmental Disorders* 34,151–161.

Brady K (2008) Cambridge Framework for Risk Assessment (CAMRA), in Towl GJ, Farrington DP, Crighton DA, Hughes G (eds) *Dictionary of Forensic Psychology*. Cullompton: Willan Publishing.

Breakwell G (2007) *The Psychology of Risk*. Cambridge: Cambridge University Press.

Bregin PR (2004) Suicidality, violence and mania caused by selective serotonin reuptake inhibitors (SSRIs): A review and analysis. *International Journal of Risk and Safety in Medicine* 16(1), 31–49.

Bridgwood A, Malbon G (1995) *Survey of the physical health of prisoners*. London: HMSO.

Brinded P, Fairley N, Malcolm F, Stevens I, Mulder R (1999) The Christchurch Prisons Psychiatric Epidemiology Study: methodology and prevalence rates for psychiatric disorders. *Criminal Behaviour and Mental Health* 9, 131–143.

Brinded P, Simpson A, Laidlaw TM, Fairley N, Malcolm F (2001) Prevalence of psychiatric disorders in New Zealand prisons: A national study. *Australian and New Zealand Journal of Psychiatry* 35, 166–173.

Britton R (1998) *Belief and Imagination*. London: Karnac.

Brockman B (1999) Food refusal in prisoners: a communication or a method of self-killing? The role of the psychiatrist and resulting challenges. *Journal of Medical Ethics* 25, 451–456.

Broderick B (2007) Prison work: The dynamics of containment. *Therapy Today* April 2007, 37–40.

Brooke D, Taylor C, Gunn J, Maden A (1996) Point prevalence of mental disorder in unconvicted male prisoners in England and Wales. *British Medical Journal* 313, 1524–1527.

Brooker C, Repper J, Beverley C, *et al.* (2002) *Mental Health Services and Prisoners: A Review*. School of Health and Related Research, University of Sheffield.

Brown BS, Courtless TF (1971) *The Mentally Retarded Offender*. Washington, DC: U.S. Government Printing Office, Dept of Health Education and Welfare Publication No. 72–90–39.

Brugha T, Singleton N, Meltzer H, Bebbington P, Farrell M, Jenkins R, Coid J, Fryers T, Melzer D, Lewis G (2005) Psychosis in the community and in prisons: a report from the British National Survey of Psychiatric Morbidity. *American Journal of Psychiatry* 162, 774–780.

Burdon WM, Dang J, Prendergast ML, Messina NP, Farabee D (2007) Differential effectiveness of residential versus outpatient aftercare for parolees from prison-based therapeutic community treatment programs. *Substance Abuse Treatment, Prevention, and Policy* 2, 1–14.

Campbell D, Hale R (1991) Suicidal acts, in Holmes J (ed.) *A Textbook of Psychotherapy in Psychiatric Practice*. London: Churchill Livingstone.

Cantwell R, Brewin J, Glazebrook C, Dalkin T, Fox R, Medley I, Harrison G (1999) Prevalence of substance misuse in first episode psychosis. *British Journal of Psychiatry* 174, 150–153.

Caplan A (2005) Too hard to face. *Journal of the American Academy of Law & Psychiatry* 33, 394–400.

Cardone D, Dent H (1996) Memory and interrogative suggestibility: The effects of modality of information presentation and retrieval conditions upon the suggestibility scores of people with learning disabilities. *Legal and Criminological Psychology* 1, 34–42.

Casey P (2003) Expert testimony in court. 1: General principles. *Advances in Psychiatric Treatment* 9, 177–182.

Catani M, Howells R (2007) Risks and pitfalls for the management of refeeding syndrome in psychiatric patients. *Psychiatric Bulletin* 316, 209–211.

Chaiken SB, Thompson CR, Shoemaker WE (2005) Mental health interventions in correctional settings, in Scott CL, Gerbasi JB (eds) *Handbook of Correctional Mental Health*. Washington, DC: American Psychiatric Publishing, Inc.

Chao O, Taylor R (2005) Female offenders at HMP Holloway needing hospital transfer: An examination of failure to achieve hospital admission and associated factors. *International Journal of Prisoner Health* 1, 241–247.

Charlton J (1995) Trends and patterns in suicide in England and Wales. *International Journal of Epidemiology* 24, 42–45.

Chiswick D (1985) Use and abuse of psychiatric testimony. *British Medical Journal* 290, 975–977.

Chivite-Matthews N, Richardson A, O'Shea J, Becker J, Owen N, Roe S, Condon J (2005) *Drug Misuse Declared: Findings from the 2003/04 British Crime Survey England & Wales*. London: Home Office.

Cinamon H, Bradshaw R (2005) Prison health in England. *British Journal of Forensic Practice* 7(4), 8–13.

Clare E, Bottomley K (2001) *Evaluation of Close Supervision Centres.* Home Office Research Study 219, London: Home Office Publications.

Clare ICH, Gudjonsson GH (1993) Interrogative suggestibility, confabulation, and acquiescence in people with mild learning disabilities (mental handicap): Implications for reliability during police interview. *British Journal of Clinical Psychology* 32, 295–301.

Clare ICH, Gudjonsson GH (1995) The vulnerability of suspects with intellectual disabilities during police interviews: a review and experimental study of decision-making. *Mental Handicap Research* 8, 110–128.

Clare ICH, Gudjonsson GH, Harari PM (1998) Understanding of the current police caution (England and Wales). *Journal of Community and Applied Social Psychology* 8, 323–329.

Clare ICH, Murphy G (1998) Working with offenders or alleged offenders with intellectual disabilities, in Emerson E, Caine A, Bromley J, Hatton C (eds) *Clinical Psychology and People with Intellectual Disabilities.* Chichester: John Wiley & Sons.

Clarke E, Kissane DW (2002) Demoralization: its phenomenology and importance. *Australian and New Zealand Journal of Psychiatry* 36, 733–742.

Cleckley H (1988) The Mask of Sanity: An attempt to clarify some issues about the so called psychopathic personality. Augusta, GA: Emily S. Cleckley.

Cockram J, Jackson R, Underwood R (1998) People with an intellectual disability and the criminal justice system: the family perspective. *Journal of Intellectual & Developmental Disability* 23, 41–56.

Coffey C, Veit F, Wolfe R, Cini E, Patton GC (2003) Mortality in young offenders: Retrospective cohort study. *British Medical Journal* 326, 1064–1067.

Cohen P, Brook J (1987) Family factors related to the persistence of psychopathology in childhood and adolescence. *Psychiatry* 50, 332–345.

Coid J (1988) Mentally abnormal prisoners on remand – rejected or accepted by the NHS? *British Medical Journal* 296, 1779–1782.

Coid J, Petruckevitch A, Bebbington P, Brugha T, Bhugra D, Farrell M, Lewis G, Singleton N (2002) Ethnic differences in prisoners, 2: Risk factors and psychiatric service use. *British Journal of Psychiatry* 181, 481–487.

Coid J, Petruckevitch A, Bebbington P, *et. al.* (2003) Psychiatric morbidity in prisoners and solitary cellular confinement, II: special ('strip') cells. *Journal of Forensic Psychiatry & Psychology* 14(2), 320–340.

Coid J, Yang M, Tyrer P, Roberts A, Ullrich S (2006) Prevalence and correlates of personality disorder in Great Britain. *British Journal of Psychiatry* 188, 423–431.

Coles EM (2000) The emperor in the courtroom, psychology and pseudo-science. *Journal of Forensic Psychiatry* 11, 1–6.

Commission for Racial Equality (1999) *CRE Fact Sheet.* London: Commission for Racial Equality.

Committee for the Prevention of Torture (1993) *Third General Report on the CPT's activities covering the period 1 January to 31 December 1992.* Available at www.cpt.coe.int/en/annual/rep-03.htm, accessed 25 Nov 2008.

Committee for the Prevention of Torture (2006) *The CPT Standards 2006.* Strasbourg: Council of Europe.

Conley RW, Luckasson R, Bouthilet GN (eds) (1992) *The Criminal Justice System and Mental Retardation.* Baltimore, MD: Paul H. Brookes Publishing.

Connolly T, Arkes HR, Hammond KR (2000) *Judgement and Decision-making.* Second edition. Cambridge: Cambridge University Press.

Cooper CS (2003) Drug courts: current issues and future perspectives. *Substance Use and Misuse* 38, 1671–1711.

Cope R (1990) Psychiatry, ethnicity and crime, in Bluglass R, Bowden P (eds) *Principles and Practice of Forensic Psychiatry.* London: Churchill Livingstone.

Cope R, Ndegwa D (1990) Ethnic differences in admissions to a regional secure unit. *Journal of Forensic Psychiatry* 1, 365–378.

Copeland J, Chen R, Dewey M, *et al.* (1999) Community-based case-control study of depression in older people. *British Journal of Psychiatry* 175, 340–347.

Corbett JA (1979) Psychiatric morbidity and mental retardation, in James FE, Snaith P (eds) *Psychiatric Illness and Mental Handicap.* London: Gaskell.

Cortoni F, Marshall WL (2001) Sex as a coping strategy and its relationship to juvenile sexual history and intimacy in sexual offenders. *Sexual Abuse: Journal of Research and Treatment* 13, 27–43.

Craig LA, Beech A, Browne KD (2006) Cross-validation of the Risk Matrix 2000 Sexual and Violent Scales. *Journal of Interpersonal Violence* 21, 612–633.

Creese R, Bynum W, Bearn J (eds; 1995) *The Health of Prisoners.* Amsterdam: Rodopi.

Crews WD, Bonaventura S, Rowe F (1994) Dual diagnosis: prevalence of psychiatric disorders in a large state residential facility for individuals with mental retardation. *American Journal on Mental Retardation* 98, 724–731.

Crichton J (1999) Mental disorder and crime: Coincidence, correlation and cause. *Journal of Forensic Psychiatry & Psychology* 10(3), 659–677.

Crighton DA (1997) The psychology of suicide. In GJ Towl (ed.) *Suicide and self-injury in prisons.* Leicester: British Psychological Society.

Crighton DA (1999) Risk assessment in forensic mental health. *British Journal of Forensic Practice,* 1(1), 16–18.

Crighton DA (2000a) Suicide in prisons: A critique of UK research. In GJ Towl, L Snow and MJ McHugh (eds) *Suicide in Prisons.* Leicester: BPS Books.

Crighton DA (2000b) Reflections on risk assessment: Suicide in prisons. *British Journal of Forensic Practice,* 2(1), 23–30.

Crighton DA (2000c) *Suicide in Prisons in England and Wales 1988–1998: An Empirical Study.* Unpublished PhD dissertation. Anglia Ruskin University, UK.

Crighton DA (2000d) Editorial – Special issue on suicide in prisons. *British Journal of Forensic Practice* 2(1), 2–3.

Crighton DA (2006) Psychological research into reducing suicides. In GJ Towl (ed.) *Psychological Research in Prisons.* Oxford: Blackwell.

Crighton DA, Towl GJ (1997) Self inflicted deaths in England and Wales, 1988–90 and 1994–5. In GJ Towl (ed) *Suicide and Self-injury in Prisons.* Leicester: British Psychological Society.

Crighton DA, Towl GJ (2000) Intentional self-injury. In GJ Towl, L Snow and MJ McHugh (eds) *Suicide in Prisons.* Oxford: Blackwell.

Crighton DA, Towl GJ (2008) *Psychology in Prisons.* Second edition. Oxford: Wiley Blackwell.

Criminal Justice System (2005) *Inspection Reform: Establishing an Inspectorate for Justice and Community Safety. Consultation.* London: CJS Inspection Policy Unit.

Crook MA, Hally V, Panteli JV (2001) The importance of the refeeding syndrome. *Nutrition* 17, 632–637.

Crundall I, Deacon K (1997) A prison-based alcohol use education program: evaluation of a pilot study. *Substance Use and Misuse* 32, 767–777.

Cullen E (1994) Grendon: the therapeutic prison that works. *Journal of Therapeutic Communities* 15, 301–310.

Cullen E, Newell T (1999) Murderers and life imprisonment: containment, treatment, safety and risk. Winchester: Waterside Press.

Day K (1988) A hospital-based treatment programme for male mentally handicapped offenders. *British Journal of Psychiatry* 153, 635–644.

Denkowski GC, Denkowski KM (1985) The mentally retarded offender in the state prison system: identification, prevalence, adjustment and rehabilitation. *Criminal Justice and Behaviour* 12, 55–70.

Department of Corrections (2002) *Annual Report 2001–2002.* Wellington: Department of Corrections.

Department of Corrections (2005) *Statement of Intent 1 July 2005–30 June 2006.* Wellington: Department of Corrections.

Department of Health (1999a) *National Service Framework for Mental Health.* London: Department of Health.

Department of Health (1999b) *Report of the Expert Committee: Review of the Mental Health Act 1983.* London: Department of Health.

Department of Health (2001) *Changing the Outlook: A Strategy for Developing and Modernising Mental Health Services in Prisons.* London: Department of Health.

Department of Health (2003) *The NHS Confidentiality Code of Practice.* London: Department of Health.

Department of Health (2004) *The Children Act 2004.* London: HMSO.

Department of Health (2005a) *Delivering Race Equality in Mental Health Care: An Action Plan for Reform Inside / Outside Services and the Government's Response to the Independent Inquiry into the Death of David Bennett.* London: Department of Health.

Department of Health (2005b) *Prison Health: Transfer of Commissioning Responsibility to PCTs. Transfer Approval Process for April 2005.* London: Department of Health.

Department of Health (2006) *Clinical Management of Drug Dependence in the Adult Prison Setting.* London: Department of Health.

Department of Health, HM Prison Service (2002) *Guidance on Consent to Medical Treatment.* PSI 38/2002. London: HM Prison Service.

Department of Health, HM Prison Service, The National Assembly for Wales (2002) *Health Promoting Prisons: A Shared Approach.* London: Department of Health.

Department of Health, Home Office (1992) *Review of Health and Social Services for Mentally Disordered Offenders and Others Requiring Similar Services.* London: HMSO. [The Reed Report.]

Department of Health and Social Security, Home Office, Welsh Office, Lord Chancellor's Department (1978) *Review of the Mental Health Act 1959.* London: HMSO.

De Silva N (2005) *Prison Population Projections 2005–2011.* London: HMSO.

Devlin A (1996) *Prison Patter: A Dictionary of Prison Words and Slang.* Winchester: Waterside Press.

Dietz EF, O'Connell DJ, Scarpitti FR (2003) Therapeutic communities and prison management: an examination of the effects of operating an in-prison therapeutic community on levels of institutional disorder. *International Journal of Offender Therapy and Comparative Criminology* 47, 210–223.

Dillon P (2002) *The Much Lamented Death of Madam Geneva: The Eighteenth-century Gin Craze.* London: Headline.

Dolan KA, Shearer J, MacDonald M, Mattick RP, Hall W, Wodak AD (2003) A randomised controlled trial of methadone maintenance treatment versus wait list control in an Australian prison system. *Drug and Alcohol Dependence* 72, 59–65.

Dolan M, Holloway J, Bailey S, Smith C (1999) Health status of juvenile offenders. A survey of young people appearing before juvenile courts. *Journal of Adolescence* 221, 137–144.

D'Orban PT (1971) Social and psychiatric aspects of female crime. *Medicine, Science and the Law* 11, 104–116.

D'Orban PT (1972) Baby stealing. *British Medical Journal* 2, 345–349.

D'Orban PT (1976) Child stealing: a typology of female offenders. *British Journal of Criminology* 16, 275–281.

D'Orban PT (1979) Women who kill their children. *British Journal of Psychiatry* 134, 560–571.

Dove-Wilson J (1932) *Report of the Department Committee on Persistent Offenders.* London: HMSO, Cmnd 4090. [Dove-Wilson Committee.]

Downs D (1996) *More than Victims: Battered Women, the Syndrome, Society and the Law.* Chicago, IL: University of Chicago Press.

Dresser RS, Boisaubin EV (1986) Psychiatric patients who refuse nourishment. *General Hospital Psychiatry* 8, 101–106.

D'Souza RM, Butler T, Petrovesky N (2005) Assessment of cardiovascular disease risk factors and diabetes mellitus in Australian prisons: Is the prisoner population unhealthier than the rest of the Australian population? *Australian and New Zealand Journal of Public Health* 29, 318–323.

Drug Strategy Unit (2003) *The Prison Service Drug Strategy.* London: HM Prison Service.

Duggal A, Lawrence RM (2001) Aspects of food refusal in the elderly: the "hunger strike". *International Journal of Eating Disorders* 30, 213–216.

Durcan G (2008) *From the Inside: Experiences of Prison Mental Health Care.* London: The Sainsbury Centre for Mental Health.

Durcan G, Knowles K (2006) *Policy Paper 5: London's Prison Mental Health Services: A Review.* London: The Sainsbury Centre for Mental Health.

Durkheim E (1952) *Suicide.* London: Routledge, Kegan Paul.

Dyer C (2000) Force feeding of Ian Brady declared lawful. *British Medical Journal* 320, 731.

Dyer O (2004) Doctors reluctant to work on child protection, survey shows. *British Medical Journal* 328, 7435.

Earthrowl M, O'Grady J, Birmingham L (2003) Providing treatment to prisoners with mental disorders: development of a policy. *British Journal of Psychiatry* 182, 299–302.

East WN, Hubert WH de B (1939) *Report on the Psychological Treatment of Crime.* London: HMSO. [East–Hubert Report.]

Eastman N, Dhar R (2000) The role and assessment of mental incapacity: a review. *Current Opinion in Psychiatry* 13, 557–561.

Eaton LF, Menolascino FJ (1982) Psychiatric diagnosis in the mentally retarded: types, problems and challenges. *American Journal of Psychiatry* 139, 1297–1303.

Edwards A, Hurley R (1997) Prisons over two centuries, extract from *Home Office 1782–1982.* London: Home Office.

Edwards S, Tenant-Flowers M, Buggy J, Horne P, Hulme N, Easterbrook P, Taylor C (2001) Issues in the management of prisoners infected with HIV-1: the King's College Hospital HIV prison service retrospective cohort study. *British Medical Journal* 322, 398–399.

Ellis JW, Luckasson RA (1985) Mentally retarded criminal defendants. *The George Washington Law Review* 53, 414–493.

Enoch MD, Trethowan W (1991) *Uncommon Psychiatric Syndromes.* Oxford: Butterworth-Heinemann.

Everington CT, Fulero SM (1999) Competence to confess: Measuring understanding and suggestibility of defendants with mental retardation. *Mental Retardation* 37, 212–220.

Fatoye FO, Fatoye GK, Oyebanji AO, Ogunro AS (2006) Psychological characteristics as correlates of emotional burden in incarcerated offenders in Nigeria. *East African Medical Journal* 83, 545–552.

Faulk MA (1976) Psychiatric study of men serving a sentence in Winchester Prison. *Medicine, Science and Law* 16(4), 244–251.

Fawcett Society (2003) *Interim Report on Women and Offending.* Commission on Women and the Criminal Justice System. London: The Fawcett Society.

Fazel S, Bains P, Doll H (2006) Substance abuse and dependence in prisoners: a systematic review. *Addiction* 101, 181–191.

Fazel S, Danesh J (2002) Serious mental disorder in 23,000 prisoners. *Lancet* 359, 545–550.

Fazel S, Hope T, O'Donnell I, Jacoby R (2001a) Hidden psychiatric morbidity in elderly prisoners. *British Journal of Psychiatry* 179, 535–539.

Fazel S, Hope T, O'Donnell I, Jacoby R (2002) Psychiatric, demographic and personality characteristics of elderly sex offenders. *Psychological Medicine* 32, 219–226.

Fazel S, Hope T, O'Donnell I, Jacoby R (2004) Unmet needs of older prisoners: a primary care survey. *Age and Ageing* 33, 396–398.

Fazel S, Hope T, O'Donnell I, Piper M, Jacoby R (2001b) Health of elderly prisoners: worse than the general population, worse than younger prisoners. *Age and Ageing* 30, 403–407.

Fazel S, Jacoby R (2000) The elderly criminal. *International Journal of Geriatric Psychiatry* 15, 201–202.

Fazel S, Sjosdedt G, Langstrom N, Grann M (2007) Sexual offending and the risk of severe mental illness. *Journal of Clinical Psychiatry* 68, 588–594.

Fazel S, Xenitidis K, Powell J (2008) The prevalence of intellectual disabilities among 12,000 prisoners – a systematic review. *International Journal of Law and Psychiatry* 31, 369–373.

Fernandez YM (1999) *Reliable Identification of Therapist Features.* Paper presented at the ATSA (Association for the Treatment of Sexual Abusers) Annual Research & Treatment Conference, Orlando, Florida, September 1999.

Feron JM, Paulus D, Tonglet R, Lorant V, Pestiaux D (2005) Substantial use of primary health care by prisoners: Epidemiological description and possible explanations. *Journal of Epidemiology and Community Health* 59, 651–655.

Fessler DMT (2003) The implications of starvation induced psychological changes for the ethical treatment of hunger strikers. *Journal of Medical Ethics* 29, 243–247.

Finklehor D (1984) *Child Sexual Abuse: New Theory and Research.* New York: Free Press.

Finlay WML, Lyons E (2001) Methodological issues in interviewing and using self-report questionnaires with people with mental retardation. *Psychological Assessment* 13, 319–335.

Fitzgibbon DWM, Green R (2006) Mentally disordered offenders: Challenges in using the OASys risk assessment tool. *British Journal of Community Justice* 4(2), 33–45.

Floud J, Young W (1981) *Dangerousness and Criminal Justice.* London: Heinemann. [Floud Report].

Flynn A, Matthews H, Hollins S (2002) Validity of the diagnosis of personality disorder in adults with learning disabilities and severe behavioural problems. *British Journal of Psychiatry* 180, 543–546.

Ford J, Trestman R (2005) *Evidence-based enhancement of the detection, prevention, and treatment of mental illness in correctional systems.* National Institute of Justice Final Report. Available at www.ncjrs.org/pdffiles1/nij/grants/210829.pdf.

Forrester A, Henderson C, Wilson S, Cumming I, Spyrou M, Parrott J (in press) A suitable waiting room?: Hospital transfer outcomes and delays from two London prisons. *Psychiatric Bulletin.*

Foster LA, Veale CM, Fogel CI (1989) Factors present when battered women kill. *Issues in Mental Health Nursing* 10, 273–284.

Foucault M (1967) *Madness and Civilization: A History of Insanity in the Age of Reason.* London: Routledge.

Foucault M (1991) *Discipine and Punish: The Birth of the Prison.* London: Penguin.

Fox AT, Fertleman M, Cahill P, Palmer RD (2003) Medical slang in British hospitals. *Ethics and Behaviour* 13, 173–189.

French A, Brigden P, Noble S (1995) *Learning Disabled Offenders in Berkshire.* Unpublished report. East Berkshire NHS Trust.

Friendship C, Mann R, Beech AR (2003) Evaluation of a national prison based treatment program for sexual offenders in England and Wales. *Home Office Findings* 205.

Friendship C, Thornton D (2001) Sexual reconviction for sexual offenders discharged from prison in England and Wales: Implications for evaluating treatment. *British Journal of Criminology* 41, 285–292.

Fruehwald S, Frottier P, Matschnig T, Eher R (2003) The relevance of suicidal behaviour in jail and prison suicides. *European Psychiatry* 18 (4), 161–65.

Fulero SM, Everington C (1995) Assessing competence to waive Miranda rights in defendants with mental retardation. *Law and Human Behaviour* 19, 533–543.

Future Vision Coalition (2008) *A New Vision for Mental Health. Discussion paper.* Available at www.newvision-formentalhealth.org.uk/newvision/A_new_vision_for_mental_health.pdf, accessed 16 Feb 2009.

Gallagher F (1929) *Days of Fear: A Diary of the Hunger Strike.* London: Harper Bros.

Gandhi MK, Jag Parvesh Chander (1944) *The Ethics of Fasting.* Lahore: Indian Printing Works.

Gaudiano BA (2008) Cognitive-behavioural therapies: Achievements and challenges. *Evidence Based Mental Health* 11, 5–7.

Gavin N, Parsons S, Grubin D (2003) Reception screening and mental health needs assessment in a male remand prison. *Psychiatric Bulletin* 27, 251–253.

Geddes JR, Juszczak E (1995) Period trends in the rate of suicide in the first 28 days after discharge from psychiatric hospital in Scotland, 1968–92. *British Medical Journal* 311, 357–360.

Geddes JR, Juszczak E, O'Brien F, *et. al.* (1997) Suicide in the 12 months after discharge from psychiatric inpatient care, Scotland 1968–92. *Journal of Epidemiology and Community Health* 51, 430–34.

Gendreau P (1996) Offender rehabilitation: what we know and what needs to be done. *Criminal Justice Behavior* 23, 144–161.

General Medical Council (2001) *Good Medical Practice.* Second edition. London: General Medical Council.

General Medical Council (2008) *Acting as an Expert Witness.* London: General Medical Council.

Giamp JS, West ME (2003) Delivering psychological services to incarcerated men with developmental disabilities, in Schwartz BK (ed.) *Correctional Psychology: Practice, Programming, and Administration.* Kingston, NJ: Civic Research Institute.

Gibbens TCN (1971) Female offenders. *British Journal of Hospital Medicine* September, 279–286.

Gigerenzer G (2002) *Reckoning with Risk: Learning to Live with Uncertainty.* Harmondsworth: Penguin.

Gillam L (1999) Prenatal diagnosis and discrimination against the disabled. *Journal of Medical Ethics* 25, 163.

Gilvarry E (2001) *The Substance of Young Needs.* London: Health Advisory Service (HAS).

Glaser W, Deane K (1999) Normalisation in an abnormal world: a study of prisoners with an intellectual disability. *International Journal of Offender Therapy and Comparative Criminology* 43, 338–356.

Goldberg AL, Higgins BR (2006) Brief Mental Health Screening for Corrections Intake. *Corrections Today* August 2006, 82–84.

Gordon M (1922) *Penal Discipline.* London: Routledge & Kegan Paul.

Gover RM (1880) *Notes by the Medical Inspector.* Appendix No. 19. Prison Commission Annual Report. London: HMSO.

Graham A (2003) Post-prison mortality: Unnatural death among people released from Victorian prisons between January 1990 and December 1999. *Australian and New Zealand Journal of Criminology* 36, 94–108.

Green CM, Naismith LJ, Menzies RD (1991) Criminal responsibility and mental disorder in Britain and North America: a comparative study. *Medicine, Science and Law* 31, 45–54.

Griffith JD, Hiller ML, Knight K, Simpson DD (1999) A cost-effectiveness analysis of in-prison therapeutic community treatment and risk classification. *The Prison Journal* 79, 352–368.

Grounds, A (2000) The psychiatrist in court, in Gelder M, Lopez-Ibor J, Andreasen N (eds) *New Oxford Textbook of Psychiatry.* Oxford: Oxford University Press.

Grove WM (2000) Clinical versus mechanical prediction: a meta-analysis. *Psychological Assessment* 12, 19–30.

Grubin D (2008) *Validation of Risk Matrix 2000 in Scotland. Report for the Scotland Risk Management Authority.* Available at www.rmascotland.gov.uk/ViewFile.aspx?id=329, accessed 31 August 2009.

Grubin D, Carson D, Parsons S (2002) *Report on the New Prison Reception Health Screen and the Results of a Pilot Study in 10 Prisons.* London: HM Prison Service.

Gudjonsson GH (1992) *The Psychology of Interrogations, Confessions and Testimony.* Chichester: John Wiley and Sons.

Gudjonsson GH, Clare ICH, Rutter S, Pearse J (1993) *Persons at Risk During Interviews in Police Custody: The Identification of Vulnerabilities.* The Royal Commission of Criminal Justice, Research Study no. 12. London: HMSO.

Gunn J (2000) Future directions for treatment in forensic psychiatry. *British Journal of Psychiatry* 176, 332–338.

Gunn J, Maden A, Swinton M (1990) *Mentally Disordered Prisoners. Report to the Home Office.* London: Home Office.

Gunn J, Maden A, Swinton M (1991) Treatment needs of prisoners with psychiatric disorders. *British Medical Journal* 303, 338–341.

Gunn J, Robertson G, Dell S, Way C (1978) *Psychiatric Aspects of Imprisonment.* London: Academic Press.

Hagan J, Simpson JH, Gillis JR (1979) The sexual stratification of social control: a gender based perspective on crime and delinquency. *British Journal of Sociology* 30, 25–38.

Hagell A (2002) *Bright Futures: Working with Vulnerable Young People.* London: Mental Health Foundation.

Hagell A, Newburn T (1994) *Persistent Young Offenders.* London: Policy Studies Unit.

Haigh R (1999) The quintessence of a therapeutic environment, in Campling P, Haigh R (eds) *Therapeutic Communities: Past, Present and Future.* London: Jessica Kingsley Publishers.

Hall GCN (1995) Sexual offender recidivism revisited: A meta-analysis of recent treatment studies. *Journal of Consulting and Clinical Psychology* 63, 802–809.

Hall JN (1992) Correctional services for inmates with mental retardation, in Conley RW, Luckasson R, Bouthilet GN (eds) *The Criminal Justice System and Mental Retardation Defendants and Victims.* Baltimore, MD: Paul H. Brookes Publishing.

Halstead S (1997) Risk assessment and management in psychiatric practice: inferring predictors of risk. A view from learning disability. *International Review of Psychiatry* 9, 217–224.

Hammett TM, Harmon MP, Rhodes W (2002) The burden of infectious disease among inmates of, and releasees from US correctional facilities, 1997. *American Journal of Public Health* 92, 1789–1794.

Hanson RK (1997) *The Development of a Brief Actuarial Risk Scale for Sexual Offence Recidivism.* Ottawa, ON: Dept of the Solicitor General of Canada.

Hanson RK, Bussière MT (1996) *Predictors of sexual offender recidivism: a meta-analysis (User Report 96–04)*. Ottawa, Ontario: Department of the Solicitor General of Canada.

Hanson RK, Bussière MT (1998) Predicting relapse: a meta-analysis of sexual offender recidivism studies. *Journal of Consulting and Clinical Psychology* 66, 348–362.

Hanson RK, Gizzarelli R, Scott H (1994) The attitudes of incest offenders: Sexual entitlement and acceptance of sex with children. *Criminal Justice and Behavior* 21, 187–202.

Hanson RK, Harris AJR (2000) A structured approach to evaluating change among sexual offenders. *Sexual Abuse: A Journal of Research and Treatment* 13, 105–122.

Hanson R, Morton K (2003) Listening to the evidence: risk factors and treatment efficacy for sexual offenders. Presented at the NOTA (National Organisation for the Treatment of Abusers) Conference Edinburgh, September 2003.

Hanson RK, Morton-Bourgon K (2005) The characteristics of persistent sexual offenders: a meta-analysis of recidivism studies. *Journal of Consulting and Clinical Psychology* 73, 1154–1163.

Hanson RK, Thornton D (1999) *Static–99: Improving Actuarial Risk Assessment for Sex Offenders*. Ottawa, Ontario: Dept of the Solicitor General of Canada.

Hanson RK, Thornton D (2000) Improving risk assessments for sexual offenders: a comparison of three actuarial scales. *Law and Human Behaviour* 24,119–136.

Hardie KJ (1909) Letter in the *Daily News*, 27 September 1909.

Hare R (1991) *Manual for the Hare Psychopathy Checklist Revisited*. Toronto, Canada: Multi-health Systems.

Harrington R, Bailey S (2005) *Mental Health Needs and Effectiveness of Provision for Young Offenders in Custody and in the Community*. Youth Justice Board. Available at the Youth Justice Board website: www.yjb.gov.uk/ Publications

Harris GT, Rice ME, Quinsey VL, Lalumiere ML, Boer D, Lang C (2003) A multi-site comparison of actuarial risk instruments for sex offenders. *Psychological Assessment* 15, 413–425.

Harris GT, Tough S (2004) Should actuarial risk assessments be used with sex offenders who are intellectually disabled? *Journal of Applied Research in Intellectual Disabilities* 17, 235–241.

Harrison P, Beck A (2005) *Prisoners in 2004. Bureau of Justice Statistics Bulletin*, U.S. Department of Justice, NCJ210677.

Harrison T (2000) *Bion, Rickman, Foulkes and the Northfield Experiments: Acting on a Different Front*. London: Jessica Kingsley Publishers.

Hart SD, Roesch R, Corrado RR, Cox DN (1993) The Referral Decision Scale: A validation study. *Law and Human Behavior* 17, 611–623.

Harty M, Tighe J, Leese M, Parrott J, Thornicroft G (2003) Inverse care for mentally ill prisoners: Unmet needs in forensic mental health services. *Journal of Forensic Psychiatry & Psychology* 14(3), 600–614.

Hatty S, Walker J (1986) *Deaths in Australian Prisons*. Canberra: Australian Institute of Criminology.

Haveman MJ (1996) Epidemiological issues in mental retardation. *Current Opinion in Psychiatry* 9, 305–311.

Hawton K, Townsend E, Arensman E, *et al.* (2007) Psychosocial and pharmacological treatments for deliberate self-harm. *Cochrane Database of Systematic Reviews* 2, Art. No.: CD001764. Available at www.mrw. interscience.wiley.com/cochrane/clsysrev/articles/CD001764/pdf_fs.html, accessed 23 Jun 2008.

Haycock J (1989) Race and suicide in jails and prisons. *Journal of the National Medical Association* 81(4), 405–411.

Hayes S (1993) *People with an Intellectual Disability and the Criminal Justice System: Appearances Before the Local Courts*. Research Report 4. Sydney: New South Wales Reform Commission Report.

Hayes SC (1996) *People with an Intellectual Disability and the Criminal Justice System: Two Rural Courts*. Research Report 5. Sydney: New South Wales Law Reform Commission.

Heal LW, Sigelman CK (1995) Response biases in interviews of individuals with limited mental ability. *Journal of Intellectual Disability Research* 39, 331–340.

Health Advisory Committee for the Prison Service (1997) *The Provision of Mental Health Care in Prisons*. London: Prison Service.

Healthcare Commission (2006) *Guidance for Assessment Managers Involved in Implementing the Memorandum of Understanding between HM Inspectorate of Prisons (HMIP) and Healthcare Commission on Commissioning Prison Health Services.* London: Healthcare Commission.

Hinshelwood RD (1993) Locked in role: a psychotherapist within the social defence system of a prison. *Journal of Forensic Psychiatry* 4, 427–440.

Hinshelwood RD (1994) The relevance of psychotherapy. *Psychoanalytic Psychotherapy* 8, 283–294.

HM Inspectorate of Prisons (1996) *Patient or Prisoner?: A New Strategy for Health Care in Prisons.* London: Home Office.

HM Inspectorate of Prisons (1997) *Women in Prison: A Thematic Review by HM Chief Inspector of Prisons.* London: Home Office.

HM Inspectorate of Prisons (1999) *Suicide is Everyone's Concern – A Thematic Review by HM Chief Inspector of Prisons for England and Wales.* London: Home Office.

HM Inspectorate of Prisons (2005) *Annual Report of HM Chief Inspector of Prisons for England and Wales 2003–4.* London: Home Office.

HM Inspectorate of Prisons (2007a) *The Mental Health of Prisoners: A Thematic Review of the Care and Support of Prisoners with Mental Health Needs* London: HM Inspectorate of Prisons.

HM Inspectorate of Prisons (2007b) *Annual Report of HM Chief Inspector of Prisons 2005/06.* London: Home Office.

HM Inspectorate of Prisons and Probation (1999) *Lifers: A Joint Thematic Review.* London: Home Office.

HM Inspectorate of Probation (2006) *An Independent Review of a Serious Further Offence Case: Anthony Rice.* London: Home Office.

HM Prison Service (1996) *Management of Disruptive Prisoners: CRC Review Project Final Report.* Unpublished. [Spurr Report.]

HM Prison Service (2001) *The Comprehensive Review of Parole and Lifer Processes.* London: Home Office.

HM Prison Service (2002) *Guidance on the Protection and Use of Confidential Health Information in Prison and Inter-agency Information Sharing.* London: Home Office.

HM Prison Service (2004a) *Category A Prisoners, Review of Security Category.* Prison Service Order 1010. London: Home Office.

HM Prison Service (2004b) *Death in Custody Investigations by the Prisons and Probation Ombudsman.* Prison Service Order 1301. London: HM Prison Service.

HM Prison Service (2004c) *Regimes for Juveniles.* Prison Service Order 4950. London: HM Prison Service.

HM Prison Service (2006a) *Lifer Manual.* Prison Service Order 4700. London: HM Prison Service.

HM Prison Service (2006b) *Continuity of Health Care for Prisoners.* Prison Service Order 3050. London: HM Prison Service.

HM Prison Service (2007a) *The ACCT Approach – Caring for People at Risk in Prison.* London: Safer Custody Group. Available from www.hmprisonservice.gov.uk/assets/documents/10000C1BACCTStaffGuide.pdf, accessed 30 Jun 2008.

HM Prison Service (2007b) *Suicide Prevention and Self-harm Management.* Prison Service Order 2700. London: HM Prison Service.

HM Prison Service, NHS Executive (1999) *The Future Organisation of Prison Health Care. Report by the Joint Prison Service and National Health Service Executive Working Group.* London: Department of Health.

Hobbs M, Krazlan K, Ridout S, Mai Q, Knuiman M, Chapman R (2006) *Mortality and Morbidity in Prisoners After Release from Prison in Western Australia 1995–2003.* Research and Public Policy Series Number 71. Canberra: Australian Institute of Criminology. Available at www.aic.gov.au/documents/6/7/3/{6731BD68-AD7F-48CF-B527-2D3C4FA71E13}tandi320.pdf, accessed 30 August 2009.

Hodgins S (1992) Mental disorder, intellectual deficiency and crime: evidence from a birth cohort. *Archives of General Psychiatry* 49, 476–483.

Hodgins S, Mednick SA, Brennan PA, Schulsinger F, Engberg M (1996) Mental disorder and crime. *Archives of General Psychiatry* 53, 489–496.

Hodgins S, Müller-Isberner R (2004) Preventing crime by people with schizophrenic disorders: the role of psychiatric services. *British Journal of Psychiatry* 185, 245–250.

Hollins S, Clare ICH, Murphy G, Webb B (1997a) *You're Under Arrest.* London: Gaskell Press.

Hollins S, Murphy G, Clare ICH, Webb B (1997b) *You're On Trial.* London: Gaskell Press.

Holloway K, Bennett T, Farrington D (2005) *The Effectiveness of Criminal Justice and Treatment Programmes in Reducing Drug Related Crime: A Systematic Review.* Home Office Online Report 26/05. London: Home Office.

Home Office (1895) *Report from the Departmental Committee on Prisons.* London: HMSO, C. 7702. [Gladstone Committee.]

Home Office (1964) *The Organisation of the Prison Medical Service.* London: HMSO.

Home Office (1966) *Report of the Inquiry into Prison Escapes and Security.* London: HMSO, Cmnd 3175. [Mountbatten Report.]

Home Office (1971) *Habitual Drunken Offenders: Report of the Working Party.* London: HMSO.

Home Office (1979) *Committee of Inquiry into UK Prison Services.* London: HMSO, Cmnd 7673. [May Report.]

Home Office (1984) *Managing the Long-term Prison System: The Report of the Control Review Committee.* London: Home Office.

Home Office (1990a) *Report of an Efficiency Scrutiny of Prison Medical Services.* London: Home Office.

Home Office (1990b) *Home Office Circular 66/90: Provision for Mentally Disordered Offenders.* London: Home Office.

Home Office (1991a) *Prison Disturbances 1990.* London: HMSO. [Woolf Report.]

Home Office (1991b) *Custody, Care and Justice: The Way Ahead for the Prison Service in England and Wales.* London: HMSO, Cm 1647.

Home Office (1994) *Report of the Enquiry into the Escape of Six Prisoners from the Security Unit at Whitemoor Prison.* London: HMSO. [Woodcock Report.]

Home Office (1995a) *Review of Prison Service Security in England and Wales and the Escape from Parkhurst Prison on Tuesday 3rd January 1995.* London: HMSO. [Learmont Report.]

Home Office (1995b) *Police and Criminal Evidence Act 1984. Codes of Practice.* Revised edition. London: HMSO.

Home Office (1995c) *Tackling Drugs Together: A Strategy for England 1995–1998.* London: HMSO.

Home Office (1995d) *Criminal Careers of Those Born Between 1953 and 1973. Statistical Bulletin 14/95.* London: Home Office.

Home Office (1997) *Managing Courts Effectively: The Reasons for Adjournments in Magistrates Courts.* Home Office Research Study 168. London: Home Office.

Home Office (2000a) *A Guide to the Criminal Justice System in England and Wales.* London: Home Office.

Home Office (2000b) *Prison Statistics England and Wales 1999.* London: HMSO.

Home Office (2003a) *Prison Statistics England and Wales 2002.* London: HMSO.

Home Office (2003b) *Statistics on Women and the Criminal Justice System. A Home Office publication under Section 95 of the Criminal Justice Act 1991.* London: Home Office.

Home Office (2004a) *Statistics of Mentally Disordered Offenders, England and Wales. Statistical Bulletin 16/04.* Home Office: London.

Home Office (2004b) *Violent Crime in England and Wales.* London: Home Office.

Home Office (2005) *Prison Statistics 2004: England and Wales.* London: Home Office.

Home Office (2006a) *Statistics on Race and the Criminal Justice System – 2005.* London: Home Office.

Home Office (2006b) *Violent Crime Overview, Homicide and Gun Crime 2004/2005.* London: Home Office.

Home Office (2007) *Expectations.* London: HMSO.

Home Office (2008) *British Crime Survey, 2007–2008.* London: Home Office.

Home Office, Department of Health and Social Security (1975) *Report of the Committee on Mentally Abnormal Offenders.* London: HMSO. [Butler Report.]

Home Office, HM Inspectorate of Prisons for England and Wales (1997) *Young Prisoners: A Thematic Review by HM Chief Inspector of Prisons for England and Wales.* London: Home Office.

Howard J (1784) *The State of the Prisons in England and Wales.* Third edition. Warrington: William Eyres.

Howard League for Penal Reform (2002) *Children in Prison: Barred Rights.* London: Howard League for Penal Reform.

Howard LM (2006) The psychoses, in Henderson C, Smith C, Smith S, Steven A (eds) *Women and Psychiatric Treatment: A comprehensive Text and Practical Guide*. London: Routledge.

Humphreys M (2000) Aspects of basic management of offenders with mental disorders. *Advances in Psychiatric Treatment* 6, 22–32.

Hurd, Rt Hon The Lord of Westwell (2004) Are prison reformers winning the arguments? 2004 Prison Reform Trust Lecture. *Prison Service Journal* 154, 3.

Hyatt Williams A (1998) *Cruelty, Violence and Murder: Understanding the Criminal Mind*. London: Karnac.

Inquest (2008) Inquest website www.inquest.gn.apc.org, accessed 12 November 2008.

Institute of Alcohol Studies (2007) *Factsheet*. London: Institute of Alcohol Studies.

International Centre for Prison Studies (2008) *World Prison Brief*. Available at www.kcl.ac.uk/depsta/law/research/icps/worldbrief/wpb_country.php?country=169, accessed 24 Nov 2008.

Isherwood S, Parrott J (2002) Audit of transfers under the Mental Health Act from prison: The impact of organisational change. *Psychiatric Bulletin* 26, 368–370.

James D, Farnham F, Moorey H, Lloyd H, Hill K, Blizard R, Barnes TRE (2002) *Outcome of Psychiatrist Admission through the Courts*. Home Office RDS Occasional Paper No.79. London: Home Office.

James DJ, Glaze LE (2006) Mental health problems of prison and jail inmates. *Bureau of Justice Statistics Special Report*, U.S. Department of Justice, NCJ 213600.

Janoff Bulman R (1985) The aftermath of victimisation: rebuilding shattered assumptions, in Figley C (ed.) *Truam and its Wake Vol. 1*. New York: Brunner Mazel.

Jenkins R (1974) Hansard *877 H.C. Debs.*, column 451 (17 July).

Jenkins R, Bebbington P, Brugha TS, Farrell M, Lewis G, Meltzer H (1998) British psychiatric morbidity survey. *British Journal of Psychiatry* 173, 4–7.

Jenkins R, Bhugra D, Meltzer H, *et al.* (2005) Psychiatric and social aspects of suicidal behaviour in prisons. *Psychological Medicine* 35(2), 257–269.

Jenkins R, Singh B (2000) Policy and Practice in Suicide Prevention. *British Journal of Forensic Practice* 2(1), 3–11.

Johannes Weir Foundation for Health and Human Rights (1995) *Assistance in Hunger Strikes*. Amersfoort: Johannes Weir Foundation.

Johnston SJ (2002) Risk assessment in offenders with intellectual disability: the evidence base. *Journal of Intellectual Disability Research* 46, 47–56.

Joint Committee on Human Rights (2004) *Joint Committee on Human Rights – Third Report*. London: House of Lords and House of Commons.

Jolliffe D, Farrington D (2004) Empathy and offending: a systematic review and meta-analysis. *Aggression and Violent Behavior* 9, 441–476.

Jones D (2006) Psychopathological considerations of prison systems, in Jones (ed.) *Humane Prisons*. Oxford: Radcliffe.

Joseph P (1992) *Psychiatric Assessment at the Magistrates' Courts*. London: Home Office.

Joseph P (1998) He who pays the piper. *Journal of Forensic Psychiatry* 9, 509–512.

Joudo J (2006) *Deaths in Custody in Australia: National Deaths in Custody Program Annual Report 2005*. Technical and background paper series, no. 21 (online only). Canberra: Australian Institute of Criminology. Available from www.aic.gov.au/documents/5/9/F/%7B59F73F5E-E045-4DF8-BA68-C8B8F14B3B52%7Dtbp021.pdf, accessed 31 August 2009.

Justice (1996) *Sentenced for Life: Reform of the Law and Procedure for Those Sentenced to Life Imprisonment*. London: Justice.

Kalk WJ, Felix M, Snoey ER, Veriawa Y (1993) Voluntary total fasting in political prisoners: clinical and biochemical observations. *South African Medical Journal* 83, 391–394.

Kanyanya IM, Othieno CJ, Ndetei DM (2007) Psychiatric morbidity among male sex offenders at Kamiti Prison, Kenya. *East African Medical Journal* 84, 151–155.

Karlan SC (1939) Symptoms and previous personality in prison psychoses. *Psychiatric Quarterly* 13, 514–520.

Katon W, Korff MV, Lin E, Walker E, Simon G, Bush T, *et al.* (1995) Collaborative management to achieve treatment guidelines: impact on depression in primary care. *Journal of the American Medical Association* 273, 1026–1031.

Kelly S, Bunting J (1998) *Trends in Suicide in England and Wales, 1982–96*. London: Office of National Statistics.

Kennedy H (1992) *Eve was Framed: Women and British Justice*. London: Vintage.

Kenney A (1924) *Memories of a Militant*. London: Edward Arnold.

Kessler RC, Nelson CB, McGonagle KA, Edlund MJ, Frank RG, Leaf PJ (1996) The epidemiology of co-occurring addictive and mental disorders: implications for prevention and service utilization. *American Journal of Orthopsychiatry* 66, 17–31.

Kesteven S (2002) *Women who Challenge: Women Offenders and Mental Health Issues*. London: Nacro.

Kirkpatrick JT, Humphrey JA (1986) *Stress in the Lives of Female Criminal Homicide Offenders*, paper presented at Second National Congress on Social Stress Research, University of New Hampshire, Durham, June 1986.

Knight K, Simpson DD, Hiller ML (1999) Three year reincarceration outcomes for in-prison therapeutic community treatment in Texas. *The Prison Journal* 79, 337–351.

Koenig H, Johnson S, Bellard J, Denker M, Fenlon R (1995) Depression and anxiety disorder among older inmates at a federal correctional facility. *Psychiatric Services* 46, 399–401.

Kohn M (1992) *Dope Girls: The Birth of the British Drugs Underground*. London: Lawrence and Wishart.

Korbonits M, Blaine D, Elia M, Powell-Tuck J (2007) Metabolic and hormonal changes during the refeeding period of prolonged fasting. *European Journal of Endocrinology* 157, 157–166.

Krajick K (1979) Growing old in prison. *Corrections Magazine* 5(1), 32–46.

Kratzer L, Hodgins S (1997) Adult outcomes of child conduct problems: a cohort study. *Journal of Abnormal Child Psychology* 25, 65–81.

Kreitman N, Philip AE, Greer S, *et al.* (1969) Parasuicide. *British Journal of Psychiatry* 115, 746–747.

Kuehn BM (2007) Mental health courts show promise. *Journal of the American Medical Association* 279, 1641–1643.

Lader D, Singleton N, Meltzer H (2000) *Psychiatric Morbidity Among Young Offenders in England and Wales*. London: Office for National Statistics.

Laming Lord (2003) *The Victoria Climbié Inquiry*. London: HMSO.

Larkin E (1991) Food refusal in prison. *Medicine, Science, and Law* 31, 41–44.

Lewinsohn P, Klein D, Seeley J (1995) Bipolar disorders in a community sample of older adolescents: Prevalence, phenomenology, comorbidity and course. *Journal of the American Academy of Child and Adolescent Psychiatry* 34, 454–463.

Lewis NA (2005) Interrogators cite doctors' aid at Guantanamo. *New York Times.*, 24 June 2005.

Liebling A (1991) *Suicide in Prisons*. Unpublished PhD dissertation. University of Cambridge, UK.

Liebling A (2004) *Prisons and their Moral Performance*. Oxford: Oxford University Press.

Lindsay WR (2002) Research and literature on sex offenders with intellectual and developmental disabilities. *Journal of Intellectual Disability Research* 46, 74–85.

Lindsay WR, Beail N (2004) Risk assessment: actuarial prediction and clinical judgement of offending incidents and behaviour for intellectual disability services. *Journal of Applied Research in Intellectual Disabilities* 17, 229–234.

Lindsay WR, Law J, Quinn K, Smart N, Smith AHW (2001) A comparison of physical and sexual abuse histories: sexual and non-sexual offenders with intellectual disability. *Child Abuse and Neglect* 25, 989–995.

Lindsay WR, Marshall I, Neilson CQ, Quinn K, Smith AHW (1998b) The treatment of men with a learning disability convicted of exhibitionism. *Research in Developmental Disabilities* 19, 295–316.

Lindsay WR, Murphy L, Smith G, Murphy D, Edwards Z, Chittock C, Grieve A, Young SJ (2004a) The dynamic risk assessment and management system: an assessment of immediate risk of violence for individuals with offending and challenging behaviour. *Journal of Applied Research in Intellectual Disabilities* 17, 267–274.

Lindsay WR, Neilson CQ, Morrison F, Smith AHW (1998a) The treatment of six men with a learning disability convicted of sexual offences with children. *British Journal of Clinical Psychology* 37, 83–98.

Lindsay WR, Olley S, Jack C, Morrison F, Smith AHW (1998c) The treatment of two stalkers with intellectual disabilities using a cognitive approach. *Journal of Applied Research in Intellectual Disabilities* 11, 333–344.

Lindsay WR, Smith A (1998) Responses to treatment for sex offenders with intellectual disability: a comparison of men with 1- and 2-year probation sentences. *Journal of Intellectual Disability Research* 42, 346–353.

Lindsay WR, Smith AHW, Law J, Quinn K, Anderson A, Smith A, Overend T, Allan R (2002) A treatment service for sex offenders and abusers with intellectual disability: characteristics of referrals and evaluation. *Journal of Applied Research in Intellectual Disability* 15, 166–174.

Lindsay WR, Smith AHW, Quinn K, Anderson A, Smith A, Allan R, Law J (2004b) Women with intellectual disability who have offended: characteristics and outcome. *Journal of Intellectual Disability Research* 48, 580–590.

Linehan MM, Armstrong HE, Suarez A, *et al.* (1991) Cognitive-behavioral treatment of chronically parasuicidal borderline patients. *Archives of General Psychiatry* 48, 1060–1064.

Lipton DS, Pearson FS, Cleland CM, Yee D (2002) The effectiveness of cognitive-behavioural treatment methods on offender recidivism, in McGuire J (ed.) *Offender Rehabilitation and Treatment: Effective Programmes and Policies to Reduce Re-offending.* Chichester: Wiley.

Lombroso C, Ferrero W (1895) *The Female Offender.* London: Fisher Unwin.

Lösel F, Schmucker M (2005) The effectiveness of treatment for sexual offenders: a comprehensive meta-analysis. *Journal of Experimental Criminology* 1, 117–146.

Lyall I, Holland AJ, Collins S (1995a) Offending by adults with learning disabilities: identifying need in one health district. *Mental Handicap Research* 8, 99–109.

Lyall I, Holland AJ, Collins S, Styles P (1995b) Incidence of persons with a learning disability detained in police custody: A needs assessment for service development. *Medicine, Science and the Law* 35, 61–71.

MacEachron AE (1979) Mentally retarded offenders: prevalence and characteristics. *American Journal of Mental Deficiency* 84, 165–176.

Mackay R (1995) *Mental Condition Defences in the Criminal Law.* Oxford: Clarendon Press.

Maden A (1996) *Women, Prisons and Psychiatry: Mental Disorder Behind Bars.* Oxford: Butterworth-Heinemann.

Maden A, Brooke D, Taylor C, Gunn J (1996) *A Survey of Mental Disorder in Remand Prisoners.* London: Home Office.

Maden A, Swinton M, Gunn J (1990) Women in prison and use of illicit drugs before arrest. *British Medical Journal* 301, 1133.

Mafullul YM, Ogunlesi OA, Sijuwola OA (2001) Psychiatric aspects of criminal homicide in Nigeria. *East African Medical Journal* 78, 35–39.

Maggia B, Martin S, Crouzet C, Richard P, Wagner P, Balmès J, Nalpas B (2004) Variation in AUDIT (Alcohol Used Disorder Identification Test) scores withing the first weeks of imprisonment. *Alcohol & Alcoholism* 39, 247–250.

Malamuth NM, Brown LM (1994) Sexually aggressive men's perception of women's communications: testing three explanations. *Journal of Personality and Social Psychology* 67, 699–712.

Mann RE, Hollin CR (2007) Sexual offenders' explanations for their offending. *Journal of Sexual Aggression* 13, 3–9.

Mann R, Webster S, Wakeling H, Marshall W (2007) The measurement and influence of child sexual abuse supportive beliefs. *Psychology, Crime and Law* 13, 443–458.

Mannuzza S, Klein RG, Bonagagura N, Malloy P, Giampino T, Addalli KA (1991) Hyperactive children almost grown up. *Archives of General Psychiatry* 48, 77–83.

Marshall P (1997) *A Reconviction Study of HMP Grendon Therapeutic Community.* Home Office Research and Statistics Directorate. Research Findings No. 53. London: Home Office.

Marshall T, Simpson S, Stevens A (2001) Use of health services by prison inmates: Comparisons with the community. *Journal of Epidemiology and Community Health* 55, 364–365.

Marshall WL, Anderson D, Fernandez Y (1999) *Cognitive Behavioural Treatment of Sexual Offenders*. New York: Wiley.

Martin C, Player E, Liriano S (2003) Results of evaluations of the RAPt drug treatment programme, in Ramsay M (ed.) *Prisoners' Drug Use and Treatment: Seven Research Studies*. Home Office Research Study 267. London: Home Office.

Martin E, Colebrook M, Gray A (1984) Health of prisoners admitted to and discharged from Bedford Prison. *British Medical Journal* 289, 965–967.

Martinson R (1974) What Works? – Questions and answers about prison reform. *The Public Interest* 10, 22–54.

Mason J, Murphy GH (2002a) People with intellectual disabilities on probation: an initial study. *Journal of Community and Applied Social Psychology* 12, 44–55.

Mason J, Murphy GH (2002b) People with an intellectual disability in the criminal justice system: developing an assessment tool for measuring prevalence. *British Journal of Clinical Psychology* 41, 315–320.

Mason K, Bennett H, Ryan E (1988) *Report of the Committee of Inquiry into procedures used in certain psychiatric hospitals in relation to admission, discharge or release on leave of certain classes of patients*. The Mason Report. Wellington: Department of Corrections.

Matthew W, Scott S (2005) Evidence-based management of conduct disorders. *Current Opinion in Psychiatry* 18, 392–396.

May C (2005) *The CARAT Drug Service in Prisons: Findings from the Research Database*. Home Office Findings 262. London: Home Office.

Mayfield D, McLeod G, Hall P (1974) The CAGE questionnaire: Validation of a new alcoholism screening instrument. *American Journal of Psychiatry* 131, 1121–1123.

Mayhew H, Binny J (1862) *The Criminal Prisons of London and Scenes of Prison Life*. London: Griffin, Bohn, and Company.

Mayr A (2004) *Prison Discourse: Language as a Means of Control and Resistance*. Hampshire: Palgrave.

McBrien J (2003) The intellectually disabled offender: methodological problems in identification. *Journal of Applied Research in Intellectual Disability* 16, 95–106.

McBrien J, Hodgetts A, Gregory J (2003) Offending and risky behaviour in community services for people with intellectual disabilities in one Local Authority. *Journal of Forensic Psychiatry* 14, 280–297.

McBrien J, Murphy G (2007) Police and carers' views on reporting alleged offences by people with intellectual disabilities. *Psychology, Crime and Law* 12 (2), 127–144.

McCabe KM, Hough R, Wood PA, Yeh M (2001) Childhood and adolescent onset conduct disorder: A test of the developmental taxonomy. *Journal of Abnormal Child Psychology* 29, 305–316.

McGrother CW, Hauck A, Bhaumik S, Thorp C, Taub N (1996) Community care for adults with learning disability and their carers: needs and outcomes from the Leicestershire register. *Journal of Intellectual Disability Research* 40, 183–190.

McGuire J, Priestley P (1995) Reviewing "What Works": Past, present and future, in McGuire J (ed.) *What Works: Reducing Reoffending. Guidelines from Research and Practice*. Chichester: John Wiley and Sons.

McKibben A, Proulx J, Lusignan R (1994) Relationships between conflict, affect and deviant sexual behaviours in rapists and pedophilies. *Behaviour Research and Therapy* 32, 571–575.

McKenzie N, Sales B (2008) New procedures to cut delays in transfer of mentally ill prisoners to hospital. *Psychiatric Bulletin* 32, 20–22.

McLaren J, Bryson SE (1987) Review of recent epidemiological studies in mental retardation: prevalence, associated disorders, and etiology. *American Journal of Mental Retardation* 92, 243–254.

McMillan D, Hastings R, Coldwell J (2004) Clinical and actuarial prediction of physical violence in a forensic intellectual disability hospital: a longitudinal study. *Journal of Applied Research in Intellectual Disabilities* 17, 255–265.

McMurran M (2007) What works in substance misuse treatments for offenders? *Criminal Behaviour and Mental Health* 17, 225–233.

McNulty C, Kissi-Deborah R, Newsom-Davies I (1995) Police involvement with clients having intellectual disabilities: A pilot study in South London. *Mental Handicap Research* 8, 129–136.

McSweeney T, Turnbull PJ, Hough M (2008) *The Treatment and supervision of drug-dependent offenders: A review of the literature prepared for the UK Drug Policy Commission.* London: Institute for Criminal Policy Research, King's College London.

Medford S, Gudjonsson G, Pearse J (2000) *The Identification of Persons at Risk in Police Custody: The Use of Appropriate Adults by the Metropolitan Police.* London: Metropolitan Police.

Melzer D, Tom B, Brugha T, Fryers T, Grounds A, Johnson T, Meltzer H, Singleton N (2002) Prisoners with psychosis in England and Wales: A one-year follow-up study. *Howard Journal* 41, 1–13.

Meltzer H, Gatward R, Goodman R, Ford T (2000) *The Mental Health of Children and Adolescents in Great Britain.* London: Office of National Statistics.

Menninger KA (1938) *Man Against Himself.* New York: Harcourt Brace.

Mental Health Foundation (1999) *Bright Futures: Promoting Children and Young People's Mental Health.* London: Mental Health Foundation.

Menzies Lyth I (1959) *Containing Anxiety in Institutions.* London: Karnac.

Miller WP (1986) The hunger-striking prisoner. *Journal of Prison and Jail Health* 6, 40–61.

Miller WR, Rollnick S (2002) *Motivational Interviewing. Preparing People for Change.* Second edition. New York: Guilford Press.

Milton J, Amin S, Singh S, Harrison G, Jones P, Croudace T, Medley I, Brewin J (2001) Aggressive incidents in first-episode psychosis. *British Journal of Psychiatry* 178, 433–440.

Ministry of Health (1961) *Report of the Working Party on Special Hospitals.* London: HMSO. [Emery Report.]

Ministry of Health (2002) *Te Puawaitanga Maori Mental Health National Strategic Framework.* Wellington: Ministry of Health.

Ministry of Justice (2007) *Offender Management Caseload Statistics 2006.* London: Ministry of Justice.

Ministry of Justice (2008a) *Offender Management Caseload Statistics 2007.* Available at www.justice.gov.uk/docs/omcs2007.pdf, accessed 24 Nov 2008.

Ministry of Justice (2008b) *Securing the Future: Proposals for the Efficient and Sustainable Use of Custody in England and Wales.* London: Ministry of Justice.

Ministry of Justice (2008c) *Population in Custody Monthly Tables April 2008 England and Wales.* London: Ministry of Justice.

Ministry of Justice (2008d) *Arrests for Recorded Crime (Notifiable Offences) and the Operation of Certain Police Powers under PACE England and Wales 2006/07.* London: Ministry of Justice.

Ministry of Justice (2009) *Statistics of Mentally Disordered Offenders 2007 England and Wales.* Ministry of Justice Statistics Bulletin. London: Ministry of Justice.

Ministry of Justice, Attorney General's Office, Home Office (2008) *Murder, Manslaughter and Infanticide: Proposals for Reform of the Law.* London: Ministry of Justice.

Møller L, Stöver H, Jürgens R, Gatherer A, Nikogsian H (2007) *Health in Prisons. A WHO Guide to the Essentials in Prison Health.* Geneva: WHO.

Monahan J (2002) The McArthur studies of violence risk. *Criminal Behaviour and Mental Health* 12, 67–72.

Monahan J, Steadman H, Silver E, *et al.* (2001) *Rethinking Risk Assessment: The MacArthur Study of Mental Disorder and Violence.* New York: Oxford University Press.

Moos RH (1986) *Group Environment Scale Manual.* Second edition. Palo Alto, CA: Consulting Psychologist's Press.

Morgan HG, Burns CC, Pococky H, *et al.* (1975) Deliberate self-harm: clinical and socio-economic characteristics of 368 patients. *British Journal of Psychiatry,* 127, 564–74.

Morris N, Rothman DJ (1998) *The Oxford History of the Prison: The Practice of Punishment in Western Society.* Oxford: Oxford University Press.

Motz A (2001) *The Psychology of Female Violence: Crimes Against the Body.* Hove, East Sussex: Routledge.

Mullen PE (2006) Schizophrenia and violence: from correlations to preventive strategies. *Advances in Psychiatric Treatment* 12, 239–248.

Müller-Isberner R, Hodgins S (2000) Evidence-based treatment for mentally disordered offenders, in Hodgins S, Müller-Isberner R (eds) *Violence, Crime and Mentally Disordered Offenders.* Chichester, West Sussex: John Wiley & Sons Ltd.

Mumola CJ, Karberg JC (2006) Drug use and dependence, state and federal prisoners, 2004. *Bureau of Justice Statistics Special Report*. U.S. Department of Justice, NCJ 213600.

Murphy G (2007) Intellectual disability and sexual abuse, in Carr A, O'Reilly G, Walsh PN, McEvoy J (eds) *Handbook of Intellectual Disability and Clinical Psychology Practice*. London: Routledge.

Murphy G, Beadle-Brown J, Wing L, Gould J, Shah A, Holmes N (2005) Chronicity of challenging behaviours in people with severe intellectual disabilities and/or autism: a total population. *Journal of Autism and Developmental Disorders* 35, 405–418.

Murphy G, Clare ICH (1991) MIETS: A service option for people with mild mental handicaps and challenging behaviour or psychiatric problems. Assessment, treatment and outcome for service users and service effectiveness. *Mental Handicap Research* 4, 180–206.

Murphy G, Clare ICH (1996) Analysis of motivation in people with mild learning disabilities (mental handicap) who set fires. *Psychology, Crime and the Law* 2, 153–164.

Murphy G, Clare ICH (2003) Adults' capacity to make legal decisions, in Bull R, Carson D (eds) *Handbook of Psychology in Legal Contexts*. Second edition. Chichester: Wiley.

Murphy G, Harnett H, Holland AJ (1995) A survey of intellectual disabilities amongst men on remand in prison. *Mental Handicap Research* 8, 81–98.

Murphy G, Holland A, Fowler P, Reep J (1991) MIETS: a service option for people with mild mental handicaps and challenging behaviour or psychiatric problems, I. Philosophy, service, and service users. *Mental Handicap Research* 4, 41–66.

Murphy GH, Sinclair N, Hays S, Offord G, Langdon P, Scott J, Williams J, Stagg J, Tufnell J, Lippold T, Mercer K, Langheit G (2004) Group cognitive-behavioural treatment for men with intellectual disabilities at risk of sexual offending. *Journal of Intellectual Disability Research* 48, 467.

Narey M (2002) Perrie Lecture 14th June – Prison Service College, Newbold Revel. Prison chief attacks CRE for hindering war on racism. Reported in the *Guardian*, Friday June 14 2002.

Nathan J, McClean D (2007) Treatment of personality disorder: Limit setting and the use of benign authority. *British Journal of Psychotherapy* 23, 231–246.

National Collaborating Centre for Mental Health (NCCMH) (2008) *Drug Misuse: Opioid Detoxification*. NICE Clinical Guideline 52. Leicester/London: The British Psychological Society/The Royal College of Psychiatrists.

National Institute for Clinical Excellence (NICE) (2007a) *Depression: Management of Depression in Primary and Secondary Care*. London: British Psychological Society/Gaskell.

National Institute for Health and Clinical Excellence (NICE) (2007b) *Drug Misuse: Psychosocial Interventions*. NICE Clinical Guideline 51. London: National Institute for Health and Clinical Excellence.

National Institute of Corrections (1987) *Guidelines for the Development of a Security Program*. Washington, DC: United States Department of Justice.

National Offender Management Service (2008a) *Safer Custody News* (May/June). London: NOMS.

National Offender Management Service (2008b) *Prison Population and Accommodation Briefing*. London: NOMS.

National Screening Committee (2003) *The UK National Screening Committee's Criteria for Appraising the Viability, Effectiveness and Appropriateness of a Screening Programme*. London: HMSO. Available at www. health.bcu.ac.uk/webmodules/PG_HPPH/GM704H%20RHP/screening/National%20Screening%20 Committee.pdf, accessed 30 August 2009.

National Treatment Agency for Substance Misuse (2009) *Integrated Drug Treatment System in Prisons (IDTS)*. London: NTA. Available at www.nta.nhs.uk/areas/criminal_justice/integrated_drug_treatment_system_in_prisons(IDTS).aspx, accessed on 30 August 2009.

Ndegwa D (2003) *Social Division and Difference: Black and Ethnic Minorities*. Liverpool: NHS National Programme on Forensic Mental Health Research and Development.

Needs A (1997) Occupational standards in applied psychology. *Forensic Update* 48, 18–23.

New York State Commission on Quality of Care For the Mentally Disabled (1991) *Inmates with Developmental Disabilities in NYS Correctional Facilities*. Available at www.cqc.state.ny.us/publications/pubinmat.htm, accessed August 20 2007.

NHS Health and Social Care Information Centre (2006) *Drug Use, Smoking and Drinking among Young People in England in 2005: Headline Figures.* London: NHS Health & Social Care Information Centre.

NHS Scotland (2005) *Alcohol Statistics Scotland 2005.* Edinburgh: NHS Scotland.

Nitsche P, Wilmanns K (1912) *The History of the Prison Psychoses.* Nervous & Mental Disease Monograph Series No. 13. New York: The Journal of Nervous & Mental Disease Publishing Company.

Niveau G (2007) Relevance and limits of the principle of "equivalence of care", in prison medicine. *Journal of Medical Ethics* 33, 610–613.

Noble JH, Conley RW (1992) Toward an epidemiology of relevant attributes, in Conley RW, Luckasson R, Bouthilet GN (eds) *The Criminal Justice System and Mental Retardation.* Baltimore, MA: Paul H. Brookes.

Norfolk, Suffolk and Cambridgeshire Strategic Health Authority (2003) *Independent Inquiry into the Death of David Bennett.* Cambridge: Norfolk, Suffolk and Cambridgeshire Strategic Health Authority.

North East London Strategic Health Authority (2003) *Report of an Independent Inquiry into the Care and Treatment of Daksha Emson M.B.B.S., MRCPsych, MSc. and her Daughter Freya.* London: North East London Strategic Health Authority.

Novick LF, Penna RD, Schwartz MS, Remmlinger E, Loewenstein R (1977) Health status of the New York City prison population. *Medical Care* 15, 205–216.

Nurse J, Woodcock P, Ormsby J (2003) Influence of environmental factors on mental health within prisons: focus group study. *British Medical Journal* 327, 480.

O'Brien G (2002) Dual diagnosis in offenders with intellectual disability: setting research priorities: a review of research findings concerning psychiatric disorder (excluding personality disorder) among offenders with intellectual disability. *Journal of Intellectual Disability Research* 46, 21–30.

O'Connor A, Johnson-Sabine E (1988) Hunger strikers. *Medicine, Science, and Law* 28, 62–64.

O'Grady J (2004) Report writing for the criminal court. *Psychiatry* 3, 34–36.

Offending Behaviour Programmes Unit (2004) *SOTP, Psychometric Assessment Battery.* London: HM Prison Service.

Office for National Statistics (1999) *Health Statistics Quarterly.* London: The Stationery Office.

Office for National Statistics (2005) *Mid-Year Population Estimates 2005.* London: Office for National Statistics.

Office for National Statistics (2007) Report: Deaths related to drug poisoning: England and Wales, 1993/2005. *Health Statistics Quarterly* 33, 82–88.

Office of Public Services Reform (2003) *The Government's Policy on Inspection of Public Services.* London: Office of Public Services Reform.

Oguz NY, Miles SH (2005) The physician and prison hunger strikes: reflecting on the experience in Turkey. *Journal of Medical Ethics* 31, 169–172.

Olds DL (2006) The nurse–family partnership: An evidence based preventative intervention. *Infant Mental Health Journal* 27, 5–25.

Owers A (2005) *Report on a full unannounced inspection of HMP/YOI Holloway 4–8 October 2004.* London: HM Inspectorate of Prisons.

Owers A (2006) Independent inspection of prisons, in Jones D (ed.) *Humane Prisons.* Oxford: Radcliffe.

Padfield N (2000) Detaining the dangerous. *Journal of Forensic Psychiatry* 11, 497–500.

Page K (2006) First Impressions, in Jones D (ed.) *Humane Prisons.* Oxford: Radcliffe.

Pailthorpe GW (1932) *What We Put in Prison and in Preventive and Rescue Homes.* London: Williams and Norgate.

Palmer J (2006) *Drug Treatment in Prisons Future Directions: Integrated Drug Treatment System (IDTS).* Presentation to the Prison Health Research Network, 20 October 2006.

Parsons S, Walker L, Grubin D (2001) Prevalence of mental disorder in female remand prisons. *Journal of Forensic Psychiatry* 12, 194–202.

Pattinson EM, Kahan J (1983) The deliberate self-harm syndrome. *American Journal of Psychiatry* 140, 867–872.

Pearse J, Gudjonsson GH (1996) How appropriate are Appropriate Adults? *Journal of Forensic Psychiatry* 7, 570–580.

Peel M (1997) Hunger strikes: understanding the underlying physiology will help doctors provide proper advice. *British Medical Journal* 315, 829–830.

Penfold C, Turnbull PJ, Webster R (2005) *Tackling prison drug markets: an exploratory qualitative study.* Home Office Online Report 39/05. London: Home Office.

Penrose LS (1939) Mental disease and crime: outline of a comparative study of European statistics. *British Journal of Medical Psychology* 18, 1–15.

Percy Commission (1957) *Report of the Royal Commission on the Law relating to Mental Illness and Mental Deficiency 1954–1957.* London: HMSO, Cmnd 169.

Perry A, Coulton S, Glanville J, Godfrey C, Lunn J, McDougall C, Neale Z (2006) Interventions for drug-using offenders in the courts, secure establishments and the community. *Cochrane Database of Systematic Reviews* 3, Art. No.: CD005193.

Perske R (1991) *Unequal Justice?* Nashville, TN: Abingdon Press.

Peters RH, Greenbaum PE, Steinberg ML, Carter CR, Ortiz MM, Fry BC, Valle SK (2000) Effectiveness of screening instruments in detecting substance use disorders among prisoners. *Journal of Substance Abuse Treatment* 18, 349–358.

Peters RH, May RL (1992) Drug treatment services in jails, in Leukefeld C, Tims F (eds) *Drug Abuse Treatment in Prisons and Jails.* Rockville, MD: U.S. Department of Health and Human Services, National Institute on Drug Abuse, Publication No. ADC 92–1884.

Petersilia J (1997) Justice for all? Offenders with mental retardation and the California corrections system. *The Prison Journal* 77, 358–381.

Petersilia, J. (2000) *Doing Justice? Criminal Offenders with Developmental Disabilities.* California Policy Research Center, University of California. Available at www.ucop.edu/cprc/documents/dojustrpt.pdf, accessed 20 August 2007.

Pizzey E (2008) *Daily Mail,* 29th July 2008.

Plutchik R (1980) *Emotion: A Psychoevolutionary Synthesis.* New York: Harper Row.

Plutchik R (1997) Suicide and violence: the two stage model of countervailing forces, in Botsis AJ, Soldatos CR and Stefanis CN (eds) *Suicide: Biopsychosocial Approaches.* Amsterdam: Elsevier.

Polaschek DLL, Hudson SM, Ward T, Siegert RJ (2001) Rapists' offence processes: A preliminary descriptive model. *Journal of Interpersonal Violence* 16, 523–544.

Polivy J, Zeitlin SB, Herman CP, Beal AL (1994) Food restriction and binge eating: a study of former prisoners of war. *Journal of Abnormal Psychology* 103, 409–411.

Pollack O (1950) *The Criminality of Women.* New York: AS Barnes/Perpetua.

Porter R (2001) *English Society in the Eighteenth Century.* London: Penguin.

Pratt D, Piper M, Appleby L, *et al.* (2006) Suicide in recently released prisoners: a population-based cohort study. *The Lancet,* 368 (9530), 119–123.

Prendergast M, Farabee D, Cartier J (1999) *The Impact of In-prison Therapeutic Community Programs on Prison Management.* Paper presented at the meeting of the American Society of Criminology, Toronto, Canada.

Prior G (1998) Self-reported health, in Prescott-Clarke P, Primatesta P (eds) *Health Survey for England 1996, volume 1: findings.* London: The Stationery Office.

Prison Reform Trust (1994) *The Report of the Committee on the Penalty for Homicide.* London: Prison Reform Trust.

Prison Reform Trust (2006) *Experiences of Minority Ethnic Employees in Prison.* London: Prison Reform Trust.

Prison Reform Trust (2007) *Bromley Briefings. Prison Factfile.* London: Prison Reform Trust.

Prison Reform Trust (2008a) *Bromley Briefings. Fact File 08.* London: Prison Reform Trust.

Prison Reform Trust (2008b) *Indefinitely Maybe: How the Indeterminate Sentence for Public Protection is Unjust and Unsustainable.* London: Prison Reform Trust.

Prochaska JO, DiClemente CC (1982) Transtheoretical therapy: Toward a more integrative model of change. *Psychotherapy: Theory, Research and Practice* 19, 276–288.

Qin P, Nordentoft M (2005) Suicide risk in relation to psychiatric hospitalisation: evidence based on longitudinal registers. *Archives of General Psychiatry* 62, 427–432.

Quinsey VL, Harris GT, Rice ME, Cromier CA (1998) *Violent Offenders: Appraising and Managing Risk.* Washington, DC: American Psychological Association.

Ramsbotham D (2003) *Prisongate: The Shocking State of Britain's Prisons and the Need for Visionary Change.* London: Free Press.

Rapoport R (1960) *Community as Doctor.* London: Tavistock.

Reber A (1985) *Penguin Dictionary of Psychology.* London: Penguin.

Reed J (2002) Delivering psychiatric care to prisoners. *Advances in Psychiatric Treatment* 8, 117–127.

Reed J, Department of Health, Home Office (1994) *Working Group on Psychopathic Disorder. Report.* London: Department of Health.

Reed J, Lyne M (2000) Inpatient care of mentally ill people in prison: Results of a year's programme of semi-structured inspections. *British Medical Journal* 320, 1031–1034.

Reid AH, Ballinger BR (1987) Personality disorder in mental handicap. *Psychological Medicine* 17, 983–987.

Reiss D, Meux C (2000) Education and training in forensic psychiatry. *Journal of Forensic Psychiatry* 11, 501–505.

Reiss S (1988) *Reiss Screen Test Manual.* Orland Park, IL: International Diagnostic Systems.

Reiss S (1990) Prevalence of dual diagnosis in community based day programmes in the Chicago metropolitan area. *American Journal of Mental Retardation* 94, 578–585.

Reiss S (1994) Psychopathology in mental retardation, in Bouras N (ed.) *Mental Health in Mental Retardation: Recent Advances and Practices.* Cambridge: Cambridge University Press.

Resnick PJ (1969) Child murder by parents: a psychiatric review of filicide. *American Journal of Psychiatry* 126, 325–334.

Reyes H (1998) Medical and ethical aspects of hunger strikes in custody and the issue of torture, in Oehmichen M, *Maltreatment and Torture.* Lübeck: Verlag Schmidt-Römhild. Published on the website of the International Committee of the Red Cross, www.icrc.org/eng, accessed 30 May 2008.

Reza B, Magill C (2006) *Race and the Criminal Justice System: An overview to the complete statistics 2004–2005.* London: Criminal Justice System Race Unit.

Richardson A, Budd T, Engineer R, Phillips A, Thompson J, Nicholls J (2003) *Drinking, Crime and Disorder.* Findings 185. Research, Development and Statistics Directorate. London: Home Office.

Richardson SA, Koller H (1985) Epidemiology, in Clarke AM, Clarke ADB, Berg JM (eds) *Mental Deficiency: The Changing Outlook.* London: Methuen.

Robbins I, Mackeith J, Davison S, Kopelman M, Meux C, Ratnam S, Somekh D, Taylor R (2005) Psychiatric problems of detainees under the Anti-Terrorism Crime and Security Act 2001. *Psychiatric Bulletin* 29, 407–409.

Roberts J (ed.; 1994) *Escaping Prison Myths: Selected Topics in the History of Federal Corrections.* Washington, DC: American University Press.

Robertson G, Dell S, James K, Grounds A (1994) Psychotic men remanded in custody to Brixton Prison. *British Journal of Psychiatry* 164, 55–61.

Robertson M, Waller G (2007) Overview of psychiatric ethics1: professional ethics and psychiatry. *Australasian Psychiatry* 15, 201–206.

Rogers R, Sewell KW, Ustad K, Reinhardt V, Edwards W (1995) The referral decision scale with mentally disordered inmates: A preliminary study of convergent and discriminant validity. *Law and Human Behavior* 19, 481–491.

Rose J, Jenkins R, O'Connor C, Jones C, Felce D (2002) A group treatment for men with intellectual disabilities who sexually offend or abuse. *Journal of Applied Research in Intellectual Disabilities* 15, 138–150.

Rose J, West C, Clifford D (2000) Group interventions for anger in people with intellectual disabilities. *Research in Developmental Disabilities* 21, 171–181.

Rosenberg DA (1987) Web of deceit: a literature review of Munchausen syndrome by proxy. *Child Abuse and Neglect* 11, 547–563.

Roy A (1982) Risk factors for suicide in psychiatric patients. *Archives of General Psychiatry* 39, 1089–1095.

Royal College of Psychiatrists (2000) *Good Psychiatric Practice: Confidentiality.* Council Report CR85. London: Royal College of Psychiatrists.

Royal College of Psychiatrists (2001) *Curriculum for Basic Specialist Training and the MRCPsych Examination.* Council Report CR95. London: Royal College of Psychiatrists.

Royal College of Psychiatrists (2002) *Suicide in Prisons.* Council Report CR99. London: Royal College of Psychiatrists.

Royal College of Psychiatrists (2004a) *A competency based curriculum for higher specialist training.* Second edition. London: Royal College of Psychiatrists.

Royal College of Psychiatrists (2004b) *Psychiatrists and Multi-Agency Public Protection Arrangements.* London: Royal College of Psychiatrists.

Royal College of Psychiatrists (2004c) The psychiatrist, courts and sentencing: the impact of extended sentencing on the ethical framework of forensic psychiatry (Council Report 129). *Psychiatric Bulletin* 29(2), 73–77.

Royal College of Psychiatrists (2005) *Statement of the Royal College of Psychiatrists in Respect of the Psychiatric Problems of Detainees Held under the 2001 Anti-Terrorism Crime & Security Act.* London: Royal College of Psychiatrists.

Royal College of Psychiatrists (2008a) *Alcohol: Our Favourite Drug.* London: Royal College of Psychiatrists.

Royal College of Psychiatrists (2008b) *Council Report on Risk Assessment.* London: Royal College of Psychiatrists.

Russell O (1997) *The Psychiatry of Learning Disabilities.* London: Gaskill.

Rutherford H, Taylor P (2004) The transfer of women offenders with mental disorder from prison to hospital. *Journal of Forensic Psychiatry & Psychology* 15, 108–123.

Rutter M, Giller H, Hagell A (1998) *Antisocial Behavior by Young People.* Cambridge: Cambridge University Press.

Rycroft C (1968) *A Critical Dictionary of Psychoanalysis.* London: Penguin.

Ryrie N, Lawrence C, Miller A (eds; 2006) Young offending and youth justice. *Special Issue of Educational and Child Psychology* 23, 2.

Sabol WJ, Harrison PM (2007) Prison and jail inmates at midyear 2006. *Bureau of Justice Statistics Bulletin,* U.S. Department of Justice, NCJ 217675.

Sacks S, Sacks JY, McKendrick K, Banks S, Stommel J (2004) Modified TC for MICA inmates in correctional settings: crime outcomes. *Behavioural Sciences and the Law* 22, 477–501.

Sainsbury Centre for Mental Health (2008) *Short Changed. Spending on Prison Mental Health Care.* London: Sainsbury Centre for Mental Health.

Sales B, McKenzie N (2007) Time to act on behalf of mentally disordered offenders. *British Medical Journal* 334, 1222.

Santamour MB (1987) The offender with mental retardation. *The Prison Journal* 66, 3–18.

Santamour MB, West B (1982a) The mentally retarded offender: presentation of the facts and a discussion of issues, in Santamour MB, Watson PS (eds) *The Retarded Offender.* New York: Praeger Publishers.

Santamour MB, West B (1982b) Retarded offenders: habilitative program development, in Santamour MB, Watson PS (eds) *The Retarded Offender.* New York: Praeger Publishers.

Sattar G (2001) *Rates and Causes of Death among Prisoners and Offenders under Community Supervision.* Home Office Research Study 231. London: Home Office.

Saunders P, Copeland J, Dewey M, *et al.* (1993) The prevalence of dementia, depression and neurosis in later life: the Liverpool MRC-ALPHA study. *International Journal of Epidemiology* 22, 838–847.

Schuman J (1999) The ethnic minority populations of Great Britain: latest estimates. *Population Trends* 33–43.

Scobie IN (1987) *A study of the inter-relationships between ketosis and leucine, alanine, and glucose metabolism in normal and obese fasted human subjects using tracer methodology.* MD thesis, University of Glasgow, Glasgow.

Scotland, Baroness of Asthal (2004) Hansard, column 9, 28 June 2004.

Scott P (1953) Psychiatric reports for magistrates courts. *British Journal of Delinquency* 4, 82–98.

Scott PD (1973) Parents who kill their children. *Medicine, Science and the Law* 13, 120–126.

Scott PD (1974) Commentary on SJH Ganser, in Hirsch SR, Shepheard H (eds) *Themes and Variations in European Psychiatry.* Charlottesville, VA: University of Virginia Press.

Scott S (2002) Parent training programmes, in Rutter M, Taylor E (eds) *Child and Adolescent Psychiatry: Modern Approaches.* Oxford: Blackwell Science.

Scott S, Spender Q, Doolan M, Jacobs B, Aspland H (2001) Multicentre controlled trial of parenting groups for childhood antisocial behaviour in clinical practice. *British Medical Journal* 323, 194–203.

Seaman SR, Brettle RP, Gore SM (1998) Mortality from overdose among injecting drug users recently released from prison: Database linked study. *British Medical Journal 316*, 426–428.

Seddon T (2007) *Punishment and Madness. Governing Prisoners with Mental Health Problems.* Basingstoke: Routledge-Cavendish.

Seidman BT, Marshall WL, Hudson S, Robertson PJ (1994) An examination of intimacy and loneliness in sex offenders. *Journal of Interpersonal Violence* 9, 518–534.

Seligman MEP (1975) *Helplessness.* San Francisco, CA: Freeman.

Sharp C, Budd T (2005) *Minority Ethnic Groups and Crime: Findings From the Offending, Crime and Justice Survey 2003.* Home Office Online Report 33/05. London: Home Office.

Shaw J, Appleby L, Baker D (2003a) *National Confidential Inquiry into Suicide and Homicide by People with Mental Illness.* London: Department of Health. Available at www.dh.gov.uk/prod_consum_dh/groups/dh_digitalassets/@dh/@en/documents/digitalasset/dh_4034301.pdf, accessed 22 June 2008.

Shaw J, Appleby L, Baker D (2003b) *Safer Prisons: A National Study of Prison Suicides. The National Confidential Inquiry into Suicides and Homicides by People with Mental Illness.* London: Department of Health.

Shiekh J, Yesavage J (1986) Geriatric Depression Scale: recent findings in development of a shorter version, in Brink J (ed.) *Clinical Gerontology: A guide to assessment and interventions.* New York: Howarth Press.

Silove D, Curtis J, Mason C, Becker R (1996) Ethical considerations in the management of asylum seekers on hunger strike. *Journal of the American Medical Association* 276, 410–415.

Silverman IJ (2001) The correctional process, in Silverman IJ (ed.) *Corrections: A Comprehensive View.* Second edition. Belmont, CA: Wadsworth/Thomson Learning.

Sim J (1990) *Medical Power in Prisons: The Prison Medical Service in England 1774–1989.* Milton Keynes: Open University Press.

Simpson AIF, Brinded P, Fairley N, Laidlaw TM, Malcolm F (2003) Does ethnicity affect need for mental health service among New Zealand prisoners? *Australian and New Zealand Journal of Psychiatry* 37(6), 728–734.

Singleton N, Bumpstead R, O'Brien M, Lee A, Meltzer H (2003a) Psychiatric morbidity among adults living in private households. *International Review of Psychiatry* 15, 65–73.

Singleton N, Meltzer H, Gatward R. (1998) *Psychiatric Morbidity Among Prisoners in England and Wales.* London: The Stationery Office.

Singleton N, Pendry E, Taylor C, Farrell M, Marsden J (2003b) *Drug-related Mortality among Newly Released Offenders.* Findings 187. London: Home Office.

Sjostedt G, Langstrom N (2002) Assessment of risk for criminal recidivism among rapists: a comparison of four different measures. *Psychology, Crime and Law* 8, 25–40.

Smallbone SW, Dadds MR (1998) Childhood attachment and adult attachment in incarcerated adult male sex offenders. *Journal of Interpersonal Violence* 13, 555–573.

Smith A (1998) Psychiatric evidence and discretionary life sentences. *Journal of Forensic Psychiatry* 9, 17–38.

Smith C, Algozzine B, Schmid R, Hennly T (1990) Prison adjustment of youthful inmates with mental retardation. *Mental Retardation* 28, 177–181.

Smith LA, Gates S, Foxcroft D (2006) Therapeutic communities for substance related disorder. *Cochrane Database of Systematic Reviews* 1, Art. No.: CD005338.

Smith R (1984) *Prison Health Care.* London: British Medical Association.

Smith R (1999) Prisoners: an end to second class health care? *British Medical Journal* 318, 954–955.

Smith SA (1993) Confusing the terms "guilty" and "not guilty": Implications for alleged offenders with mental retardation. *Psychological Reports* 73, 675–678.

Snow L (2006) Intentional self-injury. In GJ Towl (ed.) *Psychological Research in Prisons.* Oxford: Blackwell.

Social Exclusion Unit (2002) *Reducing Re-offending by Ex-prisoners.* London: Social Exclusion Unit, Office of the Deputy Prime Minister.

Solomka B (1996) The role of psychiatric evidence in passing "longer than normal" sentences. *Journal of Forensic Psychiatry* 7, 239–255.

Sournia JC (1990) *A History of Alcoholism.* Oxford: Wiley Blackwell.

Southall D, Plunkett MCB, Banks MW, Falkov AF, Samuels MP (1997) Covert video recordings of life threatening child abuse: lessons for child protection. *Pediatrics* 100, 735–760.

Sovner R (1986) Limiting factors in the use of DSM–III criteria with mentally ill/mentally retarded persons. *Psychopharmacology Bulletin* 22, 1055–1059.

Sovner R, Hurley AD (1983) Do the mentally retarded suffer from affective illness? *Archives of General Psychiatry* 40, 61–67.

Special Hospitals Service Authority (1993) *Report of the Committee of Inquiry into the Death in Broadmoor Hospital of Orville Blackwood and a Review of the Deaths of Two Other Afro-Caribbean Patients. 'Big, Black and Dangerous?'* London: Special Hospitals Service Authority.

Stavis PF (1991) Doing justice? The criminal justice system and persons with mental retardation. *Quality of Care Newsletter*, New York State Commission on Quality of Care for the Mentally Disabled, Issue 47. Available at www.cqc.state.ny.us/counsels_corner/cc47.htm, accessed 21 January 2005.

Steadman HJ, Scott JE, Osher F, Agnese TK, Robbins PC (2005). Validation of the brief jail mental health screen. *Psychiatric Services* 56, 816–822.

Stone JH, Roberts M, O'Grady J, Taylor A (2000) *Faulk's Basic Forensic Psychiatry.* Third edition. Oxford: Blackwell Science.

Sutherland E (1947) *Criminology.* Philadelphia, PA: JB Lippincott Company.

Taylor J (2002) A review of the assessment and treatment of anger and aggression in offenders with intellectual disability. *Journal of Intellectual Disability Research* 46, 57–73.

Taylor JL, Novaco RW, Gillmer B, Robertson A (2004a) Treatment of anger and aggression, in Lindsay WR, Taylor JL, Sturmey P (eds) *Offenders with Developmental Disabilities.* Chichester: John Wiley & Sons.

Taylor JL, Novaco RW, Gillmer B, Thorne I (2002b) Cognitive-behavioural treatment of anger intensity among offenders with intellectual disabilities. *Journal of Applied Research in Intellectual Disabilities* 15, 151–165.

Taylor J, Thorne I, Robertson A, Avery G (2002a) Evaluation of a group intervention for convicted arsonists with mild and borderline intellectual disabilities. *Criminal Behaviour and Mental Health* 12, 282–293.

Taylor JL, Thorne I, Slavkin ML (2004b) Treatment of fire-setting behaviour, in Lindsay WR, Taylor JL, Sturmey P (eds) *Offenders with Developmental Disabilities.* Chichester: John Wiley & Sons.

Taylor P, Parrott J (1988) Elderly offenders: a study of age-related factors among custodially remanded prisoners. *British Journal of Psychiatry* 152, 340–346.

Taylor R (2000) A seven year reconviction study of HMP Grendon Therapeutic Community, in Shine J (ed.) *HMP Grendon, A Compilation of Grendon Research.* Aylesbury: Leyhill Press.

Teplin LA (1990) Detecting disorder: The treatment of mental illness among jail detainees. *Journal of Consulting and Clinical Psychology* 58, 233–236.

Teplin LA, Abram KM, McClelland GM (1996) Prevalence of psychiatric disorder among incarcerated women. *Archives of General Psychiatry* 53, 505–512.

Teplin LA, Swartz J (1989) Screening for severe mental disorder in jails: The development of the referral decision scale. *Law and Human Behavior* 13, 1–18.

Thomas SDM (2005) *Inverse Care? Comparing needs and satisfaction with services between prisoners in health care centres and patients in forensic medium secure units.* Unpublished PhD thesis, Institute of Psychiatry, King's College, London.

Thompson C, Kimmonth A, Stevens L, Peveler R, Stevens A, Osler K, *et al.* (2000) Effects of a clinical-practice guideline and practice-based education on detection and outcome on depression in primary care: Hampshire Depression Project randomised controlled trial. *Lancet* 355, 185–191.

Thornton D (2002) Constructing and testing a framework for dynamic risk assessment. *Sexual Abuse: A Journal of Research and Treatment* 14, 139–153.

Thornton D, Beech A, Marshall WL (2004) Pretreatment self-esteem and posttreatment sexual recidivism. *International Journal of Offender Therapy and Comparative Criminology* 48, 587–599.

Thornton D, Mann R, Webster S, Bludd L, Travers R, Friendship R, Erikson M (2003) Distinguishing and combining risks for sexual and violent recidivism. *Annals of the New York Academy of Sciences* 989, 225–235.

Topp DO (1979) Suicide in prison. *British Journal of Psychiatry* 134, 24–27.

Torhorst A, Moller HJ, Kurz A, Schmid-Bode KW, Lauter H (1988) Comparing a 3-month and a 12-month-outpatient aftercare program for parasuicide repeaters. In Moller HJ, Schmidtke A and Welz R (eds) *Current Issues of Suicidology*. Berlin: Springer-Verlag.

Torrey EF (1999) Reinventing mental health care. *City Journal* 5.4.

Towl GJ (1991) Nursing practice: scrutinising the power complex. *Nursing Standard* 5, 45–46.

Towl GJ (1996) Homicide and suicide: Assessing risk in prisons. *The Psychologist* 9.

Towl GJ (2000) Suicide in prisons. In Towl GJ, Snow L and McHugh MJ (eds) *Suicide in Prisons*. Leicester: BPS Books.

Towl GJ (2002) Working with offenders: The ins and outs. *The Psychologist* 15 236–239.

Towl GJ (2004) Applied psychological services in HM Prison Service and the National Probation Service, in Needs A, Towl GJ (eds) *Applying Psychology to Forensic Practice*. Oxford: Blackwell.

Towl GJ (2005) Risk Assessment. *Evidence-Based Mental Health* 8, 91–93.

Towl GJ (ed.; 2006) *Psychological Research in Prisons*. Oxford: Blackwell.

Towl GJ (2008a) Introduction and overview, in Towl GJ, Farrington DP, Crighton DA, Hughes G (eds) *Dictionary of Forensic Psychology*. Cullompton: Willan Publishing.

Towl GJ (2008b) In response. *The Psychologist* 21, 444–449.

Towl GJ (2008c) Psychology in prisons, in Jewkes Y, Bennett J (eds) *Dictionary of Prisons and Punishment*. Cullompton: Willan Publishing.

Towl GJ, Bailey J (1995) Group work in prisons: An overview, in Towl GJ (ed.) *Groupwork in Prisons. Issues in Criminological and Legal Psychology No.23*. Leicester: The British Psychological Society.

Towl GJ, Crighton DA (1997) Risk assessment with offenders. *International Review of Psychiatry* 9, 187–193.

Towl GJ, Crighton DA (1998) Suicide in prisons in England and Wales from 1988 to 1995. *Criminal Behaviour and Mental Health* 8, 184–192.

Towl GJ, Crighton DA (2007) Psychological services in English and Welsh prisons, in Ax RK, Fagan TJ (eds) *Corrections, Mental Health and Social Policy*. Springfield, IL: Charles C. Thomas.

Towl GJ, McDougall C (1999) What Do Forensic Psychologists Do? *Issues in Forensic Psychology*. Division of Forensic Psychology, BPS, Leicester.

Towl GJ, Snow L, McHugh MJ (eds) (2000) *Suicide in Prisons*. Leicester: BPS Books.

Travers R (1996) Treatment of women in forensic settings, in Henderson C, Smith C, Smith S, Stevens A (eds) *Women and Psychiatric Treatment: A Comprehensive Text and Practical Guide*. London: Routledge.

Tumim S (1990) *Report of a Review by Her Majesty's Chief Inspector of Prisons for England and Wales of Suicide and Self-harm in Prison Service Establishments in England and Wales*. London: HMSO.

Turley A, Thornton T, Johnson C, Azzolino S (2004) Jail drug and alcohol treatment program reduces recidivism in nonviolent offenders: a longitudinal study of Monroe County, New York's jail treatment drug and alcohol program. *International Journal of Offender Therapy and Comparative Criminology* 48, 721–728.

UK Drug Policy Commission (2008) *Reducing Drug Use, Reducing Reoffending: Are programmes for problem drug-using offenders in the UK supported by the evidence?* London: The UK Drug Policy Commission (UKDPC).

University of the Witwatersrand (1989) Voluntary Total Fasting – ethical–medical considerations. *South African Medical Journal* 76, 235–236.

Uzoaba J (1998) *Managing Older Offenders: Where Do We Stand?* Ottawa: Correctional Service of Canada.

Vandereycken W, van Houdenhove V (1996) Stealing behavior in eating disorders: characteristics and associated psychopathology. *Comprehensive Psychiatry* 37, 316–321.

Van der Helm-van Mil AHM, van Vugt JPP, Lammers GJ, Harinck HIJ (2005) Hypernatraemia from a hunger strike as a cause of osmotic myelinolysis. *Neurology* 64, 574–575.

Vaughan P (2004) An evaluation of psychiatric support to the magistrates courts. *Medicine Science and the Law* 44(3), 193–196.

Vaughan PJ, Pullen N, Kelly M (2000) Services for mentally disordered offenders in community psychiatry teams. *Journal of Forensic Psychiatry* 11, 571–586.

Vega M, Silverman M (1988) Stress and the elderly convict. *International Journal of Offender Therapy and Comparative Criminology* 32, 153–162.

Verkes RJ, Van der Mast RC, Hengeveld M, *et al.* (1998) Reduction by paroxetine of suicidal behavior in patients with repeated suicide attempts but not major depression. *American Journal of Psychiatry* 55, 543–547.

Vermeiren R, Clippele A, Deboutte D (2000) A descriptive survey of Flemish delinquent adolescents. *Journal of Adolescence* 23, 277–285.

Veysey BM, Steadman HJ, Morrissey JP, Johnsen M, Beckstead JW (1998) Using the referral decision scale to screen mentally ill jail detainees: Validity and implementation issues. *Law and Human Behavior* 22, 205–215.

Wahadin A (2003) Doing hard time. Older women in prison. *Prison Service Journal* 145, 25–29.

Walker LE (1984) *The Battered Woman Syndrome.* New York: Springer.

Walker N (1968) *Crime and Insanity in England, Volume one: The Historical Perspective.* Edinburgh: Edinburgh University Press.

Walker N, McCabe S (1973) *Crime and Insanity in England, Volume two: New Solutions and New Problems.* Edinburgh: Edinburgh University Press.

Walker T, Cheseldine S (1997) Towards outcome measurements: monitoring effectiveness of anger management and assertiveness training in a group setting. *British Journal of Learning Disabilities* 25, 134–137.

Walsh BT (2001) Eating disorders, in Braunwald E, Fauci AS, *et al.* (eds) *Harrison's Principles of Internal Medicine.* Fifteenth edition. New York: McGraw-Hill.

Walsh BW, Rosen PM (1988) *Self-mutilation: Theory, Research and Treatment.* New York: Guildford Press.

Walsh CE (1989) The older and long term inmate growing old in the New Jersey prison system, in Chaneles S, Burnett C (eds) *Older Prisoners: Current Trends.* New York: The Haworth Press.

Ward T, Gannon T (2006) Rehabilitation, etiology, and self-regulation: The Good Lives Model of rehabilitation for sexual offenders. *Aggression and Violent Behavior* 11, 77–94.

Ward T, Keenan T (1999) Child molesters' implicit theories. *Journal of Interpersonal Violence* 14, 821–838.

Ward T, Siegert RJ (2002) Towards a comprehensive theory of child sexual abuse: a theory knitting perspective. *Psychology, Crime, and Law* 9, 125–143.

Waterhouse J, Platt S (1990) General hospital admission in the management of parasuicide: A randomised controlled trial. *British Journal of Psychiatry* 156, 236–242.

Watts C (2001) The history of the prison system, Chapter 2 in Bryans S, Jones R (eds) *Prisons and the Prisoner. An Introduction to the Work of Her Majesty's Prison Service.* London: The Stationery Office.

Webster SD, Mann RE, Thornton D, Wakeling HC (2007) Further validation of the short self-esteem scale with sexual offenders. *Legal and Criminological Psychology* 12, 207–216.

Wechsler D (1944) *The Measurement of Adult Intelligence.* Third edition. Baltimore, MD: Williams & Wilkins.

Welldon E (1988) *Mother, Madonna, Whore: The Idealisation and Denigration of Motherhood.* London: Free Association Books.

Welldon E, Van Velsen C (eds) (1988) *A Practical Guide to Forensic Psychotherapy.* London: Jessica Kingsley Publishers.

Werthem F (1927) *The Show of Violence.* New York: New York University Press.

Wessex Consortium (2003) *Protocol for accessing psychiatric information by magistrates' courts.* Available at www. hants.gov.uk/wessexconsortium, accessed 25 Nov 2008.

Wexler HK, DeLeon G, Thomas G, Kressel D, Peters J (1999) The Amity prison TC evaluation – reincarceration outcomes. *Criminal Justice and Behavior* 26, 147–167.

Whitaker S (2001) Anger control for people with learning disabilities: a critical review. *Behavioural and Cognitive Psychotherapy* 29, 277–293.

White A, Nicolaas G, Foster K, Browne F, Carey S (1992) *Health Survey for England 1991*. London: Office of Population Censuses and Surveys.

White DL, Wood H (1988) The Lancaster County mentally retarded offenders, in Stark JA, Menolascino FJ, Albarelli MH, Gray VC (eds) *Mental Retardation and Mental Health: Classification, Diagnosis, Treatment, Services*. New York: Springer-Verlag.

White M, Nichols C, Cook R, *et al.* (1995) Diagnostic overshadowing and mental retardation: a meta-analysis. *American Journal of Mental Retardation* 100, 293–298.

Whynes DK, Bean PT (1991) *Policing and Prescribing: The British System of Drug Control*. London: Macmillan.

Williams F, Wakeling H, Webster S (2007) A psychometric study of six self-report measures for use with sexual offenders with cognitive and social functioning deficits. *Psychology, Crime and Law* 13, 505–522.

Williamson M (2006) *Improving the Health and Social Outcomes of People Recently Released from Prisons in the UK: A Perspective from Primary Care*. London: The Sainsbury Centre for Mental Health.

Willner P, Jones J, Tams R, Green G (2002) A randomised controlled trial of the efficacy of a cognitive-behavioural anger management group for clients with learning disabilities. *Journal of Applied Research in Intellectual Disabilities* 15, 224–235.

Wilmott Y, Foot V (2001) Healthcare in prison, Chapter 21 in Bryans S, Jones R (eds) *Prisons and the Prisoner. An Introduction to the Work of Her Majesty's Prison Service*. London: The Stationery Office.

Wilson DJ (2000) *Drug Use, Testing, and Treatment in Jails* (NCJ 179999). Washington, DC: Office of Justice Programs, Bureau of Justice Statistics, US Department of Justice.

Wilson RM (2000) Screening for breast and cervical cancer as a common cause for litigation. *British Medical Journal* 320, 1352–1353.

Wilson S (2004) The principle of equivalence and the future of mental health care in prisons. *British Journal of Psychiatry* 184, 5–7.

Wilson S (2005) Terrorist detainees – psychiatry or morals? *Psychiatric Bulletin* 30, 75.

Wilson S, Forrester A. (2002) Too little, too late? The treatment of mentally incapacitated prisoners. *Journal of Forensic Psychiatry* 13, 1–8.

Winter N, Holland AJ, Collins S (1997) Factors predisposing to suspected offending by adults with self-reported learning disabilities. *Psychological Medicine* 27, 595–607.

Wong SCP (2000) *Violence Reduction Program: Program Management Manual*. Saskatchewan, Canada: Department of Psychology, University of Saskatchewan.

Wong SCP, Hare RD (2005) *Guidelines for a Psychopathy Treatment Program*. Toronto, Ontario: Multi-Health Systems.

Woodward M (1955) The role of low intelligence in delinquency. *British Journal of Delinquency* 5, 281–303.

Wool R (1996) *Food Refusal, Advance Directives, and Mental Capacity*. DDL (96) 1.

World Health Organisation (1992) *ICD10 Classification of Mental and Behavioural Disorders*. Geneva: WHO.

World Health Organisation (2007) *ICD 10 Online*. Available at www.who.int/classifications/apps/icd/icd10online, accessed 22 June 2008.

World Medical Association (1975) *Declaration of Tokyo*. Adopted by the World Medical Association, Tokyo, Japan. October 1975. Available at www.wma.net/e/policy/c18.htm, accessed on 9 September 2009.

World Medical Association (1992) *World Medical Association Declaration on Hunger Strikers*. Adopted by the 43rd World Medical Assembly, Malta, November 1991 and editorially revised at the 44th World Medical Assembly, Marbella, Spain, September 1992. Available at www.wma.net/e/policy/h31.htm, accessed on 9 September 2009.

Wykes M (1995) Passion, marriage and murder, in Dobash RE, Dobash RP, Noaks L (eds) *Gender and Crime*. Cardiff: University of South Wales Press.

Xenitidis K, Henry J, Russell A, *et al.* (1999) An inpatient treatment model for adults with mild intellectual disability and challenging behaviour. *Journal of Intellectual Disability Research*, 43, 128 –134.

Yakeley J (2009) Violent women, in *A Psychoanalytic Approach to Violence*. London: Palgrave MacMillan (in press).

Yellowlees A (1987) The role of the psychiatrist in the penal system, Chapter 6 in Backett S, McNeill J, Yellowlees A (eds) *Imprisonment Today: Current Issues in the Prison Debate.* London: Macmillan.

Youth Justice Board (2004) *Substance Misuse and Juvenile Offenders.* Youth Justice Board. Available at the Youth Justice Board website: www.yjb.gov.uk/Publications

Youth Justice Board (2005) *Strategy for the Secure Estate for Children and Young People,* published by the Youth Justice Board available at the Youth Justice Board website on www.yjb.gov.uk/Publications.

Youth Justice Board (2009) *Youth Justice System. Custody Figures.* Youth Justice Board available at www.yjb.gov.uk/engb/yjs/Custody/CustodyFigures.

Zeitlin H (1999) Psychiatric comorbidity with substance misuse in children and teenagers. *Drug and Alcohol Dependence* 55, 225–234.

Legal Cases

Attorney General for Jersey v Holley [2005] UKPC 23.
Bolam v Friern Hospital Management Committee [1957] 1 W.L.R. 582; 101 S.J. 357; [1957] 2 All E.R. 118.
Bolitho (administratrix of the estate of Bolitho (deceased)) v City and Hackney Health Authority [1997] 3 W.L.R. 1151; [1997] 4 All E.R. 771; [1997] 2 C.L.Y. 3789.
Campbell and Fells v United Kingdom [1984] 7 EHRR 165.
Clark v State of California [1998] U.S. Ninth Circuit Court of Appeals, No. 9616952.
Conway v Rimmer [1968] AC 910, 952.
Cornelius v De Taranto [2000] EWCA Civ 1511.
Ezeh v United Kingdom [2003] 39 EHRR 1.
Freeman v Home Office [1984] 1 All ER 1036.
HL v United Kingdom [2004] no. 45508/99.
Leigh v Gladstone (1909) 46 TLR 139.
McNaughten Rules [1848] 10 CI + F200.
R v Ahluwalia [1992] 4 AER 889.
R v Avon Coroner, ex parte Bentley [2002] 166 JP 297.
R v Bournewood Community and Mental Health NHS Trust, ex parte L [1998] 2 WLR 764, [1999] AC 458.
R v HM Coroner for Coventry, ex parte O'Reilly [1996] 160 JP 749.
R v HM Coroner for East Kent, ex parte Spooner [1987] 152 JP 15.
R v HM Coroner for Inner North London, ex parte Linnane [1989] 1 WLR 395.
R v HM Coroner for North Humberside, ex parte Jamieson [1995] QB 1 and [1994] 3 All ER 972.
R v HM Coroner for Western District of East Sussex, ex parte Homberg [1994] 158 JP 357.
R v Hodgson [1968] 52 Cr App R (s) 113.
R v Kelly [1999] 2 All ER 13.
R v Poplar Coroner, ex parte Thomas [1993] QB 610; sub nom: R v HM Coroner for Greater London, ex parte Thomas.
R v Pritchard [1836] 7 C + P 303.
R v Secretary of State for the Home Department, ex parte Anderson [2002] UKHL 46.
R v Secretary of State for the Home Department, ex parte Doody [1994] 1 AC 531.
R v Secretary of State for the Home Department, ex parte Hickey [1995] 1 WLR 734.
R v Smith [2000] 4 All E R 289.
R v Thornton [1996] 2 All ER 1023.
R v Turner [1975] QB 834 Cr App R 80.
R (Brady) v Ashworth Hospital Authority [2000] Lloyd's Med R 355; (2001) 58 BMLR 173.
Re C. (Adult: Refusal of Medical Treatment) [1994] 1 W.L.R. 290; [1994] 1 All E.R. 819; [1994] 1 F.L.R. 31; [1994] F.C.R. 151.

Re F. v West Berkshire Health Authority, sub nom. F. [1990] 2 A.C. 1; [1989] 2 W.L.R. 1025; [1989] 2 All E.R. 545; (1989) 133 S.J. 785; [1989] 2 F.L.R. 376; (1989) 139 New L.J. 789, HL; [1989] L.S. Gaz. March 8, 42, CA.

Re H. (Mental Patient) [1992] 8 B.M.L.R. 71.

Re M.B. (Medical Treatment) [1997] 2 F.L.R. 426, CA.

Re T. (Adult: Refusal of Medical Treatment) [1992] 4 All E.R. 649, CA.

Re W. (Adult: Refusal of Medical Treatment) [2002] EWHC 901 (Fam).

Re Y. (Mental Incapacity: Bone Marrow Transplant) [1996] 2 F.L.R. 787.

Secretary of State for the Home Department v Robb [1995] 1 All ER 677.

Secretary of State for Justice v David Walker and Brett James [2008] EWCA Civ 30.

Stafford v United Kingdom [2002] no. 46295/99, ECHR 2002–IV.

W v Egdell & Others [1990] 1 All ER CA.

Subject Index

ADHD (Attention Deficit
Hyperactivity Disorder)
117
alcohol use 68–9
see also substance misuse
antisocial personality disorder
(ASPD) 210–12
Assessment, Care in Custody,
and Teamwork (ACCT) 60,
267–8
Asylum and Immigration Act
(1999) 232
AUDIT (Alcohol Use Disorder
Identification Test) 37
autism 117

Baby P 91
Bennett, David 127
Bethlem Royal Hospital 10
Biggs, Ronnie 17
Birmingham prison 13
Blackwood, Orville 127
Blake, George 13, 17, 18
bridewells 10, 65–6
Brief Jail Mental Health Screen
(BJMHS) 36–7
Bright Futures (Hagell) 78
Brinsford YOI and Remand
Centre 83–4
Broadmoor Hospital 11
Butler Report 13

Canarvon Committee 11
Carter Report 23
child abduction 92
child abusers, women as 91–2

child psychiatry 77–8
Children Act (1989) 81, 82–3,
91
amendment (2004) 91
CIS–R (Clinical Interview
Schedule – Revised) 41
Climbié, Victoria 91
*Clinical Management of Drug
Dependence in the Adult Prison
Setting* (Department of
Health) 73, 74
Close Supervision Centres (CSC)
221–2
cognitive behavioural therapy
(CBT) 62, 72, 121, 122,
123
Coldbath Fields House of
Correction 12
Control Review Committee
system 14
Core Sex Offender Treatment
Programme (SOTP) 134
Coroners Act (1988) 227
Counselling, Assessment,
Referral, Advice and
Throughcare (CARAT) 72,
73
County Asylums Act (1808) 10
Crime Sentences Act (1997)
182–3
Criminal Justice Act (1991) 134,
189, 201
Criminal Justice Act (2003) 80,
183, 185, 195, 196, 200
Criminal Lunatics Act (1800) 10
Criminal Lunatics Asylums Act
(1860) 11

Crime and Disorder Act (1998)
80

Dangerous and Severe
Personality Disorder
programmes (DSPD)
219–21
Dartmoor prison 11
death in custody
agencies involved in 225–7
and Coroners' courts 226–7
and Human Rights Act (1998)
223–4
inquest into 227–9
and National Health Service
225
number of 224
and Prisons and Probation
Ombudsman (PPO) 226
Defence of the Realm Act
(1917) 67
*Delivering Race Equality in Mental
Health Care* (Department of
Health) 129
Detention and Training Orders
80–1
dialectical behaviour therapy
(DBT) 62–3
domestic violence 93–5
Domestic Violence, Crime and
Victims Act (2004) 180,
181
Dove-Wilson Committee 13
Dovegate prison 51, 215
*Drug Dependants within the Prison
System* (Advisory Council on
the Misuse of Drugs) 67

drug management in prisons 70–6
Drug Misuse: Opioid Detoxification (National Collaborating Centre for Mental Health) 73
Drug Misuse: Psychosocial Interventions (NICE) 73
drug usage see substance misuse
Du Cane, Sir Edmund 11, 12, 230

East–Herbert Report 13
education in prisons 21
Effective Regime Interventions (Drug Strategy Unit) 73
elderly prisoners
  crimes committed 99
  demographic information on 99–101
  and ethnicity 99
  and food refusal 163–4
  and gender 99
  and mental health disorders 101–3
  mental health services for 104–5
  morbidity of 101
  rise in 98–9
  services for 104–6
  sex offenders 104
  substance abuse 104
Emery Report 13
Emson, Daksha 127
epilepsy 118
ethnic minority prisoners
  and elderly prisoners 99
  foreign nationals 128
  and mental health disorders 126–7
  numbers of 125–6
  and personality disorders 127
  and prisoners with intellectual disabilities 115
  provision for 129–30
  psychiatric morbidity amongst 126
  reducing numbers of 129–30
  research into 131
  and substance misuse 68, 69–70, 131

and suicide in prisons 57
and young offenders 79
Expectations (HM Inspectorate of Prisons) 233

F2052SH system 60
Feltham YOI 84
Floud Report 14
food refusal
  and elderly prisoners 163–4
  and mental health disorders 161–4
  see also hunger striking
Food Refusal, Advance Directives, and Mental Capacity (Wool) 161
foreign national prisoners 128
Fry, Elizabeth 11
Fry, Margery 13
Future Organisation of Prison Health Care (HM Prison Service & NHS Executive) 24, 44

Ganser's syndrome 43
Gaols Act (1823) 11
gender
  and crimes committed 86–7
  and elderly prisoners 99
  and intellectual disabilities 115
  and mental health disorders 89–90
  substance misuse 68, 69
  suicide 54, 57
  youth offending 79, 81
  see also women
Gin Act (1736) 66
Gin Act (1743) 66
Gladstone Committee 12
Grendon prison 13, 14, 51, 213–17
Guidance on Consent to Medical Treatment (Department of Health and HM Prison Service) 161
Gwynn Committee 13

Habitual Drunkard Offenders (Home Office) 67
Habitual Drunkards Act (1878) 66

Health in Prisons Project (World Health Organisation) 44
Health of Prisoners Act (1774) 10
health screening
  conditions screened 35–6
  current situation 32–3
  disease markers 36–7
  false negatives and positives in 35, 36–7
  historical 32
  and mental health 36–7, 38, 41
  and morbidity in prisons 30–1
  new screening process 37–9
  principles of 33–4
  risk factors 36–7
  and substance misuse 37
  screening tools 36–7
Holloway prison 87–9
Homicide Act (1957) 94, 181–2
hospital transfers 45–8, 62
Howard League for Penal Reform 13
Howard, Michael 17
Human Rights Act (1998) 223–4
hunger striking
  assessment of 164–6, 169
  force-feeding 157–8
  guidelines for managing 159–61
  history of 155–7
  management of 166–9, 170–1
  and mental health disorders 158–9, 169
  physical status of ongoing 167–9
  see also food refusal
Huntercombe YOI 84

imprisonment levels 16
Independent Monitoring Board (IMB) 22
indeterminate detention for public protection (IPP) 22, 23
infanticide 92–3, 182
Infanticide Act (1922) 92
  amendment (1938) 93, 182
Insane Prisoners Act (1840) 10

intellectual disabilities
aggression reduction 123
and arson 122
assessment of prisoners with
119–20
autism 117
characteristics of prisoners
with 115
crimes committed 118
definition of 107–8
drug treatments for prisoners
with 121
epilepsy 118
ethnicity of prisoners with
115
figures on 110–15
and gender 115
and mental health disorders
108–10
mortality rates 109
psychological treatment for
prisoners with 121–3
risk assessment and
management 123–4
and sex offences 122
and substance misuse 117
treatments for prisoners with
121–4
and United States of America
243–5
vulnerabilities of prisoners
with 115–16

Kennet prison 23

Learmont Report 14, 18
Lewis, Derek 17
life imprisonment
automatic life sentences 197
discretionary life sentences
195–6
imprisonment for public
protection (IPP) 196–7,
205–6
mandatory life sentences 195,
197
and Mental Health Act (1983)
201
and National Offender
Management Service
(NOMS) 199

numbers of 194
and Parole Board 199–201
release from 198–9
structure of 197–9
types of 194
Lifers: A Joint Thematic Review
(HM Inspectorate of Prisons
and Probation 1999) 186
local prisons 18, 19
Lowdham Grange open prison
13
Lucy Faithfull Foundation 84

May Report 14
McNaughten Rules 181
medical care in prisons 14–15,
20–1, 24–5
Mental Capacity Act (2005)
and treatment in prison
147–53
Mental Deficiency Act (1913)
66
Mental Health Act (1959) 10
Mental Health Act (1983) 10,
45–6, 48, 59, 81, 120,
121, 127, 148, 173, 180,
182–3, 196, 259
2007 amendment 51, 120,
259
and transfer from prison to
hospital 144–6
mental health disorders amongst
prisoners
and food refusal 161–4
and Foucault's theories 44
and hunger striking 158–9,
169
management of 48–50
in New Zealand 248–9
and offending 42–3
Penrose's law 42
prevalence of 41
"prison psychosis" 43–4
reasons for prevalence 42–4
and suicide risk 57
treatment of 41–2, 50–1
Mental Health Inreach Initiative
29
mental health services in prisons
assessment of 26–7
challenges to 27–9

commissioning services 25
equivalence of care 44–5
and ethnicity 28
identification of need 26
management of prisoners
48–50
and Mental Health Act (1983)
148
models of 26–7
need for 25–6
political support for 40
screening 36–7
and substance misuse 28–9
transfer to hospitals 45–8
treatment of prisoners 41–2,
50–1
unmet needs 25–6
and young offenders 83–4
morbidity amongst prisoners
30–1, 42
Mountbatten Report 13, 17,
18, 19

National Adolescent Forensic
Network 84–5
*National Confidential Inquiry into
Suicides and Homicides by
People with Mental Illness*
(Shaw, Appleby and Baker)
224
National Health Service Act
(1977) 145
National Offender Management
Service (NOMS) 20, 23,
134, 143, 199
New Vision for Mental Health, A
(Future Vision Coalition) 40
New Zealand
forensic psychiatric services in
246–7
and mental health services
248–51
prisons in 247–8
*NHS Confidentiality Code of
Practice* (Department of
Health) 258

Owers, Anne 238

Parkhurst prison 17, 18
Paterson, Sir Alexander 12–13

Patient or Prisoner? (HM Inspectorate of Prisons) 21, 24
Paxman, Jeremy 17
Penitentiary Act (1779) 10
Penrose's law 42
Pentonville prison 12
Percy Commission 10
Powers of Crinminal Courts (Sentencing) Act (2000) 197
Prison Act (1865) 32
Prison-Addressing Substance-Related Offending (P-ASRO) 71, 72
prison conditions
  between 1750-1800 9–10
  in the 19th century 11–12
  and Elizabeth Fry 11
prison inspections
  current inspection regime 232–5
  future of 238
  health care inspections 235–6
  history of 230–2
  outcomes of 236–8
prison language
  and authority 268–9
  as cultural defence 261–2, 264
  and depersonalisation 264–6
  and distinction from "outsiders" 266–7
  and distress avoidance 267–8
  prison-specific terms 264
  replacement for "outside" language 263–4
  type of 262–3
  volume of 262–3
Prison Medical Service
  founded 10
  renamed 14
"prison psychosis" 43–4
Prison Service
  amalgamated with the Probation Service 20
  objectives of 16–17
prisoners
  categories 17–18
  and drug usage 20–1
  education for 21
  escapes from prisons 17–18

and infectious disease 30
life for 21–2
medical care for 14–15, 20–1, 24–5
and morbidity 30–1, 42
number of 16, 22–3
and psychiatric disorders 30–1
remand 19, 25
suicide risk 31
prisons
  as communities 253–4
  disturbances in 14
  education in 21
  escapes 17–18
  life in 21–2
  local prisons 18
  medical care in 14–15, 20–1, 24–5
  organisation of 20
  as places of punishment 11–12
  as places for rehabilitation 12–13
  prison-building programme 23
  prisoner numbers 16, 22–3
  security in 13–14, 17–18
  as therapy 212–13
Prisons Act (1835) 11
Prisons Act (1877) 11
Pritchard criteria 120
psychiatric reports
  and adjudication reports 188
  and Category A prisoners 187–8
  and confidentiality 190–1
  and ethics 188–9
  and the expert witness 183–4
  legal issues 178
  and Multi-Agency Public Protection Arrangement (MAPPA) 188
  and Parole Board reviews 185–7
  partiality of 191
  qualities of 174–7
  and sentencing 182–3, 189–90
  training for preparation of 191–3
  and trial process 178–83
  types of 172–3
  within prison 185–8
psychiatry in prisons

history of 9–14
participation in punishments 257–8
and prison as community 253–4
risk management 259–60
role of psychiatrists 254–6
psychology in prisons
  ethics of 204–5
  group work 207–9
  numbers of psychologists 203–4
  policy developments 204
  risk assessments 205–7
psychotherapy
first used in prisOns 13
punishment
  and the role of prison 11–12

Radzinowicz Report 13
Ramsbotham, Sir David 24, 231–2
Rapid Risk Assessment of Sexual Offence Recidivism 123
Referral Decision Scale (RDS) 36
Regional Offender Managers (ROMS) 20
rehabilitation
  and the role of prison 12–13
Rehabilitation of Addicted Prisoners Trust (RAPt) 71, 72, 73–4
Regimes for Juveniles (HM Prison Service) 82
remand prisoners 19, 25
Ruggles-Brise, Sir Evelyn 12

SCID (Structured Clinical Interview for DSM Disorders) 41
Secure Accommodation Orders 81
secure training centres (STCs) 81, 82
security
  in prisons 13–14, 17–18
self-injury
  causes of 60
  definition of 53

and dialectical behaviour
therapy (DBT) 62–3
and hospitalisation 62
public health research models
56–61
reducing 61–4
research models 54–5
role of psychologists 59–60
use of anti-depressant drugs
63–4
and women 90–1
Sex Offender Treatment
Programme (SOTP) 122,
135–7, 140–1, 142
Sex Offender Treatment Service
Collaborative programme
(SOTSEC-ID) 122
sex offenders
assessment of treatment of
141–3
and elderly prisoners 104
housing 132–4
numbers of sex offenders 132
and prisoners with intellectual
disabilities 122
provision for 134
risk factors for 134–6
and Sex Offender Treatment
Programme (SOTP) 122,
135–7, 140–1, 142
and Structured Assessment of
Risk and Need (SARN)
138–9
treatment of 139–41
and young offenders 84
Spurr Report 14
State of the Prisons, The
(Howard) 9
Structured Assessment of Risk
and Need (SARN) 138–9
substance misuse
age profile 68
alcohol use 65–7, 104
Counselling, Assessment,
Referral, Advice and
Throughcare (CARAT)
72, 73
drug management 70–6
drug usage 67
and elderly prisoners 104
and ethnicity 68, 69–70, 131

figures on 69–70
future developments 74–6
and gender 68, 69
history of 65–7
illicit drug usage 67–8
Integrated Drug Treatment
System (IDTS) 74–6
and mental health services in
prisons 28–9
and mortality rates 70
and Prison-Addressing
Substance-Related
Offending (P-ASRO) 71,
72
and prisoners with intellectual
disabilities 117
and Rehabilitation of Addicted
Prisoners Trust (RAPt) 71,
72, 73–4
screening for 37
standards for treatment 73
treatment for 71–2
in the United States of
America 242–3
Substance of Young Needs, The
(Gilvarry) 84
suicide 31
age profile 54–5
epidemiological research in
53–4
and ethnicity 57
figures on 52–3, 56–7
and gender 54, 57
and length of sentence 58
and mental health disorders 57
period in custody 58–9
public health research models
56–61
reducing 61–4
research models 54–5
role of psychologists 59–60
use of anti-depressant drugs
63–4
in young offender institutions
55

Tackling Drugs Together (Home
Office) 67
therapy in prisons
and antisocial personality
disorder (ASPD) 210–12

Close Supervision Centres
(CSC) 221–2
cognitive therapy 217–19
Dangerous and Severe
Personality Disorder
programmes (DSPD)
219–21
and Grendon prison 213–17
prison as therapy 212–13
"What works" movement
217–19
Tumim, Sir Stephen 231

United States of America
and the death penalty 257
and intellectual disabilities
243–5
and mental health disorders
241–2
number in prison 239
and substance misuse 242–3
types of correctional facilities
239–41

Wakefield prison 13
Wandsworth prison 17
Whitemoor prison 17, 18
Wilson, Charles 17
Winson Green prison 17
Woking prison 11
women
age profile 87
as child abductors 92
as child abusers 91–2
crimes committed by 86–7
and domestic violence 93–5
as drug mules 95–6
future developments 96–7
and Holloway prison 87–9
and infanticide 92–3
and mental health disorders
87–8, 89–90
and murder of violent partners
94–5
profile of in prison 87–8
and self-injury 90–2
as sex offenders 133–4
Woodcock Report 14, 18
Woolf Report 14, 134, 231
Wormwood Scrubs prison 13,
17

Young Offender Institutions
    (YOIs) 81, 82–3
young offenders
  and child protection 82–3
  and child psychiatry 77–8
  and the Children Act (1989)
    82
  Detention and Training Orders
    80–1
  and ethnicity 79
  and gender 79, 81
  mental health of 78–80
  mental health services for
    83–4
  and The National Adolescent
    Forensic Network 84–5
  reasons for mental disorders
    and offending 79–80
  routes to detention 80–2
  numbers in detention 77
  Secure Accommodation Orders
    81
  secure training centres (STCs)
    81, 82
  sex offenders 84
  Young Offender Institutions
    (YOIs) 81, 82–3
  and the Youth Justice Board 81

Author Index

Abram, K.M. 115
Aday, R. 105
Adesanya, A. 128
Adshead, G. 91, 255, 259
Advisory Council on the Misuse of Drugs 67
Advisory Council on the Penal System 13
Agbahowe, S.A. 128
Ahmad, M. 69
Aiyegbusi, A. 90
American Psychiatric Association 78, 107, 178
Anderson, J.C. 105, 134
Andrews, D.A. 134
Annas, G.J. 156
Appelbaum, P. 259
Appleby, L. 54, 59, 224
Archbold 179
Arendt, M. 131
Arensman, E. 62
Arkes, H.R. 56
Armstrong, D. 63, 261
Arndt, S. 104
Arrigo, B.A. 44
Arscott, K. 121
Arsenault, L. 78, 131
Ashworth, A. 195, 196, 197
Attorney General's Office 95
Australian Institute of Health and Welfare 31

Babor, T.F. 37
Bailey, S. 78, 79, 84, 207
Bains, p. 69
Baker, D. 54, 224
Banerjee, S. 83

Banes, J. 115
Baroff, G. 116
Barratt, A. 34
Barron, P. 115, 117, 118, 121
Basoglu, M. 168
Bateman, A. 271
Beail, N. 123
Bean, P. 67, 116
Bearn, J. 66
Bebbington, P. 57
Beck, A.J. 98, 106, 240
Beckett, R.C. 139, 140
Beech, A.M. 135, 138, 139, 140, 141
Belenko, S. 242
Bennett, H. 246
Bennett, T. 72
Benson, B.A. 120, 121, 123
Berridge, V. 67
Beverley, c. 26
Birmingham, L. 30, 31, 32, 33, 36, 38, 57, 111, 152, 185, 255, 268, 269
Black, L. 123
Bland, J. 90
Bluglass, R. 105, 174, 176
Boer, D.P. 124
Bogue, J. 54
Bonaventrua, s. 109
Bonta, J. 134
Borrill, J. 69, 70
Borthwick-Duffy, S.A. 109
Boudreaux, M.C. 92
Bouthilet, G.N. 244
Bowden, P. 145, 174, 176, 189, 254, 257
Bowers, P.E. 43

Boyington, J. 236
Brady, K. 206
Bradley, E.A. 117
Bradshaw, R. 60
Breakwell, G. 206
Bregin, P.R. 64
Brettle, R.P. 30
Brigden, p. 112
Brinded, P. 30, 31, 248
British Medical Association 157
Britton, R. 267, 269
Brockman, B. 166
Brook, J. 78
Brooke, D. 24, 25, 111, 145
Brooker, C. 26
Brown, B.S. 111, 135
Browne, K.D. 138
Brugha, T. 41, 43, 56
Bryson, S.E. 109
Budd, T. 126
Bullock, J.L. 44
Bunting, J. 52
Burdon, W.M. 243
Burns, C.C. 53
Bussière, M.T. 135, 137
Butler, T. 31

Campbell, D. 268
Cantwell, R. 78
Caplan, A. 254
Cardone, D. 116
Carson, D. 38
Cartier, J. 243
Casey, P. 192
Catani, M. 168
Chaiken, S.B. 241
Chao, O. 87, 88, 89, 96

Chen, R. 103
Cheseldine, S. 120
Chiswick, D. 188, 189
Chivite-Matthews, N. 68
Cinamon, H. 60
Clare, I.C.H. 116, 120, 121, 123
Clarke, E. 158
Cleckley, H. 212
Clifford, D. 121
Clippele, A. 80
Cockram, J. 244
Coffey, C. 30
Cohen, P. 78
Coid, J. 28, 57, 111, 131, 211
Coldwell, J. 123
Colebrook, M. 30
Coles, E.M. 191
Collins, S. 115
Commission for Racial Equality 129
Committee for the Prevention of Torture 160
Conley, R.W. 244
Connolly, T. 56
Cook, R. 110
Cooper, C.S. 242
Cope, R. 127
Copeland, J. 102, 103
Corbett, J.A. 109
Cortoni, F. 135
Courtless, T.F. 111
Craig, L.A. 138
Creese, R. 66
Crews, W.D. 109
Crighton, J. 52, 53, 54, 56, 57, 58, 59, 60, 61, 62, 64, 203, 205, 206, 208
Crook, M.A. 168
Crundall, I. 104
Cullen, E. 194, 198, 200, 217

Dadds, M.R. 135
Dagnan, D. 121
Danesh, J. 14, 25, 30, 41, 102, 253
Day, K. 110, 115
De Silva, N. 262
Deacon, K. 104, 118
Deboutte, D. 80
Denkowski, G.C. 111
Denkowski, K.M. 111

Dent, H. 116
Department of Corrections 247, 248
Department of Health 15, 25, 40, 73, 74, 91, 127, 129, 145, 149, 154, 253, 256, 258
Department of Health and Social Security 13, 145
Devlin, A. 263
Dewey, M. 102, 103
Dhar, R. 149
DiClemente, C.C. 218
Dietz, E.F. 243
Dillon, P. 65, 66, 67
Dolan, K.A. 90
Dolan, M. 72
Doll, H. 69
D'Orban, P.T. 87, 92, 93
Downs, D. 94
Drug Strategy Unit 73
D'Souza, R.M. 31
Duggal, A. 163
Durcan, G. 26, 49, 50
Dyer, C. 161
Dyer, O. 258

Earthrowl, M. 152
East, W.N. 13
Eastman, N. 149
Edwards, A. 11, 12, 13, 14
Edwards, S. 67, 271
Enoch, M.D. 43
Everington, C.T. 116

Farabee, D. 243
Farrington, D.P. 72, 117
Fatoye, F.O. 128
Faulk, M.A. 110
Fawcett Society 87
Fazel, S. 14, 25, 30, 41, 69, 101, 102, 103, 104, 105, 112, 128, 253
Fernandez, Y.M. 134, 140
Feron, J.M. 31
Ferraro, W. 87
Fessler, D.M.T. 163
Finklehor, D. 218
Finlay, W.M.L. 116
Fisher, D. 139, 140
Fitzgibbon, D.W.M. 61

Flaum, M. 104
Floud, J. 14
Fogel, C.I. 94
Fonagy, P. 271
Foot, V. 14
Ford, J. 37
Forrester, A. 42, 48, 49, 152
Foster, L.A. 94
Foucault, M. 15, 44
Fox, A.T. 268
Foxcroft, D. 72
French, A. 112
Friendship, C. 141, 142
Fruehwald, S. 60
Fulero, S.M. 116
Fuller Torrey, E. 241
Future Vision Coalition 40

Gandhi, M.K. 155
Gannon, T. 137
Gates, S. 72
Gatward, R. 25, 30, 41, 111
Gavin, N. 28, 38
Geddes, J.R. 59
Gendreau, P. 243
General Medical Council 183–4, 190
Giamp, J.S. 244
Gibbens, T.C.N. 87
Gigerenzer, G. 61
Gillam, L. 109
Giller, H. 78
Gillis, J.R. 87
Gilvarry, E. 84
Gizzarelli, R. 135
Glaser, W. 118
Glaze, L.E. 241
Goldberg, A.L. 37
Gordon, M. 11
Gore, S.M. 30
Gover, R.M. 12
Graham, A. 30
Gray, V.C. 30
Green, C.M. 10, 61
Greer, S. 53
Gregory, J. 114
Grounds, A. 174, 176
Grove, W.M. 123
Grubin, D. 28, 30, 31, 38, 111, 138
Gudjonsson, G.H. 112, 116

Gunn, J. 10, 11, 13, 24, 41, 42, 88, 111, 116, 145, 217, 249

Haaven, J. 124
Hagan, J. 87
Hagell, A. 78, 80
Hale, R. 268
Hall, G.C.N. 37, 134
Hall, J.N. 244
Hally, V. 168
Halstead, S. 123
Hammett, T.M. 30
Hammond, K.R. 56
Hanson, R.K. 134, 135, 137, 142
Harari, P.M. 115, 116
Hare, R. 211, 221
Harmon, M.P. 30
Harnett, H. 111
Harrington, R. 79, 84
Harris, G.T. 123, 134
Harrison, T. 98, 213, 239, 240
Hart, S.D. 36
Harty, M. 25
Hassiotis, A. 115
Hastings, R. 123
Hatty, S. 54
Haveman, M.J. 108
Hawton, K. 62, 63
Haycock, J. 57
Hayes, S. 112, 115, 116
Heal, L.W. 116
Health Advisory Committee for the Prison Service 145
Healthcare Commission 237
Hengevald, M. 63
Higgins, B.R. 37
Hiller, M.L. 243
Hinshelwood, R.D. 166, 261, 265, 267, 270
HM Inspectorate of Prisons 14, 15, 21, 24, 26, 50, 51, 60, 78, 87, 110, 125, 186, 224, 231, 233
HM Inspectorate of Probation 200
HM Prison Service 14, 24, 44, 55, 60, 82, 145, 161, 187, 190, 197, 225, 226, 231, 270

Hobbs, M. 30
Hodgetts, A. 114
Hodgins, S. 113, 118, 131
Holland, A.J. 111, 115
Hollin, C.R. 135
Hollins, S. 110
Holloway, K. 72
Home Office 12, 13, 14, 15, 17, 18, 40, 67, 69, 78, 86, 87, 95, 96, 98, 99, 116, 125, 127, 134, 145, 161, 199, 231, 264
Hough, R. 69
Howard, J. 9, 10
Howard, L.M. 89–90
Howard League for Penal Reform 82
Howells, R. 168
Humphrey, J.A. 94
Humphreys, M. 185
Hurd, D. 238
Hurley, A.D. 11, 12, 13, 14
Hyatt Williams, A. 266

Inquest 224
Institute of Alcohol Studies 68
International Centre for Prison Studies 16
Isherwood, S. 26, 27, 47
Ivins, J. 120

Jackson, R. 244
Jacoby, R. 104
James, D. 45, 241
Janoff Bulman, R. 253
Jenkins, R. 52, 54, 56, 157
Johannes Weir Foundation for Health and Human Rights 167, 170
Joint Committee on Human Rights 224
Johnson Rice, C. 121
Johnson-Sabine, E. 162
Johnston, S.J. 123
Joliffe, D. 117
Jones, D. 269
Joseph, P. 191
Joudo, J. 55
Justice 195
Juszczak, E. 59

Kahan, J. 53
Kalk, W.J. 163, 165, 168, 170
Kanyanya, I.M. 128
Karberg, J.C. 242
Katon, W. 105
Keenan, T. 135
Kelly, S. 52, 114
Kennedy, R.C. 87
Kenney, A. 156
Kessler, R.C. 131
Kesteven, S. 15
Kirkpatrick, J.T. 94
Kissane, D.W. 158
Kissi-Deborah, R. 114
Klein, D. 78
Knight, K. 243
Knowles, K. 26, 50
Koenig, H. 102
Kohn, M. 67
Koller, H. 109, 113
Krajick, K. 105
Kratzer, L. 78
Kreitman, N. 53
Kroese, B. 121
Kuehn, B.M. 242

Laming, Lord 91
Langstrom, N. 123
Larkin, E. 158, 162
Lawrence, C. 205
Lewinsohn, P. 78
Lewis, N.A. 257
Lidz, C. 259
Liebling, A. 55, 268
Lindsay, W.R. 110, 115, 120, 121, 122, 123, 124
Linehan, M.M. 63
Lipton, D.S. 72
Liriano, S. 73
Lombroso, C. 87
Lösel, F. 134, 143
Luckasson, R. 244
Lusignan, R. 135
Lyall, I. 112
Lyne, M. 145, 146
Lyons, E. 116

MacEachron, A.E. 111, 115, 118, 244
Mackay, R. 178, 182
Maden, A. 24, 41, 88, 96, 111

Mafullul, Y.M. 128
Magill, C. 125
Maggia, B. 37
Malamuth, N.M. 135
Mann, R. 135, 141
Mannuzza, S. 117
Marchsall, S. 78
Marshall, P. 214, 217
Marshall, T. 31
Marshall, W.L. 134, 135
Martin, C. 30, 73
Martinson, R. 217
Mason, J.111, 112
Mason, K. 30, 246
Matthew, W. 131
May, C. 73, 242
Mayfield, D. 37
Mayhew, H. 12
Mayr, A. 263
McBrien, J. 110, 112
McCabe, K.M. 10, 11, 118, 131
McClean, D. 271
McClelland, G.M. 115
McDougall, C. 205
McGrother, C.W. 109
McGuire, J. 217
McHugh, M.J. 56
McKenzie, N. 26, 27
McKibben, A. 135
McLaren, J. 109
McLeod, G. 37
McMillan, D. 123
McMurran, M. 72
McNulty, C. 114
McSweeney, T. 69, 72
Medford, S. 116
Meltzer, D. 54, 77, 78, 131
Meltzer, H. 25, 30, 31, 41, 111
Menninger, K.A. 55
Mental Health Foundation 80
Menzies, R.D. 10
Menzies Lyth, I. 261, 264, 265, 267, 268, 269
Meux, C. 192
Mezey, G. 90, 95
Miles, S.H. 166
Miller, W. 167, 205, 220
Milton, J. 78
Ministry of Health 13
Ministry of Health (New Zealand) 249
Ministry of Justice 16, 23, 46,

47, 86, 95, 132, 194, 196, 199
Miranti, S.V. 121
Møller, L. 44
Monahan, J. 56, 123
Moos, R.H. 140
Morgan, H.G. 53, 127
Morris, N. 9
Morton, K. 137
Morton-Bourgon, K. 134, 135
Motz, A. 90, 91, 93, 94
Mullen, P.E. 43
Müller-Isberner, R. 131
Mumola, C.J. 242
Murphy, G. 110, 111, 112, 113, 120, 121, 122, 123
Mwenda, I. 69

Naismith, L.J. 10
Narey, M. 57
Nathan, J. 271
National Collaborating Centre for Mental Health 73
National Institute for Clinical Excellence (NICE) 62, 73
National Institute of Corrections 240
National Offender Management Service 60, 224
National Treatment Agency for Substance Misuse 74
Ndegwa, D. 127, 131
Ndetei, D.M. 128
Needs, A. 205
Nemitz, T. 116
New York State Commission on Quality of Care for the Mentally Disabled 244
Newburn, T. 80
Newell, T. 194, 198, 200
Newsom-Davies, I. 114
NHS Executive 14, 24, 44, 145, 231, 270
NHS Health & Social Care Information Centre 68
NHS Scotland 68
Nichols, C. 110
Nitsche, P. 43
Niveau, G. 44
Noble, J.H. 112, 244
Nordentoft, M. 59
Novaco, R.W. 123

Novick, L.F. 30
Nurse, J. 262, 266

O'Brien, G. 59, 110
O'Connell, D.J. 243
O'Connor, A. 162
Office for National Statistics 68, 69, 99, 101, 126
Office of Public Services Reform 233
O'Grady, J. 152, 176
Ogunlesi, O.A. 128
Oguz, N.Y. 166
Olds, D.L. 131
Ormsby, J. 262
Othieno, C.J. 128
Owers, A. 89, 267

Padfield, N. 190
Page, K. 266
Palmer, J 70
Panteli, J.V. 168
Parrott, J. 26, 27, 47, 101, 104
Parsons, S. 28, 31, 38
Pattison, E.M. 53
Pearse, J. 116
Peel, M. 168
Penfold, C. 70
Penrose, L.S. 42
Perry, A. 71, 72
Perske, R. 116
Peters, R.H. 37, 242
Petersilia, J. 244
Petrovesky, N. 31
Petruckevitch, A. 57
Peugh, J. 242
Philip, A.E. 53
Piper, M. 59
Pizzey, E. 95
Platt, S. 62
Player, E. 73
Plutchik, R. 60
Pococky, H. 53
Polaschek, D.L. 135
Polivy, J. 162
Pollack, O. 87
Porter, R. 66
Power, K. 54
Pratt, D. 59
Prendergast, M. 243
Prison Reform Trust 19, 20,

22–3, 72, 128, 205
Probation 1999 186
Prochaska, J.O. 218
Proulx, J. 135
Pullen, N. 114

Qin, P. 59
Quinsey, V.L. 123

Ramsbotham, D. 89
Rapoport, R. 214
Reber, A. 269
Reed, J. 127, 145, 146, 185
Reiss, J. 109, 192
Repper, J. 26
Resnick, P.J. 93
Reyes, H. 165
Reza, B. 125
Rhodes, W. 30
Richardson, A. 69
Richardson, S.A. 109, 113
Robbins, I. 44, 258
Roberts, J. 65
Robertson, G. 145, 254
Rogers, R. 36
Rollnick, S. 220
Rose, J. 121, 122, 123
Rosefield, H.A. 105
Rosen, P.M. 53
Rosenberg, D.A. 91
Rothman, D.J. 9
Rowe, F. 109
Roy, A. 59
Royal College of Psychiatrists
    59–60, 68, 188, 190, 192,
    224, 256, 258
Rutherford, H. 88
Rutter, M. 78
Ryan, E. 246
Rycroft, C. 262, 267, 269
Ryrie, N. 205

Sabol, W.J. 239
Sacks, S. 71
Sainsbury Centre 44
Sales, B. 26, 27
Santamour, M.B. 244, 245
Sattar, G. 43, 60
Saunders, P. 102
Scarpitti, F.R. 243
Schmucker, M. 134, 143

Schuman, J. 99
Scobie, I.N. 167
Scott, P. 43, 93, 131, 135
Scott, S. 189
Seaman, S.R. 30
Seddon, T. 15, 44
Seeley, J. 78
Seidman, B.T. 135
Seligman, M.E.P. 94
Sharp, C. 126
Shaw, J. 54, 60, 224, 268
Shiekh, J. 105
Shipley, B. 105
Shoemaker, W.E. 241
Siegert, R.J. 134
Sigelman, C.K. 116
Sijuwola, O.A. 128
Silove, D. 165, 166, 170
Silver, E. 56
Silverman, I.J. 106, 239
Sim, J. 10, 11, 65, 188
Simpson, A. 31, 87, 243
Singh, B. 52, 54
Singleton, N. 25, 30, 41, 70,
    88, 99, 110, 111, 145, 253
Sjostedt, G. 123
Slavkin, M.L. 120
Smallbone, S.W. 135
Smith, A. 10, 14
Smith, R. 72
Smith, S. 105, 121, 122
Snow, L. 56, 60
Social Exclusion Unit 21
Solomka, B. 189, 259
Sovner, R. 109
Steadman, H.J. 32, 36, 56
Stevens, L. 31
Stone, J.H. 174, 176
Suarez, A. 63
Summers, J.A. 117
Sutherland, E. 87
Swartz, J. 36
Swinton, M. 24, 41, 88, 111

Taylor, J. 87, 88, 89, 96, 101,
    104
Taylor, P. 120, 121, 122, 123,
Taylor, R. 217
Teplin, L.A. 31, 36, 115
Thomas, S.D.M. 25
Thompson, C. 105
Thompson, J. 241

Thorne, I. 120
Thornton, D. 135, 138, 142
Topp, D.O. 58
Tough, S. 123, 124
Towl, G.J. 52, 53, 54, 56, 58,
    59, 60, 61, 62, 203, 205,
    206, 207, 208
Townsend, E. 62
Travers, R. 90
Trestman, R. 37
Trethowan, W. 43
Turley, A. 242
Turnbull, P.J. 69, 70
Turvey, C.L. 104

UK Drug Policy Commission
    72, 74
Underwood, R. 244
Uzoaba, J. 98, 99

Van der Mast, R.C. 63
van Houdenhove, V. 162
Van Velsen, C. 266, 270
Vandereycken, W. 162
Vaughan, P. 114, 185
Veale, C.M. 94
Vega, M. 106
Verkes, R.J. 63
Vermeiren, R. 80
Veysey, B.M. 36

Wahadin, A. 99, 100
Wakeling, H. 142
Walker, N. 10, 11, 31, 54, 94
Walker, T. 118, 120
Waller, G. 254
Walsh, B. 53, 105, 168
Ward, T. 134, 135, 137
Waterhouse, J. 62
Watts, C. 10, 12
Webster, S.D. 70, 135, 142
Wechsler, D. 108
Welldon, E. 87, 90, 91, 266,
    270
Werthem, F. 217
West, C. 121
Wexler, H.K. 71
Whitaker, S. 123
White, D.L. 110
Whynes, D.K. 67
Williams, F. 142

Williamson, M. 50
Willner, P. 121, 123
Wilmanns, K. 43
Wilmott, Y. 14
Wilson, D.J. 34, 44, 45, 49
Wilson, R. 144, 152
Wilson, S. 255, 258, 271
Winter, N. 115
Wong, S.C.P. 221, 222
Wood, H. 110, 117
Woodcock, P. 262
Woodward, M. 110
Wool, R. 161
World Health Organisation 44,
    178
World Medical Association
    159–60, 164
Wykes, M. 86, 94

Xenitidis, K. 122

Yakeley, J. 87
Yellowlees, A. 11
Yesavage, J. 105
Young, W. 14
Youth Justice Board 77, 80, 81